REVISED AND UPDATED

International
Diabetes
Center

Learning to
LIVE
WELL
with
Diabetes

Editorial Committee

Marion J. Franz,
R.D.,M.S.,C.D.E

Donnell D. Etzwiler, M.D.

Judy Ostrom Joynes,
M.A.,R.N.,C.D.E.

Pricilla M. Hollander,
 M.D.,Ph.D.

Editor
Cheryl Weiler

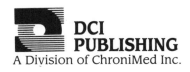
DCI PUBLISHING
A Division of ChroniMed Inc.

Library of Congress Cataloging-in-Publication Data
Learning to live well with diabetes / [edited by] Marion J. Franz... [et al.]. — [Updated and rev. ed.]
     p. cm.
   At head of title: International Diabetes Center.
   Includes index.
   ISBN 0-937721-79-4 : $24.95
   1. Diabetes—Popular works. I. Franz, Marion J. II. International Diabetes Center.
   RC660.4.L43 1991
   616.4'62—dc20   91-15874
                                                                                   CIP

Editor: Cheryl Weiler
Cover and Text Design and Production: MacLean & Tuminelly
Illustrations: Doug Oudekerk
Medical Illustrations: Andrew Grivas, MA
Chapter 30 Illustrations: Tom Foty Advertising Art
Photography: Hilary N. Bullock Photography
Production Manager: Wenda Johnson
Printed in the United States of America

10 9 8 7 6 5 4 3 2 1

Published by:
DCI Publishing
A Division of ChroniMed Inc.
PO Box 47945
Minneapolis, MN 55447-9727

CONTENTS

Acknowledgements...viii

Foreword...ix

Authors...xiv

Introduction..1
Ready for the Challenge?
Joe Nelson, MA, LP

SECTION I

Getting Started: The Basics

1 ▪ Diabetes: The Light Grows Brighter 7
Donnell D. Etzwiler, MD

2 ▪ Nutrition: The Cornerstone 21
Marion J. Franz, MS, RD, CDE

3 ▪ Exercise: The Advantage Is Yours 49
Marion J. Franz, MS, RD, CDE
Jane Norstrom, MA

4 ▪ Monitoring: The Secret to Control 65
Judy Ostrom Joynes, MA, RN, CDE
Lucy Mullen, RN, BS, CDE

5 ▪ Insulin: A Message to the Cells...83
Lucy Mullen, RN, BS, CDE
Judy Ostrom Joynes, MA, RN, CDE

6 ▪ Emotional Adjustment: The Key to Living Well 101
Randi S. Birk, MA, LP

SECTION II

Living Well: Controlling Diabetes With Insulin

7 ▪ Your Health Care Plan: Individualized for Your Lifestyle 124
Martha L. Spencer, MD

8 ▪ Nutrition: The Key Is Consistency 137
Marion J. Franz, MS, RD, CDE
Diane Reader, RD, CDE
Gay Castle, RD, CDE

9 ▪ Exercise: Clues for Safe Participation 147
Marion J. Franz, MS, RD, CDE
Jane Norstrom, MA

10 ▪ Pattern Control: Monitoring Your Way to Better Blood Glucose 161
Judy Ostrom Joynes, MA, RN, CDE

11 ▪ Acute Complications: The Ups and Downs of Blood Glucose........................177
Martha L. Spencer, MD

SECTION III

Living Well: Managing Diabetes With Meal Planning, Exercise, and/or Oral Agents

12 ▪ Your Health Care Plan: "Meal Planning- and
Exercise-Dependent" Diabetes...197
Priscilla M. Hollander, MD

13 ▪ Nutrition: In Search of a Reasonable Weight 209
Arlene Monk, RD, CDE
Marion J. Franz, MS, RD, CDE

14 ▪ Routine Exercise: The Answer to Improved Blood Glucose Control 221
Marion J. Franz, MS, RD, CDE
Jane Norstrom, MA

SECTION IV

Long-Term Problems: Education and Prevention

15 ▪ Long-Term Problems: Three Links in the Chain of Prevention 239
   Richard M. Bergenstal, MD

16 ▪ Heart Problems: Steps to Reduce Risk Factors...249
   Priscilla M. Hollander, MD
   Leonard Nordstrom, MD

17 ▪ Nerve Problems: Protecting the Body's Communication System....................259
   Priscilla M. Hollander, MD

18 ▪ Foot Problems: Keeping Feet for a Lifetime...267
   Janet Swenson Lima, RN, MPH
   Stephen H. Powless, DPM
   Ellie Strock, RN,C, CDE

19 ▪ Eye Problems: Improving the Outlook by Early Detection 277
   William J. Mestrezat, MD

20 ▪ Kidney Problems: Using the Prevention and Treatment Threesome 287
   Donald A. Duncan, MD

21 ▪ Sexual Problems: Communicating and Seeking Help 295
   Clyde E. Blackard, MD
   Joe Nelson, MA, LP
   Janet Swenson Lima, RN, MPH
   Ellie Strock, RN,C, CDE

SECTION V

Advanced Management and Special Concerns

22 ▪ Meal Planning: Adding Flexibility 305
   Marion J. Franz, MS, RD, CDE
   Nancy Cooper, RD, CDE

23 ▪ Stress Management: Learning to Cope With External
   and Internal Stressors..321
   Randi S. Birk, MA, LP

24 ▪ Medications: How They Can Affect Diabetes 333
   Dean E. Goldberg, PharmD, CDE

25 ▪ Insulin Intensification: Fine-Tuning Blood Glucose Control............................341
   Priscilla M. Hollander, MD

26 ▪ Pregnancy: Careful Planning and Control 349
Priscilla M. Hollander, MD
Leslie Pratt, MD

27 ▪ Athletes: Juggling Insulin, Food, and Activity........................363
Marion J. Franz, MS, RD, CDE
Jane Norstrom, MA

28 ▪ Planning Travel: Your Ticket to Opportunity.........................375
Jan Pearson, RN, BAN, CDE

29 ▪ Healthful Habits: Strategies for Living Well 383
Helen Bowlin, RN, BSN

SECTION VI

Diabetes and Youth

30 ▪ For Kids: Taking Care of Me 393
Barbara Balik, RN, MS
Becky Clasen, RN, BA, CDE
Gretchen Kauth, RD, CDE

31 ▪ For Parents: What You Should Know About Normal
Growth and Development..413
Patricia M. Moynihan, RN, MPH

32 ▪ For Parents: Meals, Not Military Maneuvers 427
Marion J. Franz, MS, RD, CDE
Broatch Haig, RD, CDE

33 ▪ For Teens: Answers to Your Questions About Health,
Growing Up, and Sexuality..445
Broatch Haig, RD, CDE
Martha L. Spencer, MD

SECTION VII

Finding the Light at the End of the Tunnel

34 ▪ Research: Can You Help? 461
LeAnn McNeil, RN, MS

35 ▪ Technology: Its Role in Research and Diabetes Management.......................467
Roger S. Mazze, PhD

36 ▪ Research: Providing Pieces for the Diabetes Puzzle 473
Donnell D. Etzwiler, MD

APPENDIX

A ▪ Exchange Lists for Meal Planning 481

B ▪ Blood Glucose Monitoring Equipment Guide 495

C ▪ Exchange Lists for Infant Foods..497

Resource List for Additional Information 501

Index 505

Acknowledgements

The Editorial Committee and the International Diabetes Center gratefully acknowledge and extend our sincere thanks to the following people, whose skills and efforts helped make this book possible.

OUR PATIENTS AND FRIENDS

People with diabetes who share with us their life experiences and help us learn the realities of living well with diabetes.

OUR COLLEAGUES

The authors for their dedication to diabetes education, their willingness to go that extra mile to share their knowledge, and their acquired respect for deadlines.

The entire IDC and Park Nicollet Medical Foundation staff that have provided encouragement when the task of completing this book seemed overwhelming.

Mary Ann Roeder for typing the manuscript.

Sylvia Timian for her excellent and thoughtful copy editing.

George Cleveland, David Wexler, Steve Crees, and our other friends and colleagues at Diabetes Center, Inc for their support and encouragement.

OUR DESIGN TEAM

Wenda Johnson, production manager, for coordinating and managing the mammoth task of producing the manual.

Nancy MacLean Tuminelly, art director, for her creative and insightful design and for her superior management skills that helped get this book done well and on time.

Hilary N. Bullock, photographer, for her flair with a camera.

Doug Oudekerk, illustrator, for his clever and talented visual interpretations of the ideas presented in this book.

Andrew Grivas, medical illustrator, for his skillfully rendered medical drawings that give clarity to the workings of the human body.

Tom Foty, illustrator, for his warm and user-friendly illustrations in the children's chapter.

NOT TO BE FORGOTTEN...

The Editorial Committee and IDC are extremely grateful and appreciative of Cheryl Weiler's talents and editorial skills. Without her sacrifices of time and effort, this manual would not be a reality. Thanks.

Foreword

A WORD ABOUT THE MANUAL

There's a lot to know about diabetes! When you first pick up this manual, it may look overwhelming. You may have had that same feeling when you learned you had diabetes. The key to successfully handling any large task is to break it down into smaller, more manageable tasks. We recommend the same approach for reading and using this manual, and we've organized the book to help you do so.

The manual is divided into sections to help you break down the wealth of information here. Each section covers a category in diabetes care and management. As you read, use the open space on the sides of the pages to jot down questions or make notes about information that isn't clear to you. Use these notes to ask questions at your next visit with your health care team. They should be able to clear up any of your misunderstandings.

The first three sections of the book are written for people who have just learned they have diabetes or for anyone who wants to learn or review the basics of diabetes and its management. These sections can also be helpful if you've had diabetes for some time but want to know the latest and most up-to-date information available on diabetes and its management. Or maybe you need to refresh your memory about why it's important to do what you can to keep your diabetes in excellent control.

Section I contains the basic information you need to start managing your diabetes. If you take injected insulin to manage your diabetes, go on to read

Section II. It will help you with information you need to *live well*. If you manage your diabetes with meal planning, exercise, and/or diabetes pills (oral agents), read Section III instead. It will help you understand why it's important to do these things and manage your diabetes as well as you can. Each chapter in these three sections ends with "Monitoring Your Knowledge" questions to help you remember the important points of each chapter.

Section IV covers long-term problems associated with diabetes. These chapters are not meant to scare you. They're meant to provide information that we hope will help you prevent the development of these problems. Each chapter ends with two checklists for preventing the development of long-term problems—one listing things you can do, and one listing things your health care team can do.

After you've mastered the basics of diabetes management, you'll be ready to read Section V. It addresses special problems related to diabetes. It also covers advanced management skills that can help you fine-tune your diabetes control and add flexibility to your lifestyle.

Section VI is a very special section. It's written specifically for families who have children or adolescents with diabetes. If you have a child with diabetes, take some time to read and discuss Chapter 30. It will help your child better understand diabetes and, more importantly, will help them begin to identify their feelings about diabetes. The next two chapters in this section are for parents, and the final chapter is for teens.

The manual ends with information about research and the future. We hope that after reading Section VII, you'll feel that now is, indeed, an exciting time for persons who have diabetes.

As you can see, this manual is not meant to be read in one sitting. Read what is important for you at this time, then come back to the manual again and again. Come back to it for additional information, for reminders about what you should be doing, and for motivation to continue all the important daily diabetes management tasks.

A WORD ABOUT THE INTERNATIONAL DIABETES CENTER

The goal of the International Diabetes Center (IDC) and its affiliates is to help persons with diabetes have fulfilling and active lifestyles. We strive to achieve this goal through excellence in diabetes care, education, and research, using planned systems of care and the most modern techniques available. We believe that the road to successful diabetes management is paved with informed persons with diabetes working alongside concerned, knowledgeable diabetes health professionals. You will want to find a team like this in your community to help you manage your diabetes.

Nearly thirty years ago, Dr Donnell D. Etzwiler recognized that persons with diabetes were responsible for about 99% of their own care. With that in mind, he founded the IDC in 1967 to help persons with diabetes learn to skillfully and confidently take control of their own lives, and thus live *well* with diabetes. The IDC, a division of Park Nicollet Medical Foundation, provides the professional resources that enable them to do it.

At the IDC and its affiliated centers, we conduct education programs for persons with diabetes and their families, helping them learn to manage their diabetes. More than 8,000 persons with diabetes and their families have attended our five-day, in-depth education program. As the days and weeks go by, we learn more and more from them about the effects of living with diabetes on a day-to-day basis. We are grateful for the lessons they teach us.

The IDC has also trained more than 8,000 health professionals from around the world through seminars, workshops, consultations, and postgraduate courses. Research by the IDC evaluates the latest discoveries and technological advances and translates them into effective health care delivery systems that can help persons with diabetes cope.

The IDC Affiliate Program includes centers of excellence in the United States as well as consulting contracts with centers in Austria, Taiwan, and the Soviet Union. In 1985, the IDC was designated by the United Nations' World Health Organization (WHO) as its Collaborating Center for Diabetes Education and Training. In 1988, the WHO Collaborating Center for Behavioral Medicine and Computer Science was added.

A WORD ABOUT THE EDITORIAL COMMITTEE

Marion J. Franz, RD, MS, CDE, is director of nutrition and publications at the IDC. She has a master's degree in nutrition from the University of Minnesota and is a registered dietitian (RD) and certified diabetes educator (CDE). She joined the IDC in 1977 and now coordinates its nutrition services and directs the development of its education materials.

Ms Franz has written about diabetes, nutrition, exercise, and wellness in several books, in numerous articles in professional and lay journals, and in chapters in manuals and books for both the public and health professionals. She has been active in the American Diabetes Association, serving on its Board of Directors, committees, and task forces. Recent honors include the 1985 American Diabetes Association Award for Outstanding Health Professional Educator in the Field of Diabetes and the 1987 American Dietetic Association Foundation Award for Excellence in the Practice of Clinical Nutrition. She has lectured all over the United States and in Great Britain, France, New Zealand, Australia, Saudi Arabia, and the Soviet Union.

Donnell D. Etzwiler, MD, is the founder of the IDC and is a pediatric diabetologist at Park Nicollet Medical Center, which he joined in 1955. He received his medical training at Yale and at the New York Hospital-Cornell Medical Center. He is an internationally recognized leader in diabetes education and patient care and has published more than 100 articles and chapters.

Dr Etzwiler was president of the American Diabetes Association in 1976-1977. He is chairperson of the World Health Organization Diabetes Collaborating Centers and was vice president of the International Diabetes Federation from 1977 to 1986. He was a commissioner on the National Commission on Diabetes and has served on the Advisory Committee of the National Diabetes Advisory Board, the Centers for Disease Control Diabetes Program. He has received the following honors from the American Diabetes Association: Banting Medal, Becton Dickinson Award for Diabetes and Camping, Upjohn Award for Education, and the Award for Diabetes in Youth. He is also an honorary member of the American Dietetic Association and a member of the Institute of Medicine of the National Academy of Science. Dr Etzwiler is a principal investigator in the Diabetes Control and Complications Trial.

Judy Ostrom Joynes, MA, RN, CDE, is director of education at the IDC. She received her master's degree in education from the University of St Thomas in St Paul, Minnesota. She joined the IDC in 1973 and directs both the patient and health professional programs. Through her efforts, many persons have learned to *live well* with diabetes.

Ms Joynes has written articles and educational materials both for persons with diabetes and for health professionals and has lectured locally, regionally, nationally, and internationally to both lay and professional audiences. She has served on local and state boards of the American Diabetes Association and the national board of the American Association of Diabetes Educators (AADE). In 1988 she was honored by the AADE as Diabetes Educator of the Year.

Priscilla M. Hollander, MD, PhD, is an adult endocrinologist at the IDC. She joined Park Nicollet Medical Center in 1980 as an endocrinologist specializing in the care of persons with diabetes. She has an MD degree from Harvard Medical School, a PhD from Yale University, and training in endocrinology and diabetes from the University of Washington in Seattle.

Dr Hollander has been president of the Minnesota affiliate of the American Diabetes Association and has served on its national committees. She is co-investigator for the National Institutes of Health Diabetes Control and Complications Trial Study. She has been principal investigator for various research studies and medical consultant for intensification and pump programs, has written extensively in the field of diabetes, and lectures locally and nationally.

A WORD ABOUT THE AUTHORS AND YOU

Our authors are equally well qualified in their fields. All are involved in patient care and in patient and professional education, and many are involved in research. They serve as volunteers for the American Diabetes Association, the American Association of Diabetes Educators, The American Dietetic Association, the Juvenile Diabetes Foundation, and many other professional organizations.

We have all enjoyed meeting the challenge of planning, writing, and editing this manual. We hope you find our efforts worthwhile and helpful. More importantly, we hope that through our efforts you will learn to *live well* with your diabetes. If you do, we'll feel that our efforts have been successful. Let us know.

Cheryl Weiler

Authors

Barbara Balik, RN, MS
Pediatric Nurse Practitioner
Minneapolis Children's
Medical Center

Richard M. Bergenstal, MD
Adult Endocrinologist
International Diabetes Center
Park Nicollet Medical Center

Randi S. Birk, MA, LP
Psychosocial Services
International Diabetes Center

Clyde E. Blackard, MD
Urologist
Park Nicollet Medical Center

Helen Bowlin, RN, BSN
Administration and Outreach
International Diabetes Center

Gay Castle, RD, CDE
Diabetes Nutrition Specialist
Pediatric Diabetes Clinics
Park Nicollet Medical Center

Becky Clasen, RN, BA, CDE
Pediatric Diabetes Nurse Specialist
Supervisor, Pediatric Endocrinology
Park Nicollet Medical Center

Nancy Cooper, RD, CDE
Diabetes Nutrition Specialist
International Diabetes Center

Donald A. Duncan, MD
Nephrologist
Park Nicollet Medical Center

Donnell D. Etzwiler, MD
Founder
International Diabetes Center
Pediatric Diabetologist
Park Nicollet Medical Center

Marion J. Franz, MS, RD, CDE
Nutrition and Publications
International Diabetes Center

Dean E. Goldberg, PharmD, CDE
Manager, Clinical Pharmacy Services
Diversified Pharmaceutical Services
Minneapolis

Broatch Haig, RD, CDE
Minnesota Diabetes in Youth Program
International Diabetes Center

Priscilla M. Hollander, MD
Adult Endocrinologist
International Diabetes Center
Park Nicollet Medical Center

Judy Ostrom Joynes, MA, RN, CDE
Patient and Health
Professional Education
International Diabetes Center

Gretchen Kauth, RD, CDE
Health Education
Park Nicollet Medical Foundation

Janet Swenson Lima, RN, MPH
Diabetes Nurse Specialist
Park Nicollet Medical Center

LeAnn McNeil, RN, MS
Research
International Diabetes Center

Roger S. Mazze, PhD
Research and Development
International Diabetes Center

William J. Mestrezat, MD
Ophthalmologist
Retina-Vitreous Surgeon
Flint, Michigan

Arlene Monk, RD, CDE
Diabetes Nutrition Specialist
International Diabetes Center

Patricia M. Moynihan, RN, MPH
Clinical Nurse Specialist
Department of Pediatrics
University of Minnesota Hospital
and Clinics

Lucy Mullen, RN, BS, CDE
Diabetes Nurse Specialist

Joe Nelson, MA, LP
Family Counselor
International Diabetes Center

Leonard Nordstrom, MD
Cardiologist
Park Nicollet Medical Center

Jane Norstrom, MA
Exercise Physiologist
Health Education
Park Nicollet Medical Foundation

Jan Pearson, RN, BAN, CDE
Diabetes Nurse Specialist
International Diabetes Center

Stephen H. Powless, DPM
Podiatrist, Foot Clinic
Park Nicollet Medical Center

Leslie Pratt, MD
Obstetrician/Gynecologist
Park Nicollet Medical Center

Diane Reader, RD, CDE
Diabetes Nutrition Specialist
Adult Diabetes Clinics
Park Nicollet Medical Center

Martha L. Spencer, MD
Pediatric Endocrinologist
International Diabetes Center
Park Nicollet Medical Center

Ellie Strock, RN, C, CDE
Research and Development
International Diabetes Center

Joe Nelson, MA, LP

Ready for the Challenge?

More than 100 million people in the world have diabetes. They are sports heroes, dancers, mothers, fathers, scholars, scientists, movie stars, and now you.

Having diabetes isn't the end of the world. It's the beginning of a new chapter in your life. To be happy and to successfully take care of your diabetes, you'll need to know all about it—just like millions of others. This manual will help you form your own beliefs about diabetes based on facts and realities. It will help you develop philosophies about *living well* with diabetes. In the end, it will help you control diabetes so diabetes doesn't control you.

What do you know, believe, and feel about having diabetes? Who is responsible for diabetes care? What are you willing to do to take care of yourself and live well with diabetes?

Whether you're newly diagnosed or you've known about your diabetes for 25 years, you may not have clear answers to these basic questions about yourself and your relationship with diabetes. Many people are reading this manual, not for casual information, but for answers to these questions. They want to discover how they can take better care of themselves and *live well* with diabetes.

WHO IS THIS MANUAL FOR?

This manual is for many different people who must deal with diabetes. If you've just been diagnosed with diabetes within the last year, hopefully you are opening this book with an open mind and are hungry for information. If you've had diabetes for a while, you may be reading this book to get new information and renewed motivation. If you're one of the millions of people who have Type II diabetes, you may be looking for more information about diabetes and how to make better decisions about your health. Perhaps you were diagnosed as a child and now, as an adolescent, are becoming more interested in taking care of yourself and being less dependent on your parents. In that case, the information in this manual will be vital for developing your independence. You may be a young adult preparing for a career, in which case it is essential that your diabetes is well managed so it doesn't interfere. Perhaps you are about to get married or to begin sharing your life with another person and you want to take care of your diabetes and share information about it. Maybe your child or a family member has diabetes, and you want to learn more about it. More than likely, you're at a point in your life where you need new information, renewed information, or motivation to help you use it.

WHAT WILL THIS MANUAL DO FOR YOU?

It's obvious this manual is written by experts in the field of diabetes. It focuses on the most current information available to help people manage their diabetes. What isn't so obvious is that this is an opportunity. It's an opportunity for you to gain the knowledge necessary to take charge of a very important part of your life. This manual invites you to underline, highlight, make notes in the margin, and ask questions pertinent to your lifestyle and your diabetes. We invite you to take what you need right now, and the rest will be available another time when you feel you need it.

This manual challenges you to do the best you can with what you have available and use the information in these chapters to meet your personal needs. This manual is not magic. When most of us are struggling with something in our lives, we look for a light bulb to go on or some kind of outside magic that will create change without effort. Some people seek a new doctor, some attend many different classes, and some read numerous books. But overall, there is no magic that will automatically bring us a sense of accomplishment, help us feel better, or fix what's wrong. This manual is not magic, but it's a step in the right direction. It will help you make some choices that will have a positive influence on your ability to take care of yourself. In that sense, it may be the nearest thing to magic available.

HOW SHOULD YOU USE THIS MANUAL?

Use it for information. The information here is current and taught by experts in the field, and it will assure that you're on the cutting edge of diabetes knowledge. By learning new ideas and using new strategies to manage your diabetes, you'll find renewed motivation to keep taking good care of yourself.

Share this manual with people who care about you and people you care about. Having people around that provide the kind of support you want is a very important part of living well with diabetes. Use this manual as your main reference for diabetes information. The wealth of information here will be essential in years to come when you need information and/or motivation to re-ignite your investment in yourself.

If you're not ready to help yourself, put this manual down. However, if you're ready for the opportunity, the invitation, and the challenge this manual presents—continue reading. As you read, keep a few things in mind:

1. Change is hard work—just because we want something to change doesn't mean it will automatically. It will take time to establish the control of your diabetes you'd like to have.

2. You're only human, so perfection or perfect diabetes control is probably not attainable at all times. What you can hope for is improvement and the best control you're able to achieve. But you

don't need to beat yourself up for not having a blood glucose in the normal range, and you certainly don't need to punish yourself if you decide to go off your meal plan. You do need to make a commitment to yourself to make wise choices and move in the direction of doing well. The fact is, you may set a goal with diabetes but never quite reach it because diabetes is ever changing and with you forever.

3. Learn to appreciate and enjoy the changes involved in the process of good diabetes care. You'll increase your odds of staying motivated and building a lifestyle that fits you and your diabetes management goals.

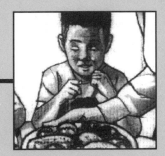

Getting Started

The Basics

CHAPTER 1

Donnell D. Etzwiler, MD

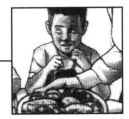

Diabetes:
The Light Grows Brighter

If you have diabetes, you are not alone. Diabetes affects almost 14 million people in the United States, and the number is growing daily throughout the entire world. On the other hand, if you or someone you know develops diabetes, there has never been a better time throughout history.

Although diabetes has no cure at this time, a tremendous amount of research is being done, and yes, there does seem to be light at the end of the tunnel. This thought should not be used as an excuse to ignore your diabetes. It's meant to encourage you to achieve the best possible control of it so you can take full advantage of future breakthroughs.

Only within the past century have we been able to control diabetes. In this chapter you'll learn why it's now more important than ever to carefully manage your diabetes and be aggressive in controlling it.

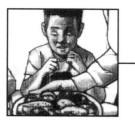

Diabetes is a serious disease that has been known for thousands of years. It was actually described in some of the earliest Egyptian medical writings. But only recently have we realized the seriousness of the disease and its complications.

In the mid-1970s, the US Congress established the National Commission on Diabetes. The Commission spent almost a year researching diabetes, its impact on the nation, and any efforts being made to control and conquer it. It was found that diabetes contributed significantly to coronary heart disease, stroke, amputations, blindness, and kidney failure.

The Commission also discovered that the public knew relatively little about diabetes. The common belief was that most people with diabetes were overweight and that treatment consisted of watching what you eat and perhaps losing weight. If this wasn't effective, diabetes pills could be taken or, for some people, insulin could be injected. In general, the public believed if people with diabetes followed these guidelines, they could live a normal life.

The Commission's report impressed Congress enough that it recommended and funded a National Diabetes Advisory Board. This Board continues to constantly monitor the impact of diabetes on our nation's health. It helps coordinate diabetes efforts among the government, academic groups, patients, organizations, professional associations, the medical field, and volunteer health groups.

The Center for Disease Control, Division of Diabetes Translation, now informs us that:

- Diabetes affects an estimated 14 million people in the United States. About seven million people have been diagnosed with diabetes and an additional seven million may unknowingly have the disease.
- Each year about 700,000 more people are diagnosed with diabetes.
- Diabetes is a leading cause of death by disease.
- Annually, more than 200,000 deaths in the United States are directly or indirectly attributed to diabetes.
- Diabetes cost this nation more than $20.4 billion in 1987.
- Each year, diabetes is responsible for 12,000 cases of new blindness among people 20 to 74 years old, making it the leading cause of new blindness.
- People with diabetes are twice as likely as others to develop heart disease or have heart attacks.
- Risk of stroke is six times greater in people with diabetes.
- People with diabetes are four times more likely to have amputations.

To avoid becoming part of these statistics, it's important that people

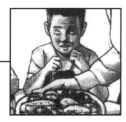

with diabetes get control of their disease early in its course and continue to manage it carefully. This can mean changes in lifestyle and may conflict with the idea of a totally "normal" life, but good diabetes control enhances quality of life and increases the chance of having a longer, more productive life.

The good news from the report is that total mortality (death) rate among persons with diabetes decreased, as did mortality rates from heart disease and diabetic ketoacidosis. We know more and more people with diabetes are living longer lives. The challenge is to help you continue to live well with diabetes!

Studies continue to suggest that good control of diabetes is the first, and most vital, step toward preventing possible problems. To carry out the responsibilities necessary for your care, you must be informed and willing to participate in a carefully planned management program. Being informed about diabetes and its history can help you understand why it's important for you to take control of your diabetes.

A BRIEF HISTORY OF DIABETES

Diabetes was described in the Egyptian manuscript Ebers Papyrus, written in about 1500 BC. Later, Arabic and Chinese literature described people who drank large amounts of water and urinated excessively as suffering from this disease. The earliest literature even describes tests in which urine from patients was poured near anthills. If ants were attracted to the urine, sugar was present and the diagnosis of diabetes was made.

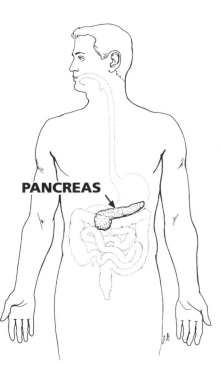

PANCREAS

The Greek doctor Aretaeus (AD 120-200) was the first to call the disease "diabetes," which means to syphon or flow through. The Latin word "mellitus," which means honeyed, was later added. The condition is referred to in medical literature as *diabetes mellitus*, which indicates the presence of sugar in the urine.

In 1860, a German doctor named Paul Langerhans examined under a microscope pieces of the pancreas, a pistol-shaped organ that lies behind the stomach. He noted certain cells took up different colored dyes. Some of these cells seemed to be clustered together in groups, or islands, throughout the pancreas. Since these islands make up only about 1% of the entire pancreas, he referred to them simply as the *islets of Langerhans*, but their function was a mystery.

Today we know these islets contain beta cells that make, store, and release the body's supply of a hormone called *insulin*. Insulin lowers the amount of glucose (sugar) in the blood. The islets also contain alpha cells,

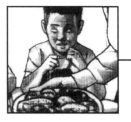

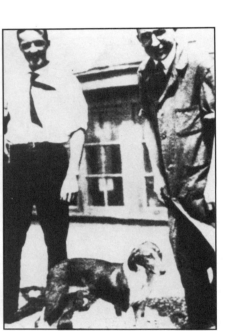

Charles Best (left) and Dr Frederick Banting with the first dog to be kept alive by insulin (August 1921)

which produce and release another hormone called *glucagon*. Glucagon raises the amount of glucose in the blood. Both insulin and glucagon will be discussed in detail later in the book.

Perhaps one of the most significant diabetes experiments occurred in the 1880s, when Oscar Minkowski and Joseph von Mering discovered that the pancreas is closely involved with diabetes. These scientists were not interested in diabetes. They wanted to know what the various organs in the abdomen contributed to the digestion and use of food. They discovered that when the pancreas of a dog was removed, the animal began urinating frequently and the amount of glucose in the blood increased. Ultimately, the animal died. This experiment drew the scientific world's attention to the pancreas and its relationship to diabetes.

Before 1921, the life expectancy of a young person with diabetes was limited to days, weeks, or months. But that year a major breakthrough occurred. Two researchers in Toronto spent the summer trying to isolate a substance from the pancreas they thought would be helpful in treating diabetes. The senior researcher, Dr Frederick Banting, had no special training or experience with diabetes. He was assisted by a young medical student named Charles Best. They were an unlikely pair of diabetes researchers, but together they succeeded in extracting and isolating a substance from the pancreas of a dog. When the substance was injected into diabetic dogs, their blood glucose was lowered and the amount of glucose in their urine decreased. This extract came from the islet cells of the pancreas and was first referred to as isletin. It later became known as insulin. Banting received the Nobel Prize for Medicine in 1923 for his discovery of insulin.

The commercial development and sale of insulin changed the outlook for young people with diabetes. The entire world rejoiced in the belief that a cure for diabetes had been found. It was naively thought that if people with diabetes took their insulin regularly and ate properly, they could live a normal life. In the 1930s, however, the medical literature began to report problems occurring in people who had been treated with insulin since the onset of diabetes. These problems included loss of eyesight, poor blood supplies to the lower legs and feet, increased numbers of heart attacks, and severe damage to the nervous system.

Despite these alarming findings, extensive diabetes research was not resumed until after World War II. At that time, Drs Saul Berson and Rosalyn Yalow, two researchers in New York, attempted to measure the amount of insulin in the blood. Since the amount is extremely small (about one part per billion), this was a very difficult task. When they devised a method of measuring these small quantities of insulin, to their surprise they found there was not always an absence of insulin in people with diabetes. Some had little or no insulin in the blood, others had normal amounts, and

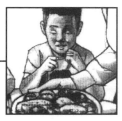

Before insulin, the effects of diabetes and starvation diets were obvious (Sara Hughes before [above] and after [below] insulin treatment)

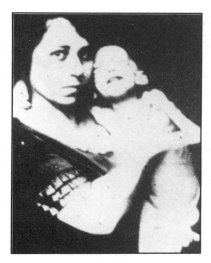

many overweight persons with diabetes frequently had more insulin than persons who did not have the disease. These amazing discoveries stimulated increasing amounts of diabetes research, and Yalow received the Nobel Prize for Medicine in 1977.

This work caused some scientists to question the accepted cause of diabetes. For a long time it had been thought that diabetes was caused by the pancreas not producing a sufficient *quantity* of insulin. Researchers then began to wonder if some people might have diabetes because they were not able to produce a good *quality* of insulin.

In the early 1950s in England, other research unrelated to diabetes also resulted in the development of some new and important information in the field. Dr Frederick Sanger, a scientist, was trying to determine the structure of a protein molecule. He needed a source of a small protein that could be obtained easily in a highly purified state. Insulin is such a protein, and it could be purchased inexpensively at the corner drug store, so he used it in his experiments. Sanger found that the insulin molecule resembles two lengths of chains bound together. He also found that the individual links in the chains varied in different animal species. Insulin from pigs differed from human insulin in only one of the 51 tiny links that make up the two chains, whereas insulin from cattle differed in three sites. Insulin from whales and other animals had other variations, so it was apparent that not all insulin was exactly the same.

In the late 1960s, Dr Donald Steiner of the University of Chicago found a substance that is apparently first made in the islets of the pancreas and then changed into insulin. This substance, proinsulin (pro means "before"), was found to be about 1/20th as effective in lowering blood glucose as insulin. The discovery of proinsulin helped researchers understand how insulin is formed and changed in the pancreas. It also explained how diabetes could occur in some people when the amount of insulin in the blood seems normal. Thus quality, as well as quantity, of insulin is important in the prevention of the disease.

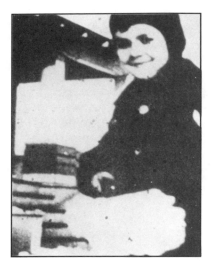

WHAT INSULIN DOES IN THE BODY

When diabetes occurs in the body of young persons and some adults, there is usually a shortage or complete lack of insulin. The insulin-producing cells in the pancreas are scarred or destroyed, so they cannot make insulin. To understand how this lack of insulin affects the body's health, it's necessary to understand how insulin normally functions in the body.

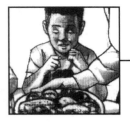

PROTEIN

CARBOHYDRATES

FATS

From the stomach, carbohydrate, protein, and fat from food enter the intestines, where tiny particles (some as glucose) pass through intestinal walls into the bloodstream to be used by the cells for energy or stored in the liver

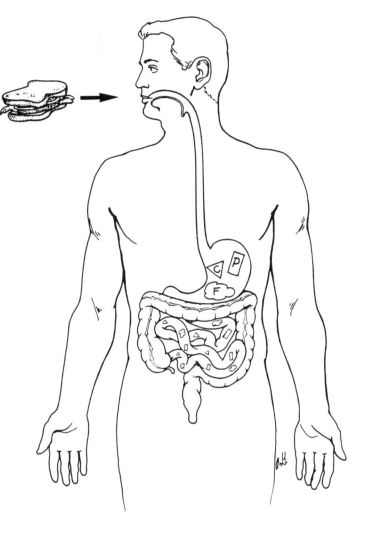

Think of the body as a complex machine. Like any machine, the body has to have energy to work. The body's three sources of energy are found in foods—carbohydrates (sugars and starches), fat (oils and fats), and protein (meat, fish, etc).

After food is chewed and swallowed, it's passed down the esophagus and into the stomach. The stomach is a very muscular organ that adds acid to the food and begins to break it into smaller particles. The particles enter the intestines, where more digestive liquids are added and the food changes into a liquid state. Here the tiny particles of food are absorbed through the walls of the intestines and into the bloodstream. Then they are carried to the trillions of cells that make up all parts of our bodies.

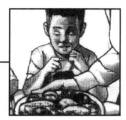

The food most readily available for energy is a carbohydrate called glucose. As the amount of glucose rises in the blood, the pancreas sends a message through the blood to all of the cells in the body in the form of a hormone called insulin. In brief, this message says: "There is a lot of glucose available, use it."

After being released into the blood, insulin is carried to the cells throughout the body and attaches itself to a specific location on the wall of each cell. These places are called insulin receptor sites. They allow insulin to signal the cell to open up its walls, take in glucose, and store it or use it for energy.

When the amount of glucose in the blood is low, the pancreas stops sending out insulin. Without insulin the cells cannot take in glucose, so they switch to using fat as their main source of energy. In this very sophisticated manner, the body is able to determine which energy fuel is available and properly use the foods we eat. When diabetes develops, either the pancreas is unable to produce a quality form of insulin or the body's cells themselves are unable to receive the insulin message. The latter is thought to be the cause of diabetes in most older adults.

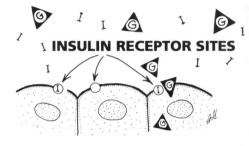

Insulin attaches to its receptor sites, allowing glucose to enter the cells

INSULIN AND BLOOD GLUCOSE LEVELS

Blood glucose (the amount of glucose in the blood) is measured in milligrams per deciliter (written as mg/dl). This measurement shows how many milligrams (thousands of a gram) of glucose are in a deciliter (approximately 1-1/2 ounces) of blood. In people who do not have diabetes, blood glucose is closely controlled at all times. When they don't eat for several hours, blood glucose rarely falls below 70 mg/dl. Even after gorging themselves on sweets, these people are able to keep their blood glucose below 140 mg/dl.

This very fine control is important because we know that if blood glucose gets too high, it can become dangerous. The kidneys must then filter the glucose from the blood and wash it out of the body in the urine. When this occurs, the person must drink large amounts of fluids to provide enough water to "wash" out the excess glucose. It's difficult to replace all of the water that's lost, and the body may quickly become dehydrated (dried out). This can be a serious threat to life.

When there is no insulin available, the body cells can't use glucose for energy and demand another source of energy to carry out their work. Since fat is the other main source of energy available, the cells switch to using it. This fuel is harder for the cells to use. Because the cells can't burn fat

13

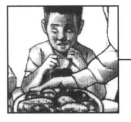

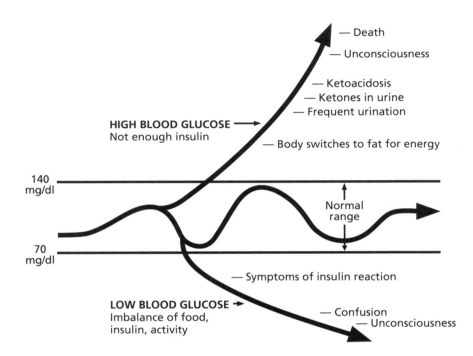

— Death

— Unconsciousness

— Ketoacidosis
— Ketones in urine
— Frequent urination

HIGH BLOOD GLUCOSE ⟶
Not enough insulin

— Body switches to fat for energy

140
mg/dl

Normal
range

70
mg/dl

— Symptoms of insulin reaction

LOW BLOOD GLUCOSE ➤
Imbalance of food,
insulin, activity

— Confusion
— Unconsciousness

completely, some of the unused material, or by-products, begin to build up in the body. These by-products are called *ketones*.

As the ketones increase, a condition called *ketoacidosis* appears. ("Osis" means "a condition of," so ketoacidosis means an acid condition resulting from ketones.) As this occurs, the person's mouth becomes dry and he or she experiences abdominal pain. If ketoacidosis is not recognized and treated promptly with insulin and fluids, the person may begin vomiting, breathing heavily, lose consciousness, and eventually may die.

Ketoacidosis is a serious threat to a person with diabetes whose body does not produce insulin. It is a preventable condition, but you must understand what it is, how to detect it, and what to do. Although ketoacidosis is preventable, it's estimated that 75,000 individuals are hospitalized with ketoacidosis each year and 4,000 die. More information about how to prevent, detect, and treat ketoacidosis can be found in Chapter 11.

It's also dangerous if blood glucose levels get too low. The brain can use only glucose for its source of energy, so when there is little glucose available, the brain begins sending out emergency signals to the rest of the body. The person then experiences hunger, headaches, confusion, and loss of consciousness and may even have convulsions. If the blood glucose is very low over many hours, brain damage may result. Therefore, it's vital that the body closely control the amount of glucose in the blood, not allowing it to become too high or low.

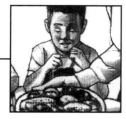

Although diabetes is sometimes referred to as "sugar diabetes," it's important to realize that whenever the way we use carbohydrate is changed, there is also a change in the use of both fat and protein. The inability to use carbohydrate properly immediately results in large amounts of fats being emptied into the bloodstream and sent to the cells as an alternate source of energy. Proper management of diabetes is an attempt to restore the normal pattern of food use and energy production.

MORE THAN ONE KIND OF DIABETES

There are different types of diabetes, and they may be treated differently. We mentioned earlier that when young people and some lean adults develop diabetes, it's usually because they've lost their ability to produce insulin. Older people, however, may have normal, low, or high levels of insulin, yet have high blood glucose levels and diabetes. This should help you understand why people with diabetes may be treated differently. It's also important to remember that each person with the disease has different medical needs, different likes and dislikes, a different lifestyle, and so on, so every diabetes treatment plan must be adapted to individual needs.

Both types of diabetes have long been recognized and basically share the same problem—the inability of the body to properly use food. They have been given separate names as the differences in the causes of diabetes have become better understood.

The type of diabetes that usually occurs in children and young adults has traditionally been called "juvenile diabetes." Since all of these people require daily insulin injections to survive, the term used for this form of the disease is *insulin-dependent diabetes mellitus (IDDM), or Type I (one) diabetes.*

The type of diabetes often referred to as "adult diabetes" is now called *noninsulin-dependent diabetes mellitus (NIDDM), or Type II (two) diabetes.* In this type of diabetes, the pancreas is still making insulin. However, the insulin is not effective in moving glucose into the cells.

Type I diabetes usually appears suddenly in children or young adults with symptoms of extreme thirst, frequent urination, tiredness, and excessive appetite. Rarely do children have these symptoms for more than three or four weeks before diabetes is diagnosed. They may have abdominal pain and vomiting at the time they first come to the doctor and are sometimes mistakenly thought to have the flu or appendicitis. However, if we could look through a microscope at the pancreas of one of these people with early symptoms of Type I diabetes, we might find that the islets are already decreased in number and show other signs of damage.

15

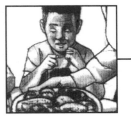

Type II diabetes differs significantly in its onset. Often a doctor may find a history of glucose in the urine or a gradual increase in the blood glucose level over months or years. In older people, diabetes is often discovered during a routine physical examination or at the time of a hospital admission for some other reason. The onset of the disease in this group is frequently not associated with any symptoms. Under a microscope, the pancreas of one of these people would probably appear normal.

The daily problems confronting people with Type I diabetes are quite different from those of people with Type II diabetes. People with Type I diabetes are likely to develop sudden problems resulting from the blood glucose being too low (insulin reactions) or too high (which can lead to ketoacidosis.) These serious disorders must be treated immediately and will be discussed in Chapter 11. These two problems seldom occur in Type II diabetes.

Even the problems that slowly arise over the years in Type I and Type II diabetes are different. People with Type I diabetes more frequently develop destruction of the small blood vessels in the eyes and kidneys. People with Type II diabetes are more prone to damage in the large blood vessels, which causes blood circulation problems, stroke, and heart disease.

Pregnant women sometimes develop a form of diabetes that is considered separate from Type I and Type II diabetes. It's called *gestational diabetes*, and it's usually discovered when the woman has a blood test for glucose done during routine visits for pregnancy. These women may or may not require insulin, but their blood glucose must be controlled very carefully during the remainder of the pregnancy if problems are to be avoided. Gestational diabetes usually goes away at the end of the pregnancy. See Chapter 22 for more information about diabetes and pregnancy. The chart on page 12 summarizes the different types of diabetes.

HOW DIABETES IS DETECTED

The diagnosis of diabetes in children (Type I) is relatively easy. The symptoms of thirst, frequent urination, and tiredness mentioned earlier should prompt the doctor to test blood glucose immediately. When Type I diabetes is present, blood glucose is usually quite high and the diagnosis can be made immediately. It's important to start treatment as soon as possible. The young person should be seen the same day by a doctor, and insulin and nutrition therapy are usually started immediately. Almost all young people with diabetes are dependent on daily injections of insulin. The kinds of insulins used in treating diabetes will be discussed in Chapter 5.

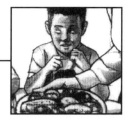

TYPES OF DIABETES

	Type I Insulin-Dependent	Type II Noninsulin-Dependent	Gestational
Onset	Usually in children or young adults.	Usually in obese adults over age 40.	Occurs in 3–5% of pregnant women.
Cause	Heredity and other factors lead to failure of pancreas' ability to produce insulin.	Inherited tendency plus obesity leads to resistance of body cells to action of insulin.	Hormonal changes lead to high blood glucose.
Symptoms	Extreme thirst and excessive appetite, tiredness, and frequent urination. May progress to ketoacidosis.	May be no obvious symptoms, or just slight fatigue and frequent thirst and urination.	Usually none; may be fatigue.
Diagnosis	High blood glucose levels.	Fasting blood glucose test.	Oral glucose tolerance test.
Treatment	Insulin injections, meal planning, and exercise.	Meal planning, exercise, and sometimes pills or insulin injections.	Meal planning, exercise, and sometimes insulin injections.
Acute Complications	Insulin reactions and ketoacidosis.	Usually none.	Usually none.
Intermediate Complications	Failure of growth and development; problems during pregnancy.	Problems during pregnancy.	Problems during pregnancy.
Long-Term Complications	Small blood vessel problems in eyes, kidneys, nerves; large blood vessel problems in heart, brain, and feet.	Large blood vessel problems in heart, brain, and feet; small blood vessel problems in eyes, feet, nerves, and kidneys.	Usually none; high blood glucose usually goes away after delivery. Woman is more likely to develop diabetes later in life.
Prevention of Problems	Diabetes education and blood glucose control.	Diabetes education, weight loss, and blood glucose control.	Blood glucose monitoring for strict control during pregnancy.

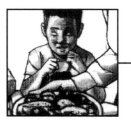

In Type II diabetes, the diagnosis may be more difficult because there is usually no obvious illness. Blood glucose levels are not always higher than normal, but a blood glucose measurement taken after eating may be high, or a measurement done first thing in the morning may be higher than normal. Sometimes a test called a *glucose tolerance test* is used to identify Type II diabetes. The idea behind this test is to give a person a large amount of a sugar drink and then test the blood glucose level after 1/2, 1, and 2 hours.

In people with newly diagnosed Type II diabetes, starting treatment is usually not an emergency, and diabetes management may start with meal planning and weight reduction. Some adults may take diabetes pills in addition to a meal plan. These medications have been available since the mid-1950s. Diabetes pills appear to lower glucose in the blood in two ways: they may stimulate the pancreas to make more insulin or they may increase the sensitivity of body cells to insulin in the blood. (These pills are not useful in Type I diabetes because the islet cells have been destroyed, so there is nothing for the pill to stimulate.) See Chapter 12 for more information about pills for Type II diabetes.

WHY CONTROL IS IMPORTANT

The main goal in treating diabetes is to restore the body's ability to properly use carbohydrates (glucose). This, in turn, results in normal fat and protein use. All experts now agree that with good control, the sudden or acute complications of diabetes (insulin reactions and ketoacidosis) may be minimized or even eliminated.

If diabetes is not controlled over weeks or months, intermediate problems may develop. Young people in poor control may fail to grow and develop. Poor control of diabetes during pregnancy can result in stillbirths and birth defects. Women with diabetes must make certain their diabetes is in very good control before becoming pregnant and then throughout the pregnancy. Some studies have shown that the risk of birth defects is eight times higher when the mother's diabetes is poorly controlled (see Chapter 22 for more details).

In the past, all diabetes experts did not agree that good control of diabetes reduces the risks of long-term complications such as heart attack, stroke, and eye and kidney problems. Increasing numbers of reports, however, suggest that good control does minimize the risk of blindness, kidney disease, and nerve damage. There are not yet any good, long-term

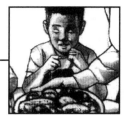

studies that prove whether disease of the large blood vessels, which can cause heart disease and stroke, occurs less often in people with good diabetes control, although most experts believe this is true.

SUMMARY

Diabetes is a serious disease that affects 14 million Americans and cannot be cured at the present time. Good diabetes control requires keeping blood glucose at normal (70-140 mg/dl) or as near-normal levels as possible, which restores the body's ability to correctly use food. To achieve such control, people with diabetes must be informed and cooperate closely with knowledgeable and concerned health professionals in a planned system of care.

The purpose of this manual is to help people with diabetes, and their family members, understand diabetes and discover how important it is to work as a part of the health care team in an individualized program of diabetes care. Indeed, there is a light at the end of the tunnel, and it grows brighter every day!

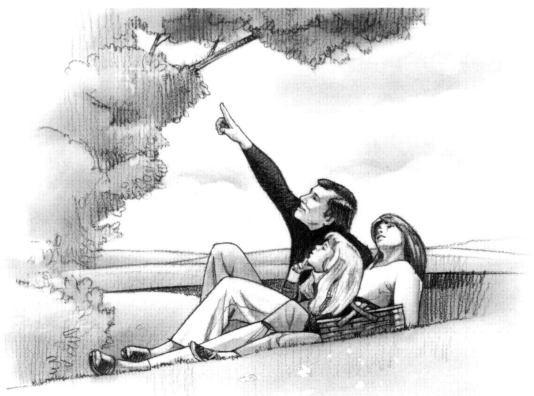

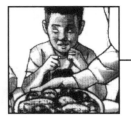

MONITORING YOUR KNOWLEDGE

1. What is diabetes?

_____

2. What is the name of the hormone that lowers blood glucose levels?

_____

3. What is the normal range for blood glucose (sugar) in people who do not have diabetes?

_____

4. What are the two main types of diabetes?

_____

_____

5. List three differences between Type I and Type II diabetes.

_____

_____

_____

6. List two parts of treatment for Type I and Type II diabetes.

_____

_____

7. The type of diabetes that develops during pregnancy is called:

_____

Answers on page 115.

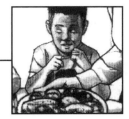

CHAPTER 2

Marion J. Franz, MS, RD, CDE

Nutrition:
The Cornerstone

Why do you have to watch what you eat if you have diabetes?

Will your efforts be worthwhile?

What's all this talk about carbohydrates, proteins, and fat?

What's so important about saturated fats, fiber, and omega-3s?

How do you determine the number of calories you need to eat in a day?

If you've ever wondered about these things, you'll find this chapter helpful. In Chapter 1 you learned that to control diabetes, you need to keep your blood glucose (sugar) level as close to the normal range for as much of the time as possible. Since diabetes affects the way your body turns food into glucose, it's easy to understand why watching what you eat is so important. Other important parts of controlling diabetes include exercise and, if necessary, medication (insulin or diabetes pills). But control of food intake has been called the "cornerstone of diabetes management."

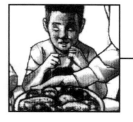

Good nutrition is important for everyone, but if you have diabetes it's even more important. Because of diabetes, your body can no longer correctly use the food you eat. If you are to control your diabetes and have a more healthful, energetic life, you'll want to keep your blood glucose level as normal as possible. To do this, you'll need to control what you eat, know how much to eat, and know when to eat.

To eat correctly, you must first understand some basic things about meal planning, such as how much food you need and how to plan meals and snacks accordingly. This chapter will not only help you do these things, it will also change any negative ideas you might have about "diabetic diets." The word "diet" often has a negative meaning of drastic caloric reduction and boring meals. It has no place in healthful meal planning for diabetes. This chapter will show you how to plan meals with more variety and better nutritional value than those eaten by most people in our society.

MEAL PLANNING AND DIABETES CONTROL

The first and major goal of meal planning is to help you keep your blood glucose level as normal as possible. To do this, you need to balance the food you eat with insulin (either the insulin you take by injection or the insulin your body is still making) and exercise or activity. You need a meal plan you can follow. A meal plan tells you what to eat and when, and it should suit your lifestyle and meet your nutritional needs.

If you take injected insulin, your insulin needs can be adjusted to your food intake. By eating consistently and monitoring your blood glucose, the amount and type of insulin you need to take can be determined. If you have Type II diabetes, controlling the amount and kinds of food you eat may help keep your blood glucose in the normal range. If you are overweight, you will find it important to try to reach a reasonable body weight. Often by losing only 10 to 20 pounds you may find your blood glucose levels returning to normal.

The second goal of meal planning is to help achieve healthy levels of blood fats (lipids). The two blood fats commonly tested for are cholesterol and triglycerides. High levels of these blood fats are associated with the development of heart and blood vessel problems. The goal is to keep blood

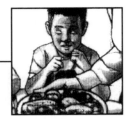

cholesterol levels below 200 mg/dl and triglycerides below 150 mg/dl. For children and adolescents, it's recommended that blood cholesterol levels be below 170 mg/dl.

The third goal is to provide a daily number of calories that will help you reach and stay at a reasonable body weight. For children, it's important that enough calories are available to provide for normal growth and development.

The fourth, and perhaps most important, goal of meal planning is to plan healthful meals that meet all your nutrition needs. The 1990 Dietary Guidelines for Americans suggest that all healthy people two years of age and older should:

1. Eat a variety of foods
2. Maintain a healthy weight
3. Choose a diet low in fat, saturated fat, and cholesterol
4. Choose a diet with plenty of vegetables, fruits, and grain products
5. Use sugar in moderation
6. Use salt/sodium in moderation
7. Use alcohol in moderation, if at all

These guidelines are similar to those recommended for people with diabetes. Watching what we eat is important for everyone!

NUTRIENTS IN FOODS

We eat and need food for a variety of reasons: for energy; for growth, maintenance, and repair of our bodies; for the regulation of body processes that keep our bodies running smoothly; and not to be forgotten, for enjoyment—food is a large part of our social lives!

These needs are provided for by six basic building blocks (nutrients) in foods: carbohydrate, protein, fat, vitamins, minerals, and water. The first three—carbohydrate, protein, and fat—supply our bodies with energy, which is measured in calories. They require insulin to be used correctly. The last three—vitamins, minerals, and water—are important to keep our bodies functioning smoothly but are not sources of energy. Therefore, they don't require insulin to be used by the body.

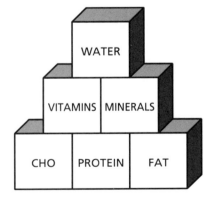

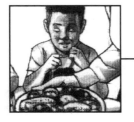

CARBOHYDRATES

Carbohydrates are our bodies' preferred source of energy or fuel and so are important in the diet. Three different types of carbohydrate are found in foods: sugar, starch, and fiber. Sugar is found in foods as either refined sugar (as found in soft drinks, jams, jellies, honey, syrup, candies, and desserts) or "naturally occurring" sugar (as found in fruits, vegetables, and milk). Starches are found in breads, cereals, pastas, and starchy vegetables. Fiber gives structure to foods and cannot be digested by our bodies. Fiber is found in whole grain breads and cereals, in fruits and vegetables, and in legumes such as dried peas, beans, and lentils.

An important question is what type of carbohydrate should people with diabetes eat? Traditionally, sugars have been restricted and starches recommended. However, recent research suggests that different carbohydrate-containing foods affect blood glucose levels differently. But this difference may not be related to the fact that one food is composed mainly of sugar and another mainly of starch.

It was commonly believed that simple carbohydrates or sugars raise blood glucose levels faster and higher than complex carbohydrates or starches. Phyllis Crapo, RD, from the University of California, San Diego, was the first investigator to challenge that belief. She and other researchers discovered that when most people eat sugar, especially in combinations with other foods, their blood glucose did not rise higher than when similar amounts of starches were eaten.

Because of this research, the advice to avoid sugar has been relaxed. But, if you want to use foods containing sugar, you have to know how to do it correctly. Sugar can be substituted only for other carbohydrates in your meal plan. It can't be eaten in addition to foods in your regular meal plan. You have to realize portion sizes are small because many of these foods are sources of concentrated or high amounts of sugar. They often contain large amounts of fat as well, making them high in calories.

How often should you substitute these foods in your meal plan? Generally, foods containing sugar are substituted for starch/bread or fruit exchanges in your meal plan. "Occasional use" is probably still the best advice. It's recommended that you limit these foods to no more than one simple dessert (frozen yogurt, ice cream, or cookies) per day. (Sucrose, which is the same thing as table sugar, may cause triglycerides to rise in some people. If you have elevated triglycerides, try to avoid eating sucrose.)

Remember, carbohydrate foods may affect each person a little differently. Blood glucose monitoring (which will be discussed in Chapters

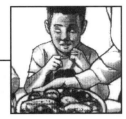

4 and 10) can help you test your response to foods and help you and your dietitian determine the meal plan most effective for you.

PROTEINS

There are both animal and vegetable sources of protein in the diet. Animal sources include meats, fish, poultry, dairy products (such as milk and cheeses), and eggs. Vegetable sources include legumes (such as dried peas, beans, lentils), soybeans, nuts and seeds, and grains, cereals, and vegetables, which contribute smaller amounts. Proteins are composed of amino acids, which are the building blocks for body tissues. Protein can also be changed into glucose.

FOOD FATS

Fats are vital for your body to function properly and are a concentrated source of energy. Fatty acids are the building blocks of fat, and there are three kinds: saturated, monounsaturated, and polyunsaturated. All foods that contain fat are made up of mixtures of these fatty acids. Food sources of fat include meats, dairy products (such as whole milk, cheese, and butter), margarines, oils, salad dressings, desserts, and many snacks and prepared foods. A diet high in fat, especially saturated fatty acids, can increase your blood cholesterol. This is a risk factor for coronary heart disease. Foods that contain fat are usually higher in calories than other foods. Consequently, it's recommended that these foods be reduced in the diet. We'll talk more about the different kinds of fat later.

HOW THE BODY USES
CARBOHYDRATE, PROTEIN, AND FAT

Carbohydrate is absorbed through the intestinal wall as glucose. It is then carried by the bloodstream to the cells, where it can be used for an immediate source of energy, or to the liver or muscles, where it can be stored

25

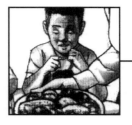

in the form of glycogen. Glycogen can later be converted back to glucose to be used for energy. Carbohydrate not needed as an immediate energy source or stored as glycogen is changed by the liver to fat and stored in fat cells for future fuel needs. Insulin is required for this whole process to take place.

How the body uses carbohydrate

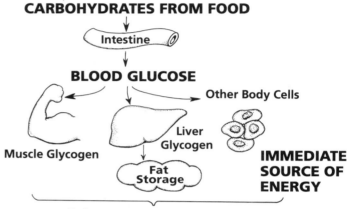

CARBOHYDRATES FROM FOOD

Intestine

BLOOD GLUCOSE

Other Body Cells

Muscle Glycogen

Liver Glycogen

Fat Storage

IMMEDIATE SOURCE OF ENERGY

All these processes require insulin

Protein from food is broken down to amino acids in the intestines. The amino acids are then absorbed through the intestinal walls into the bloodstream. Amino acids are used in forming new body tissue for growth or for repair of body tissue. They can also be used as a backup source of energy. If enough carbohydrate is not available for energy, the liver will change amino acids into glucose. Excess amino acids can also be changed to fat and stored.

Before amino acids can be used as a backup source of energy or stored as fat, insulin must be present. Insulin allows the body to use amino acids for growth and for repair of body tissue. This is one of the reasons children in poor control of their diabetes do not grow well and adults in poor control of their diabetes may not heal as rapidly as they should.

How the body uses protein

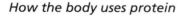

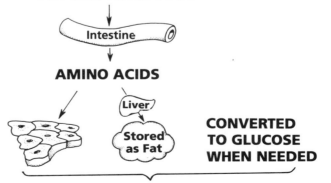

PROTEIN FROM FOOD

Intestine

AMINO ACIDS

Liver

Stored as Fat

CONVERTED TO GLUCOSE WHEN NEEDED

All these processes require insulin

26

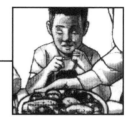

Fats in food are combinations of three fatty acids and are called triglycerides. After fat is absorbed through the intestinal wall, it's taken to the fat cells to be stored and used when necessary as a source of body fuel. Insulin allows triglycerides to enter the fat cells for storage. If enough insulin is not available, levels of triglycerides and cholesterol will often also be high. However, if too much insulin is available, stored fat is prevented from leaving the fat cells. This promotes obesity and makes it difficult to lose weight.

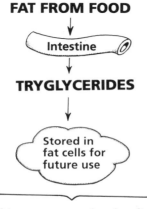

FAT FROM FOOD

Intestine

TRYGLYCERIDES

Stored in fat cells for future use

This process requires insulin

How the body uses fat

Insulin, therefore, is important in the body's use of carbohydrate, protein, and fat. The goal of diabetes management is to have the right amount of insulin available to keep blood glucose and fat levels normal.

PERCENTAGE OF CALORIES FROM CARBOHYDRATE, PROTEIN, AND FAT

Calorie values are determined by burning pure nutrients and measuring the heat they produce. One gram of carbohydrate and one gram of protein each supply 4 calories, whereas one gram of fat supplies 9 calories (approximately 30 grams equal one ounce). The average American diet gets about 35 to 40% of the calories from carbohydrate, 15 to 20% from protein, and 35 to 40% from fat.

It has been recommended that all Americans shift calories from fat sources to carbohydrate sources. The American Diabetes Association also suggests that people with diabetes get up to 50 to 60% of their calories from carbohydrate. However, this needs to be individualized depending on blood glucose and fat (lipid) levels, as well as lifestyle. Starches and

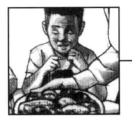

naturally occurring sugars with fiber are emphasized. The recommended percentage of calories from protein is 15 to 20%. Ideally, about 30% of the calories will come from fat, but again, this must be individualized. See the table below for general guidelines.

GENERAL NUTRITIONAL RECOMMENDATIONS FOR PEOPLE WITH DIABETES

Nutrient	Recommended Percentage of Calories	Calories Per Gram	Effect on Blood Glucose	Emphasis
Carbohydrate	50–60%	4	Main source	Eat more high fiber carbohydrates
Protein	15–20%	4	Secondary source	Plan adequate amount for growth and maintenance
Fat	30%	9	Very little	Reduce saturated fats and cholesterol

HOW TO PLAN MEALS

Some amount of thought must always go into planning meals, and this is especially true for people with diabetes. To make this easier for you, the American Diabetes Association and the American Dietetic Association have divided foods into six groups called *exchange lists*. Each list is based on the amounts of carbohydrate, protein, and fat contained in foods. Here are the six exchange lists:

> starch/bread   fruit
> meat and meat substitutes   milk
> vegetables   fat

Each list contains foods in specific serving sizes that contain approximately equal amounts of carbohydrate, protein, and fat—and therefore calories. Because of this, they can be substituted or "exchanged" for one another. It's important to use the correct serving sizes. For example:

> 1 slice bread = 3/4 cup dry cereal = 1 small potato
> 1 apple = ½ banana = 1¼ cup strawberries

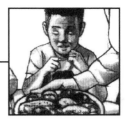

USING THE EXCHANGE LISTS EFFECTIVELY

Foods are listed on the exchange lists in serving sizes. To follow your meal plan, it's important to judge serving sizes correctly. When you begin, it may be a good idea to weigh and measure the correct serving sizes. You'll soon learn to "eyeball" serving sizes quite accurately. It's a good idea to periodically (once or twice a year) weigh and measure food to be sure you're still using correct serving sizes.

Most foods are listed in size by tablespoon or measuring cup amount, but meat is listed by ounces. One ounce of cooked meat, with the bone and fat removed, is one exchange. An average size serving will be 3 ounces of cooked meat, which will be about 1/2 inch thick and about the size of the palm of a woman's hand or a deck of cards.

The exchange lists also help you easily identify good sources of fiber. A symbol for fiber is added next to foods that have 3 or more grams of food fiber per serving. However, you will see that one serving of whole grain foods, vegetables, and fruits also averages 2 grams of food fiber per serving. A different symbol was added next to foods containing more than 400 mg of sodium, so you can see which foods contain large amounts of sodium. More about fiber and sodium later. The exchange lists are described below and printed in Appendix A.

KNOWING THE EXCHANGES

List 1. Starch/Bread: The Starch/Bread list is first because it contains foods higher in carbohydrate as well as fiber, which form the basis of a sound meal plan. Each food item in this list contains approximately 15 grams of carbohydrate, 3 grams of protein, a trace of fat, and 80 calories. Whole grain products on the list average 2 grams of food fiber per serving. Some foods are higher in fiber and have a fiber symbol next to them. This list includes cereal, grains, pasta, dried beans and peas, starchy vegetables, breads, crackers, snacks, and some starch foods prepared with fat. If in doubt about the correct portion of a starch food not on this list, a general rule is that 1/2 cup cereal, grain, or pasta or 1 ounce of a bread product is one serving.

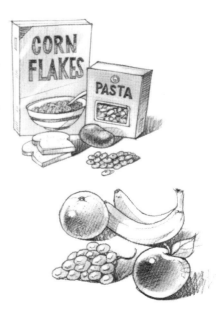

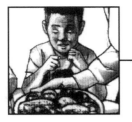

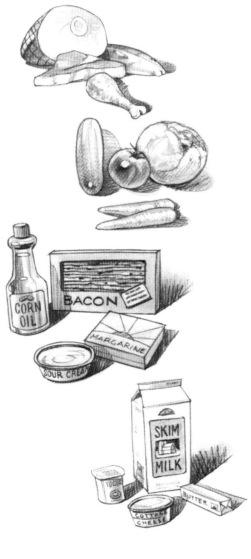

List 2. *Meat and Meat Substitutes:* The Meat and Meat Substitutes list is next for convenience in planning meals. Meats are divided into one of three lists, depending on the amount of fat they contain. One ounce of a lean meat contains about 7 grams of protein, 3 grams of fat, and 55 calories. One ounce of a medium-fat meat contains about 7 grams of protein, 5 grams of fat, and 75 calories. One ounce of a high-fat meat contains about 7 grams of protein, 8 grams of fat, and 100 calories. These are cooked meats with the bone and fat removed and no fat or flour added in preparation. You are encouraged to use more lean and medium-fat meat, poultry, and fish in your meal plan and to limit to three servings per week your choices from the high-fat group.

List 3. *Vegetable:* Vegetable exchanges contribute about 5 grams of carbohydrate, 2 grams of protein, and 25 calories. Vegetables contain 2 to 3 grams of dietary fiber per serving. The serving size is 1/2 cup cooked vegetables or vegetable juice or 1 cup raw vegetables. Starchy vegetables such as corn, peas, and potatoes are on the Starch/Bread list, and vegetables having less than 20 calories per serving are on the Free Food list.

List 4. *Fruit:* Fruit exchanges are based on the amount of fruit or fruit juice that contributes 15 grams of carbohydrate and 60 calories to a meal plan. Fresh, frozen, and dried fruits have about 2 grams of food fiber per serving. Fruit juices contain very little fiber. Fruits vary in portion sizes because they contain different amounts of water. The serving size for one fruit exchange is generally 1 small fresh fruit, 1/2 cup of canned fruit or fruit juice, or 1/4 cup of dried fruit.

List 5. *Milk:* Milk exchanges are based on foods containing 12 grams of carbohydrate and 8 grams of protein. The amount of fat in milk is measured in percent of butterfat, and the calories vary depending on what kind of milk you choose. Skim or very low-fat milk is recommended and contains a trace of fat and 90 calories.

List 6. *Fat:* Fat exchanges are based on the amount of food contributing 5 grams of fat and 45 calories. Portion sizes vary and, in general, are small.

Free Foods: Free foods contribute less than 20 calories per serving. Free foods with a specified serving size listed after the food should be limited to two or three servings per day or one at each meal or snack time, for a total of approximately 50 to 60 extra calories per day. You can eat as much as you want of items that have no serving size specified.

Combination Foods: Combination foods do not fit into only one exchange list, but are combinations of several exchanges. This list helps to fit some common combination foods into your meal plan. For additional foods, see our publication *Exchanges for All Occasions.*

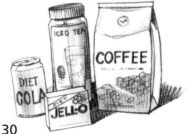

30

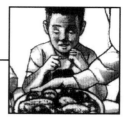

Foods for Occasional Use: If blood glucose control is maintained, moderate amounts of some foods can be used in your meal plan despite their sugar or fat content. Because they are concentrated sources of carbohydrate and fats, the portion sizes are very small. The more careful everyone can be of these foods, the better.

The complete exchange lists are reprinted in Appendix A. Nutritional content of exchanges is outlined below.

NUTRITIONAL CONTENT OF EXCHANGES

One Exchange	Serving Size	Calories	Carbohydrate Gms.	Protein Gms.	Fat Gms.
Starch/Bread	Varies	80	15	3	trace
Meat (lean)	1 oz	55	___	7	3
(medium fat)	1 oz	75	___	7	5
(high fat)	1 oz	100	___	7	8
Vegetable	1/2 cup cooked or 1 cup raw	25	5	2	___
Fruit	Varies	60	15	___	___
Milk (skim)	1 cup	90	12	8	trace
Fat	Varies	45	___	___	5

INDIVIDUALIZING YOUR MEAL PLAN

Each person with diabetes should have a meal plan designed specifically for his or her caloric and nutritional needs, as well as lifestyle. A meal plan tells you how many exchanges you can select for each meal and at snack times. A sample meal planning card is shown on the following page.

As you can see, this meal plan card tells you how many calories are planned for you; how many grams and percentages of carbohydrate, protein, and fat; times for your meals and snacks; and number of servings to select from each exchange list at each meal and snack time.

Using the exchange lists to plan your meals allows you more flexibility while helping to keep your diabetes in good control. However, different foods from the same exchange list may affect your blood glucose differently

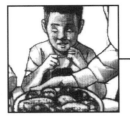

· MY MEAL PLAN ·

Meal Plan for: Jane Smith   Date: Jan. 6, 1986

Dietitian: M. Franz   Phone: 555-1234

	Grams	Percent
Carbohydrate	230	53%
Protein	80	18%
Fat	60	29%
Calories	1800	

Time	Meal Plan		Menu Ideas	Menu Ideas
7:30 a.m.	3	Starch	1 cup oatmeal	
	—	Meat	1 slice whole wheat toast	
	—	Vegetable	1/2 grapefruit	
		Fruit	1 cup skim milk	
	1 Skim	Milk	1 tsp. margarine	
	1	Fat		
12:30	2	Starch	2 slices whole wheat bread	
	2	Meat	2 oz. sliced turkey	
	0-1	Vegetable	lettuce + tomato slices	
	1	Fruit	1 apple	
	1 Skim	Milk	1 c. skim milk	
	1	Fat	1 tsp. mayonnaise	
3:30	1 Fruit or Starch		3 graham cracker squares	
6:30	2	Starch	1 baked potato with 1 tsp margarine	
	3	Meat	1 small roll with 1 tsp. margarine	
	2	Vegetable	3 oz. broiled chicken breast	
	1	Fruit	1/2 cup green beans	
	—	Milk	dinner salad with lo-cal dressing	
	2	Fat	15 grapes	
10:00	1 Fruit		1 orange	
	1 Starch		3 cups popped corn	
	0-1 Fat			

than they affect another person's blood glucose. By doing blood glucose monitoring, you can determine for yourself how each food affects you. About one-and-a-half hours after eating you will see the peak effect of food reflected in blood glucose levels. Your blood glucose should be back to what it was before the meal in about four to five hours.

Your meal plan is based on several factors:

1. Your caloric and nutrient requirements.

2. Your lifestyle—what you feel will be convenient for you to do consistently. The meal plan is worthless if you will not or cannot follow it.

3. Your diabetes therapy:

   Insulin. Food needs to be coordinated with the predictable time action of various insulins. In people who don't have diabetes, the body releases the amount of insulin needed for the amount of food

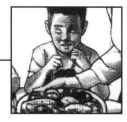

eaten at that time. Unfortunately, injected insulin cannot do this. It's important to take insulin injections at about the same time each day. This makes it essential to eat meals and snacks of about the same amount at the scheduled times.

Diabetes Pills. Some people require a diabetes pill to help control their blood glucose levels. Food must then be matched to the time action of the diabetes pills.

Diet Alone. If your diabetes is being controlled by diet only, exact timing of your meals is not as important. What will be important is the amount eaten. Eating three small meals and a few snacks to spread your food intake over the day, however, may help you control blood glucose levels.

4. Your activity level. Your normal level of physical activity will be reflected in your caloric requirements. If you take insulin, exercise causes your body to use the insulin more effectively and may lower blood glucose levels. Therefore, based on your blood glucose level before or after exercise, extra food may need to be added. Routine exercise times are planned for in the meal pattern. If you control your blood glucose levels by diet alone, exercise makes your body cells more sensitive to the insulin your body is still producing, thus helping to control your blood glucose levels.

What is most important, however, is your acceptance of the meal plan. You must feel you can follow it and live with it. If this is the case, you can learn to adjust your insulin dose (or your health care provider can advise you) on the basis of your blood glucose levels before and after meals. See pages 34 and 35 for two examples of meal plans and menus.

FIGURING OUT YOUR CALORIE NEEDS

It's important that your meal plan has the right number of daily calories to help you reach or stay at a reasonable weight. Children need enough calories to allow for normal growth and development as well.

Dietitians use general guidelines to estimate what a person's caloric needs will be. These guidelines are used to design a meal plan that should be followed for a time to see if the planned calorie level does meet your needs. During this time, weight patterns are followed in adults and growth patterns are followed in children to see if changes in the number of calories are needed.

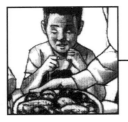

SAMPLE MEAL PLANS AND MENUS

Plan A
1,500 calories
190 grams carbohydrate (52%)
75 grams protein (20%)
45 grams fat (28%)

Meal	Exchanges	Food
Breakfast		
Starch/Bread	2	1 slice whole wheat toast, 1/2 cup Raisin Bran®
Fruit	1	1/2 grapefruit
Milk	1/2	1/2 cup skim milk
Fat	1	1 tsp margarine
Lunch		
Starch/Bread	2	2 slices whole wheat bread
Meat	2	2 oz turkey
Vegetable	0–1	carrot sticks
Fruit	1	1 apple
Milk	1	1 cup skim milk
Fat	1	1 tsp margarine
Snack		
Fruit	1	15 grapes
Dinner		
Starch/Bread	1	1 small baked potato
Meat	3	3 oz lean roast beef
Vegetable	2	1/2 cup green beans, dinner salad
Fruit	1	1/3 cup pineapple chunks
Fat	1	1 tsp margarine, low-calorie salad dressing
Evening Snack		
Starch/Bread	1	5 snack crackers
Milk	1/2	1/2 cup skim milk
Fat	0–1	(in crackers)

To determine how many daily calories an adult needs, it's first necessary to find the person's desirable body weight. The following general guidelines can be used:

Women: You should weigh 100 pounds for the first 5 feet and then add 5 pounds for each additional inch of height.

Men: You should weigh 106 pounds for the first 5 feet and then add 6 pounds for each additional inch of height.

Frame size: A person's frame size, which is the general size of the body structure, is important when figuring desirable body weight. Wrist or elbow measurements are often used to find whether a person has a large, medium, or small frame. Sometimes, however, you may just need to visually assess

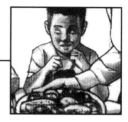

Meal	Exchanges	Food
Breakfast		
Starch/Bread	3	1 English muffin; 3/4 cup Cheerios®
Fruit	1	1 orange
Milk	1	1 cup skim milk
Fat	1	1 tsp margarine; sugar-free jelly
Snack		
Fruit or Bread	1	1 apple
Lunch		
Starch/Bread	3	1 cup vegetable beef soup; 2 slices whole wheat bread
Meat	2	2 oz lean beef
Vegetable	0–1	2 tomato slices; lettuce
Fruit	1	12 cherries
Milk	1	1 cup skim milk
Fat	1	1 tsp mayonnaise
Snack		
Starch/Bread	1	3 graham cracker squares
Fruit	1	1 fruit roll-up
Dinner		
Starch/Bread	2	1 small baked potato; 1 roll
Meat	3	3 oz broiled fish
Vegetable	2	1/2 cup carrots, dinner salad
Fruit	1	1 1/4 cup strawberries
Fat	3	1 tbsp salad dressing; 1 tsp margarine; 2 tbsp sour cream
Evening Snack		
Starch/Bread	1	1 oz small bagel
Fruit	1	1/3 canteloupe
Fat	0–1	1 tsp margarine

SAMPLE MEAL PLANS AND MENUS

Plan B
2,100 calories
280 grams carbohydrate (54%)
90 grams protein (18%)
65 grams fat (28%)

what you think is your frame size. If you have a small frame, subtract 10% from the above weight; if you have a large frame, add 10%.

An estimate of your daily caloric needs can be made once desirable weight is calculated. This is an approximate number of calories, which may change depending on activity level and lifestyle. You can estimate your caloric needs by multiplying your desirable body weight by the number of calories needed per pound:

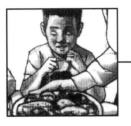

Moderately active men and very active women: 15 calories per pound of desirable body weight. Higher activity levels require additional calories, and body weight should be monitored closely to make sure needs are being met.

Moderately active women, sedentary men, or adults after age 55: 13 calories per pound of desirable body weight.

Obese or very inactive adults: 10 calories per pound of desirable body weight.

If you need to lose weight, the meal plan must include fewer calories than you use each day. About 3,500 calories are stored in each pound of body fat. So to lose one pound of fat, you must either reduce caloric intake, increase energy expenditure, or do a combination of both to equal a 3,500 calorie loss over several days. To lose one pound a week, you would need to consume 500 fewer calories per day than you need to maintain current weight, giving you a 3,500-calorie deficit after seven days. To lose two pounds per week, a 1,000-calorie-a-day deficit is needed. (To gain weight you would reverse the procedure but continue to exercise, so most of the added weight will be muscle weight rather than fat.)

The best way to lose weight is to combine extra energy expenditure with a cutback in caloric intake. The extra energy you use could come from having a regular exercise program or from changing routine activities to make them more active, such as taking the stairs instead of the elevator, walking or biking to the store instead of driving, and so on. See Chapter 3 for information about exercise and Chapter 13 for information about weight loss.

Generally, daily calorie levels below 1,200 for women and 1,500 for men are not recommended. At lower levels it's difficult to meet nutritional requirements, and the diet becomes so limited that it is difficult to follow.

Use the information you've just learned to determine your caloric needs. Complete the chart on the next page.

CALORIC NEEDS FOR CHILDREN

For children and young adults, caloric needs are based on age, height, and activity level. It's important to record height and weight on a growth chart at least every three to six months. If height or weight fails to increase in a child who should be growing, the cause must be investigated. Some possible causes are not enough calories and/or poor control of diabetes.

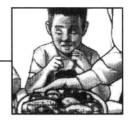

Fill in the blanks:

Your desirable body weight: _____

Add or subtract for frame size: _____

Desirable body weight (DBW): _____

Multiply desirable body weight by the number of calories needed per pound:

DBW_____ x _____cal/pound = _____

If you need to lose weight, subtract 500 calories: - 500 _____

If you need to gain weight, add 500 calories: + 500 _____

My caloric needs per day are: _____

HOW MANY CALORIES DO YOU NEED PER DAY?

An example of a height and weight chart is shown on the next page. You can see that the boy being charted was growing in the 75th percentile before developing diabetes. This means that if 100 boys his age were lined up according to height, 75 would be shorter and 25 would be taller than he is. But after this boy developed diabetes, his growth slowed to about the 25th percentile, meaning that out of 100 boys his age, 75 are now taller than he is. Such a change in growth rate should not happen. If enough insulin is not available and, as a result, blood glucose levels are high, the body cannot use food for growth and development. The growth chart allows a health professional to detect slowed growth early, when meal plan changes and/or diabetes control can still restore normal growth.

In general, children and young adults need the following number of calories each day (if they are very active or tall for their age they may need more):

Children under 12 years of age: 1,000 calories plus 100 calories per year of age. For example, a 10-year-old would need about 2,000 calories a day.

Boys age 12 to 15: 1,000 calories plus 100 calories per year of age through 11 and then 200 calories per year from 12 to 15. For example, a 13-year-old boy needs about 2,500 calories a day (1,000 + 1,100 + 400 = 2,500).

Girls age 12 to 15: This varies depending on the girl's activity level. Caloric needs often drop during the late teen years, so it is important to adjust the meal plan at this time to avoid excess weight.

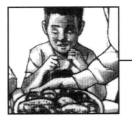

Young men age 15 to 20: Moderately active young men need about 18 calories per pound of weight per day. Very physically active young men need about 20 to 25 calories per pound. Relatively inactive young men need only about 15 calories per pound.

Young women age 15 to 20: Moderately active young women need about 14 to 16 calories per pound of weight per day.

Example of a height and weight chart

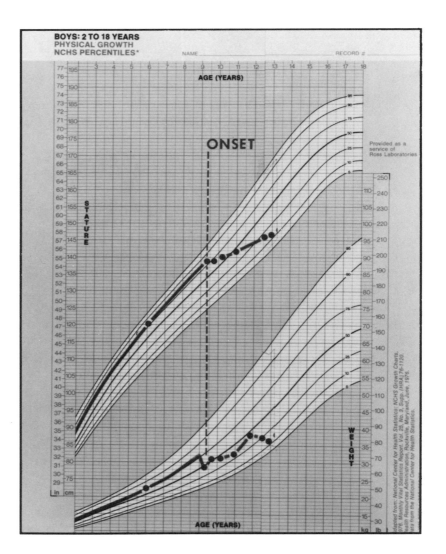

38

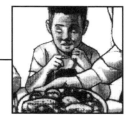

OTHER FACTS ABOUT MEAL PLANNING

We've discussed the basics of meal planning for persons with diabetes, but there are some other general concerns. It is usually recommended that you increase the amount of fiber in your diet and cut back on fat, especially saturated fats and food cholesterol. Use of salt and alcohol in moderation is also recommended.

Fiber. Fiber is the part of plant foods you can't digest or break down. There are two basic kinds of fiber—water-insoluble and water-soluble—and each has a different beneficial effect.

Water-insoluble, or more commonly known as insoluble fiber, is the type of fiber that adds bulk to the diet and has a laxative effect on the digestive system. You usually feel fuller after eating these foods. Sources of insoluble fiber are wheat bran, whole wheat or grains (such as found in some breads, cereals, and crackers), and some vegetables.

Soluble fibers appear to form a gel within the digestive system. They have been shown to lower blood cholesterol, especially when added to a low-fat diet. In some studies they've been shown to slow absorption of food, causing a lowering of blood glucose levels. Sources of soluble fiber are oat bran, legumes (dried beans and peas), barley, and some fruits and vegetables, particularly those with edible peels and seeds, such as berries, cucumbers, and so on.

Average American women consume approximately 12 grams of food fiber per day and men about 18 grams per day. Fiber intake is generally recommended to be about 20 to 35 grams per day, or double the average amount now consumed. Although the beneficial effects of dietary fiber on blood glucose and cholesterol levels are controversial, from a nutritional standpoint it's still good advice to increase fiber in your diet. Foods that contain fiber are good sources of other important vitamins and minerals, and they improve the overall nutritional quality of your diet.

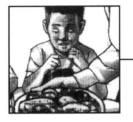

The following table summarizes average amounts of fiber per serving.

FOODS CONTAINING DIETARY FIBER

Food	Serving Size	Grams of Fiber (average)
Starches		
Breads: whole wheat, whole grain, or crackers	1 slice or 1 oz	2
Cereals: dry or cooked	varies	3
Bran	1/3–1/2 cup	8
Starchy vegetables: potatoes, brown rice, green peas	1/2 cup	3
Legumes: peas, beans, lentils	1/3 cup	4–5
Grains: kasha, couscous, bulgur, wild rice	1/2 cup	2
Fruits		
Fresh, frozen, or canned	1/2 cup	2
Fresh	1 small	2
Vegetables		
Cooked, canned, or frozen	1/2–3/4 cup	2
Raw	1–2 cups	3

To increase both types of fiber in your meal plan:

- Choose whole grain cereals, such as bran flakes, oat cereals, and other high-fiber cereals.
- Choose whole grain breads. Look for labels that say whole wheat, whole grain, stone ground, rye flour, whole oats. Dark-colored breads contain little or no whole grain, just molasses for coloring.
- Select fresh fruit and vegetables instead of juices. Eat the skin of cleaned fruits and vegetables.
- Substitute baked potatoes with skins for mashed potatoes.
- Add cooked dry beans and peas to soups, stews, and casseroles.
- Snack on vegetables, fruit, air-popped popcorn, and cereals instead of high-fat snack foods.
- Drink plenty of water as you increase your fiber intake gradually. Otherwise fiber will have a constipating effect instead of a laxative effect.
- Increase your fiber intake slowly. Intestinal gas may occur when fiber intake is increased.

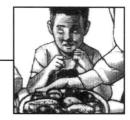

■ Eat a variety of fiber-rich foods in reasonable amounts. Fiber should come from food, not fiber supplements.

Fat. Coronary heart disease is the leading cause of death for all persons in the United States as well as for persons with diabetes. Several factors increase your chances of developing coronary heart disease. Three of the main risk factors you can help reduce are cigarette smoking, high blood pressure, and high blood cholesterol levels. Approximately half of all adult Americans have blood cholesterol levels above the recommended 200 mg/dl. What you eat, particularly the type and amount of fat in your diet, influences your blood cholesterol levels. Countries in which the people consume a high percentage of their calories from fat have a higher incidence of heart disease compared with countries in which people consume a lower percentage of their calories from fat.

Fatty acids are the building blocks of fat, and there are three kinds: saturated, monounsaturated, and polyunsaturated. All foods that contain fat are made of mixtures of these fatty acids. Americans obtain roughly 37% of their total daily calories from fat and 14% from saturated fat. It's recommended that fat intake be kept to about 30% of calories and saturated fat intake to about 10% of calories.

Food cholesterol is a fat-like substance found only in animal foods. It is also made by your body. Americans eat about 350 to 450 mg of food cholesterol each day. It is recommended that food cholesterol intake be reduced to below 300 mg daily. Your body needs cholesterol to make hormones as well as bile salts and acids, and it is an important part of cell walls. However, you don't want an elevated blood cholesterol level. The effect of food cholesterol on blood cholesterol varies from person to person.

Here are some terms you need to understand when we discuss fat:

Saturated fatty acids are generally found in animal foods, such as meat, whole milk dairy products, butter, and lard. Some plant sources of saturated fatty acids are coconut oil, palm oil, and palm kernel oil. Saturated fats are often used in baked goods and nondairy food products, such as creamers and whipped topping. Saturated fatty acids are usually solid at room temperature and raise blood cholesterol.

Unsaturated fatty acids, or ***polyunsaturated fatty acids,*** are found in oils such as safflower, sunflower, corn, and soybean. They are liquid at room temperature. The general effect of these fats is to lower blood cholesterol levels.

Monounsaturated fatty acids are found in olive oil, canola (rapeseed) oil, peanut oil, olives, peanuts, and most nuts and seeds. They also lower blood cholesterol level but have the added advantage of not lowering high-density lipoprotein (HDL), or the "good" cholesterol, levels.

41

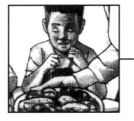

Omega 3 fatty acids, or *fish oils,* are a type of fat found in fish from cold water and in fatty fish, such as mackerel, perch, cod, salmon, tuna, and sole. Fish oils lower blood triglyceride levels and prevent blood platelets from clotting. In countries where fish intake is high and saturated fat intake is low, heart disease is low. However, taking fish oil supplements is not recommended; instead you are encouraged to eat fish two or more times a week. In persons with diabetes, fish oil supplements have been shown to worsen blood glucose control.

Hydrogenation is a chemical process that adds hydrogen to fatty acids and changes them from liquid (unsaturated) to a more solid (saturated) form. Hydrogenation lengthens the shelf life of food products, but because it also changes the unsaturated fatty acids to saturated fatty acid, it's recommended that liquid vegetable oils be used instead.

Cholesterol is a fat-like substance, and in the diet it comes from animal foods such as egg yolks, liver and other organ meats, red meat, poultry, and dairy-fat food products. Blood cholesterol levels are generally more reflective of the total amount and type of fat in the diet and cholesterol made by your body than of food cholesterol.

Lipoproteins transport cholesterol throughout the bloodstream. Since fats are not soluble in the blood, they require a carrier in order to be transported in the body. "Lipo" means fat and "protein" is the carrier. There are three main types of lipoproteins:

Low-density lipoprotein (LDL) cholesterol carries most of the cholesterol throughout the body. When too much LDL cholesterol circulates in the blood, it combines with other substances to narrow the blood vessels. A high level of LDL cholesterol increases your risk of heart disease.

High-density lipoprotein (HDL) cholesterol carries cholesterol away from the arteries back to the liver where it can be disposed. A high level of HDL cholesterol, also known as "good" cholesterol, protects against heart disease. A major factor that increases HDL cholesterol is exercise. Persons who exercise regularly have higher levels of HDL cholesterol.

Very-low-density lipoprotein (VLDL) cholesterol is the major carrier of triglycerides to the fat cells for storage.

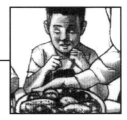

LIMITING FAT IN YOUR DIET

The following table lists grams of fat to equal 30% of the total calories in your diet. Knowing what your total grams of fat should be in a day will help you put food labels to good use. Some labels tell you how much fat is in each serving. This can help you keep track of your daily intake.

If Your Total Calories are:	Your Total Grams of Fat Should Be:
1200	40
1500	50
1800	60
2000	67
2500	83
3000	100

To reduce total fat in your meal plan:
- Limit meat portion sizes. Try to limit yourself to six meat exchanges or 6 ounces of meat per day.
- Use lean meats, such as fish, poultry, and lean beef, as often as possible. Remove skin from poultry.
- Trim visible fat from meats before and after cooking.
- Avoid high-fat meats, such as sausage, frankfurters, prime cuts of meats, and luncheon meats (cold cuts).
- Cook to get rid of as much fat as possible, for example, broil, bake, or boil. Remove fat before making gravies and sauces.
- Use a nonstick pan or nonstick vegetable cooking spray.
- Use skim milk. If you now drink whole milk, move down gradually from 2% to 1% and then to skim milk.
- Use a margarine with a liquid vegetable oil as the first ingredient. A tub margarine will be more unsaturated than a stick margarine. Be careful of portion sizes.

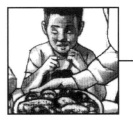

- Use liquid vegetable oils whenever possible. In recipes calling for 1 cup of solid shortening, substitute 3/4 cup of liquid vegetable oil; replace 1/2 cup shortening with 1/3 cup vegetable oil. Limit amount used.
- Use low-fat dairy products. Low-fat yogurt can be substituted for sour cream and mayonnaise. Try some of the skim milk cheeses.
- Limit intake of egg yolks to four per week.

Salt. All Americans are also encouraged to cut back on their salt intake. Obesity, inherited tendency (genetics), and high salt intake increase the risk of high blood pressure. Since people with diabetes appear to be especially susceptible to high blood pressure, and high blood pressure greatly increases the seriousness of diabetes complications, weight loss and sodium reduction are crucial. Together they can often bring high blood pressure into the normal range.

The average American daily diet contains 8 to 12 grams of salt; much more than the recommended 5 grams. Salt is approximately 40% sodium and 60% chloride. One teaspoon of salt is 5 grams (5,000 milligrams) and contains 2,300 mg of sodium. The sodium is what contributes to the development of high blood pressure.

In general, it's recommended that you try to keep your sodium intake to less than 3,000 mg per day, or about 800 to 1,000 mg per meal. Food labels list sodium in milligrams per serving.

To reduce salt in your meal plan:

- Add little or no salt to foods at the table.
- Taste foods before salting to let yourself appreciate their natural flavors, which are often obscured by salt.
- Cook with only a small amount of added salt.
- Avoid foods containing obvious amounts of salt, such as crackers and snack foods, pickles, olives, and so on.
- Limit use of processed foods such as high-salt meat products (ham, bacon, sausage, cold cuts) and convenience foods. Canned soups, other canned or packaged food, and frozen entrees or dinners are other major food sources of sodium.
- Limit intake of salty foods, such as pickles, sauerkraut, and salted snacks.
- Limit use of "fast foods."
- Experiment with herbs and spices as alternatives to salt used in cooking and to salt-based condiments such as soy sauces, steak sauces, catsup, and seasoned salts.

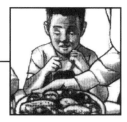

SUMMARY

The field of nutrition is changing rapidly. As facts become known and ideas change, nutritional recommendations will also undergo evaluation and change. However, with the information available to us today, it's possible to make meal planning for persons with diabetes more flexible and enjoyable while controlling blood glucose and blood fat levels as well. More nutritious eating habits can lead to improved health and a longer life for all family members who share the changes being made by the person with diabetes.

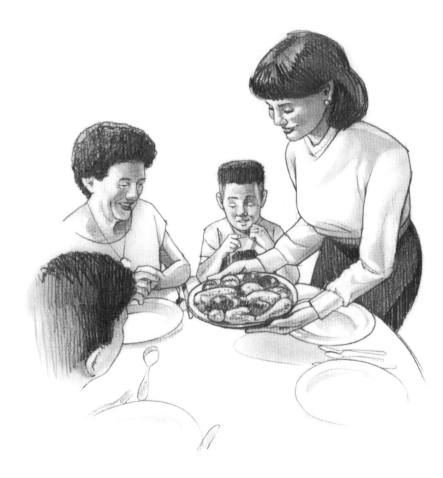

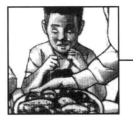

MONITORING YOUR KNOWLEDGE

1. Give two reasons why it's important to watch what you eat if you have diabetes.

_____

_____

2. Name the three nutrients found in food that need insulin for the body to use correctly.

_____

_____

_____

3.Name the six exchange lists.

_____

_____

_____

_____

_____

_____

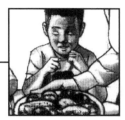

4. *Free foods contain less than how many calories per serving?*

_____

5. *What does a meal plan tell you?*

_____

6. *List three factors that will determine how many calories you need.*

_____

_____

_____

7. *Name the two types of fiber found in foods.*

_____

_____

8. *Name three types of fats found in food.*

_____

_____

_____

Answers on page 116.

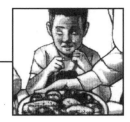

CHAPTER 3

Marion J. Franz, MS, MS, CDE
Jane Norstrom, MA

Exercise:
The Advantage Is Yours

Does exercise benefit you if you have diabetes?

Is exercise risky if you have diabetes?

How can a person get started in an exercise program?

What does "aerobic" mean?

Exercise can be fun and beneficial to everyone's health, but it may have some added benefits if you have diabetes. Exercise has the potential to lower blood glucose (sugar) levels and to help you control your weight. Overall, the fitness achieved through exercise can make many aspects of life easier and more enjoyable.

You may be interested in an exercise program but worried about precautions related to your diabetes. This chapter and Chapters 9, 14, and 27 explain those things and help you get started toward enjoying the benefits of exercise.

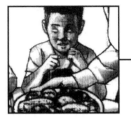

Although most people agree that exercise is important, many are reluctant to start a regular exercise program. Some argue that their daily work routine provides enough activity. However, in our mechanized society, work and home activities rarely provide enough of the type of activity that is beneficial. Others feel they don't have the time, money, or ability to exercise. Or they're reluctant because they don't know how to begin or how to put together an exercise program.

BENEFITS OF EXERCISE

Persons with diabetes will experience the same benefits and enjoyment everyone else gains from exercise: improved fitness, reduced body fat and increased muscle tone, weight control, and psychological benefits.

Exercise improves fitness. The official definition of physical fitness is: "The ability to carry out daily tasks with vigor and alertness, without undue fatigue, and with ample reserve energy to enjoy leisure pursuits and meet unforeseen emergencies." Although this seems like a long definition, the goal of an exercise program is exactly this—to help you become physically fit so you can have a healthy, active life.

Total fitness includes better flexibility, increased muscle strength and endurance, and improved heart and lung efficiency. Exercise programs should be designed to improve all three.

Flexibility keeps our bodies mobile and helps prevent injury to muscles and joints. As we age, our bodies lose flexibility. This loss of flexibility is what makes people look old. Sometimes the muscle collagen (muscle fibers) in persons with diabetes can become glycosylated (glucose becomes attached to them), resulting in decreased flexibility. Stretching exercises are important to help maintain and improve flexibility.

It's no secret that physical appearance improves as muscles become firmer. More importantly, muscle strength and endurance help us perform our daily tasks with less strain and give us increased capacity for physical work. Muscle strength also helps prevent injuries. This is important for persons with diabetes who may develop neuropathy (nerve damage), which can also weaken and damage muscles.

Improved heart and lung efficiency helps us maintain high energy levels for daily activities. It's also important because it helps reduce the risk of heart disease, which is a common long-term complication of diabetes.

Exercise reduces body fat and increases muscle. As fitness improves, you increase the amount of muscle and decrease the amount of fat stored

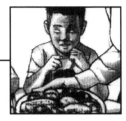

on your body. You become leaner, which improves your health. This has an added benefit for persons with diabetes, because muscle cells use and store more glucose than fat cells.

Exercise assists with weight control. If you are lean, exercise can help you maintain your weight. If you are overweight, it can help you lose weight. Weight loss can occur with exercise, but to be successful you still must decrease your food intake.

Exercise helps burn calories and increases your metabolic rate (a measure of how much energy your body uses and how fast). This means you burn more calories than a person who does not exercise. Weight loss from an exercise program will be mostly fat loss, as opposed to the losses of body water and lean body tissue (muscle) that so often occur from dieting alone.

Exercise has psychological benefits. Exercise helps people cope with stress. It builds self-confidence and improves self-image, especially if you don't think of yourself as athletic yet find you enjoy exercise. You have more energy to do things, are more relaxed, and feel less tense.

EXTRA BENEFITS OF EXERCISE IF YOU HAVE DIABETES

Diabetes is not a reason to avoid physical activity. On the contrary, it may be another reason to incorporate exercise into your lifestyle. In addition to the benefits we just listed, the person with diabetes gains other benefits from exercise.

Exercise can lower blood glucose levels. Body cells become more sensitive to insulin after exercise, which improves their ability to use and store glucose.

Exercise helps reduce risk factors for heart disease. Regular exercise (three to four times a week) has been shown to lower the incidence of coronary heart disease in persons who do not have diabetes. Exercise training can lower the amount of fat (triglycerides and cholesterol) in the blood, which are risk factors for heart disease, and increase HDL cholesterol, which protects against heart disease. Since persons with diabetes seem to develop heart and blood vessel disease at an earlier age and with greater frequency than persons who do not have diabetes, this is particularly important.

Exercise lowers blood pressure. High blood pressure (hypertension) contributes to many of the long-term problems that occur with diabetes. This lowering occurs even if you don't lose weight or decrease body fat.

Exercise combined with a reduction in daily caloric intake will often control Type II diabetes, without the need for other medication. Many

51

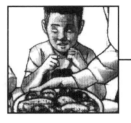

people with Type II diabetes are obese, and obesity decreases the body's ability to use insulin. Physical training, even without weight loss, can help improve the body's ability to use insulin.

RISKS FROM EXERCISE

Exercise can also pose risks to some persons with diabetes. It's important that you are aware of this and check to see if there are reasons you shouldn't exercise. Before beginning an exercise program, it's important to get your doctor's approval, especially if you're over age 40 or have had diabetes for 10 years or more.

Eye, kidney, or nerve problems may be worsened by the wrong type of exercise or strenuous exercise. Nerve damage can blunt or block the body's signals of pain or discomfort from exercise, leading to serious injury before you notice the problem. Injuries to feet can occur, especially if there is existing nerve damage or if proper precautions are not taken. High-quality, well-fitting shoes and socks appropriate for the activity are especially important.

Blood pressure during exercise may rise higher in persons with diabetes than in persons who do not have diabetes. Since persons with diabetes are at increased risk for heart problems, stop exercising and consult your doctor if you notice any of the following symptoms:

- chest pain
- dizziness
- unusual fatigue
- visual disturbances
- nausea

In addition, you'll need to know how to prevent hypoglycemia (low blood glucose) if you take insulin injections or diabetes pills. Hyperglycemia (too high a blood glucose) can also cause problems. Exercise information specific to Type I diabetes will be discussed in Chapter 9. Information specific to Type II diabetes will be discussed in Chapter 14.

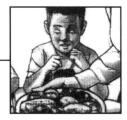

HOW TO BEGIN

Knowing how to exercise correctly and safely is important. You need to start slowly and build up endurance gradually to avoid stiff and sore muscles. Doing the right type of exercise will reduce your chances of injury while improving your health and blood glucose control.

For general fitness and blood glucose control, choose activities that are aerobic. Aerobic activities require large amounts of oxygen and involve movement of large muscle groups (such as the arms and legs). Aerobic exercise uses a lot of energy and, if done for long periods, many calories.

When performed correctly for long enough periods, aerobic exercise strengthens the heart and lungs. This occurs because the heart and lungs are required to work harder for a longer time to supply the exercising muscles with blood and oxygen. It also makes the heart and lungs more efficient at rest and when performing less strenuous tasks. You can do aerobic activities for long periods without becoming breathless because your body is able to continue using oxygen. Walking is an excellent aerobic exercise. Other examples are swimming, jogging, cycling, roller skating, cross-country skiing, dancing, and chair exercises using arms and legs.

Anaerobic activities are the opposite of aerobic exercise. (Anaerobic means without oxygen.) Anaerobic activities are performed at a high level of energy (intensity) for short periods, such as sprinting or running up a hill or stairs. These activities exceed the ability of the heart and lungs to deliver and process oxygen, and exhaustion quickly sets in.

Examples of other anaerobic activities are tennis, football, calisthenics, bowling, volleyball, and other sports in which you stop and start a lot, as well as gardening and household chores (laundry, cleaning, etc). Anaerobic activities can be fun and can increase performance, muscle strength, endurance, and agility. Some burn calories, but not nearly as many as aerobic exercise. Some anaerobic activities can become aerobic if they're done with continuous movement. Both aerobic and anaerobic activities have been shown to improve blood glucose control.

KNOWING HOW HARD TO EXERCISE

When doing aerobic exercise, it's important to exercise at a level that will improve fitness without overexerting. Since it's sometimes difficult to know exactly how hard your body is working, there are two methods you can use to figure it out: heart rate and perceived exertion.

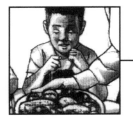

HEART RATE (PULSE RATE)

The heart is the body's only actual monitor that can give a reading as to how hard you're exercising. (Your heart, or pulse, rate tells you how many times your heart is beating.) Heart rate monitoring lets you know if you're exercising at an appropriate level (intensity).

Target heart rate is the number of times your heart should beat per minute during exercise in order for you to get the most benefit for strengthening your heart and lungs. You should exercise at a level high enough to train the heart without causing extreme tiredness and muscle stiffness. This depends on your age and level of fitness, but it should be at about 60 to 85% of your maximum heart rate, which is the fastest your heart can beat during an all-out effort. To improve fitness, your heart rate should stay within this zone during exercise.

Although the maximum heart rate varies from person to person, it can be roughly estimated by subtracting your age from 220. Multiply this number by .60 and .85 to get 60 to 85% of your maximum heart rate, which is your target heart rate. Next, divide this number by 6 to get your target heart rate for 10 seconds.

For example, if you are 40, subtract 40 from 220 to get 180. Then multiply 180 by .60 to get 108 and by .85 to get 153. Divide 108 by 6 to get 18 and 153 by 6 to get 25.5. This means you want to keep your heart rate (as measured by counting your pulse beats) in the range of 18 to 26 beats for 10 seconds. Use the table below to determine your target heart rate:

HOW TO FIGURE YOUR TARGET HEART RATE (THR)

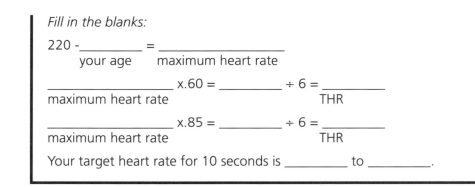

Fill in the blanks:

220 -_____ = _____
     your age   maximum heart rate

_____ x.60 = _____ ÷ 6 = _____
maximum heart rate   THR

_____ x.85 = _____ ÷ 6 = _____
maximum heart rate   THR

Your target heart rate for 10 seconds is _____ to _____.

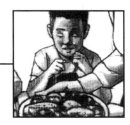

TARGET HEART RATES DURING EXERCISE

Heart Beats per 10 seconds

Intensity	Age: 15	20	25	30	35	40	45	50	55	60	65	70
60%		20	20	19	19	18	18	17	17	16	16	15	15
75%		25	25	24	23	23	22	22	21	20	20	19	19
85%		29	28	27	27	26	25	25	24	23	22	22	21

When you begin an exercise program, aim for a target heart rate at the 60% level. A more intermediate level will be a target heart rate of 75% and an advanced level will be 85%. It has been shown that you burn a higher percentage of calories from fat when you exercise at 60 to 75% of your maximum heart rate. So if weight control is a concern for you, keep your heart rate at the lower end of your zone. See the chart above for target heart rates for 60%, 75%, and 85% of maximum heart rate for different ages.

CHECKING YOUR PULSE

You can feel your pulse easily in two places. The preferred site is the radial artery, located in each wrist. To take your radial pulse, place the index and middle fingers at the base of your thumb and move them down toward your wrist and press gently (see photo). You should be able to feel your pulse beating.

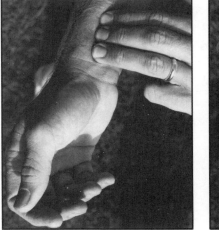

Radial pulse using index and middle fingers

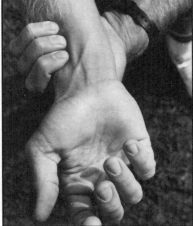

Radial pulse wrapping hand around wrist

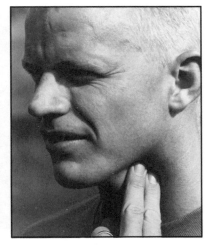

Carotid pulse

55

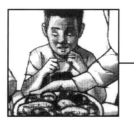

An alternate way of taking your radial pulse involves wrapping your hand around the wrist and using your fingers to find the pulse about an inch down from the wrist under the base of the thumb (see photo).

The second place is at your carotid arteries, located just under your jaw on either side of the windpipe. To take your carotid pulse, place your index and middle finger on your neck in the area of the carotid artery (see photo). Press in gently. You should be able to feel your pulse beating. Press lightly, and never press both carotid arteries at the same time. It may cause you to feel faint.

Be sure to use your fingers and not your thumb to find your pulse. Your thumb has a pulse of its own, which will confuse you. Count your pulse for 10 seconds, counting the first beat as "zero." Multiply that number by 6 to get a 1-minute pulse. For example, 20 beats in 10 seconds times 6 equals 120 beats per minute. You will want to take your pulse before, during, and immediately after you stop exercising. Count for only 10 seconds because the heart rate will slow down quickly after just 15 seconds.

Determining and using target heart rates can be very helpful when you begin an exercise program. However, it's more important for you to "listen" to your own body and take its advice while exercising. You can do this by using what is called perceived exertion, which will allow you to exercise safely and comfortably, as well as effectively, with or without a watch.

PERCEIVED EXERTION

Perceived exertion determines how hard you are working by rating how hard you "perceive," or feel, you are exercising and how tired you are. The original scale, developed by psychologist Gunnar Borg, allows persons to rate their activity from 6 to 20. In 1986, the American College of Sports Medicine (ACSM) released a revised scale ranging from 0 ("nothing at all") to 10 ("very, very strong"). This scale (shown on the next page) provides a written description for rating the degree of perceived exertion. Each level on the scale correlates with how hard you feel you're working. Exercise should be done at the 2 to 4 range, or at the "light" to "somewhat strong" level.

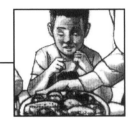

Rating	Description
0	Nothing at all
0.5	Very, very weak
1.0	Very weak
2	Weak
3	Moderate
4	Somewhat strong
5	Strong
6	
7	Very strong
8	
9	
10	Very, very strong
	Maximal

ACSM REVISED RATING OF PERCEIVED EXERTION SCALE

Reprinted, with permission, from *Guidelines for Exercise Testing and Prescription,* Figure 2-3, by American College of Sports Medicine. Philadelphia: Lea & Febiger, 1986:23.

When you exercise, remember to listen to your body, measure your intensity of exercise by using target heart rate or perceived exertion, and exercise at a level that feels "somewhat strong" to you. Slow down if you're working too hard, or work harder if necessary.

LET'S GET STARTED!

To improve, as well as maintain, your fitness level, exercise sessions should be done three to five times weekly. Fewer than three times a week is not enough to increase your fitness, help with weight control, or improve your blood glucose control. Activities should be performed continuously for at least 20 minutes while keeping your heart working at an appropriate level.

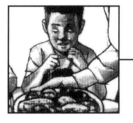

Each exercise session should have four parts: warm-up, training or aerobic exercise, muscle strengthening, and cool-down. All four are important. The pattern will look something like this.

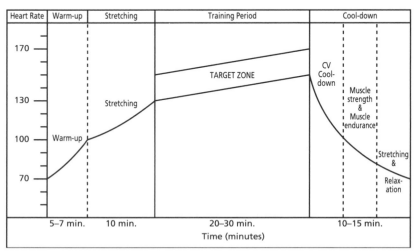

Reprinted, with permission, from Franz MJ and Norstrom J. *Diabetes Actively Staying Healthy (DASH): Your Game Plan for Diabetes and Exercise.* Minneapolis: Diabetes Center, Inc., 1990:15.

WARM-UP

The warm-up period prepares the body for exercise and should last about 5 to 10 minutes. Begin by walking or doing other movement for 5 to 10 minutes and then do a few stretches for about 5 minutes. This period of gradually increasing activity allows the heart rate and body temperature to rise in preparation for more vigorous exercise. During warm-up, your pulse should be increasing gradually.

AEROBIC ACTIVITY

As the main portion of your exercise program, aerobic activity is how you'll build endurance and overall fitness. These improvements are known as the "training effect," and three essential components are needed to achieve it—intensity, duration, and frequency.

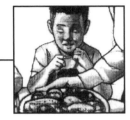

1. *Intensity* describes how hard you should work while doing a given exercise, usually using target heart rate guidelines. To improve fitness, your pulse rate must be kept within your individual target zone for at least 20 to 30 minutes of aerobic exercise. Remember that heart rate decreases with age. While doing aerobic exercise, your pulse rate should be 60 to 85% of your maximum heart rate (see chart on page 55).

Exercising at an intensity higher then the target zone will probably shorten your exercise session because you will become fatigued. It will also increase your chances of muscle injury or heart problems. You should always be able to carry on a light conversation while exercising. If you can't, you are exercising at too high a level of intensity.

2. *Duration* is how long (usually in minutes) a given exercise should be performed. Initially, the training exercise phase begins with 3- to 5-minute intervals of exercise at a target heart rate, separated by 1-minute periods of recovery (exercise at a more relaxed level). For example, you may jog 3 minutes and walk 1 minute, and so on. As your exercise tolerance increases, duration of exercise is increased and fewer recovery periods are used. The program should gradually increase from 5 to 10 minutes to 20 to 30 minutes. Increase the duration of your workouts before you increase the intensity. In other words, exercise longer, not harder.

3. *Frequency* is how many times per week exercise should be performed. To strengthen your heart and lungs, you should exercise at least three to four times during the week. To reduce your chances of injury, do different activities that use different muscle groups. For example, walking, swimming, and biking each use different muscle groups. For weight control, try to exercise five to six times per week. This way exercise becomes a part of your lifestyle. If you have diabetes and inject insulin, you should try to exercise at least every other day.

Aerobic activity is also classified according to impact—high-impact, low-impact, or non-impact. All improve heart and lung capacity by raising the heart rate. High-impact exercises are done with movements in which both feet may leave the floor at the same time, such as jumping, jogging, and some types of aerobic dance (dance routines and movement patterns done to music).

Low-impact exercises are sometimes called light-impact, or soft aerobics. They are done with at least one foot touching the floor at all times and include no jogging or jumping jacks to put a strain on joints. However, low-impact does not mean low-level exercise. Walking is an excellent example of low-impact exercise.

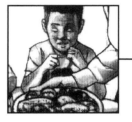

Non-impact exercises are done with neither foot touching the floor, as in swimming or cycling. Usually low- or non-impact exercises are recommended to prevent ankle, knee, or leg injuries.

It's not a good idea to do high-impact aerobic exercise every day. The risk of injury is much greater because you are putting so much stress on the same muscles. Vary your activity as often as you can. Cross training, which involves using a variety of aerobic exercises to strengthen the heart and lungs, is recommended because there is less chance of injury. For instance, you might run on Monday, bike on Tuesday, swim on Wednesday, and walk on Friday.

COOL-DOWN AND MUSCLE STRENGTHENING EXERCISES

Cool-down is a period following exercise during which activity decreases and the heart rate and body temperature gradually return to normal resting levels. Your exercise sessions should end with a cool-down period of 10 to 12 minutes.

This is the time to do muscle strengthening exercises, such as curl-ups for strengthening stomach muscles and push-ups to strengthen the upper body. Some people enjoy weight lifting or using strength-training equipment such as Nautilus or Universal, two brands available at many health clubs. This equipment is usually set up in a series of eight or more machines, each for use in strengthening a specific muscle group (hip and back machines, abdominal machines, etc). Be sure you are instructed on the proper use of this equipment by a fitness professional before using it.

Complete the cool-down with more stretching exercises. This is when stretching is really beneficial and important. Regular stretching will reduce muscle tightness and relax the body. It will help coordination, increase the range you can move your muscles and joints, and help prevent injuries such as muscle strain. Stretching also decreases stiffness and soreness that often occur after people exercise, promotes circulation, and perhaps most importantly, just plain leaves you feeling good!

By stretching correctly you'll improve your flexibility. However, improper stretching may cause problems and can actually do more harm than good. Begin by stretching the muscles that are most often the tightest—neck, shoulder, upper and lower back—and so on down to the ankles. Stretch

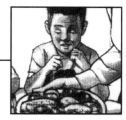

slowly, gently but firmly. Hold for 10 to 20 seconds and then relax. It's important to not hold your breath while stretching and while doing muscle strengthening exercises! Breathing should be relaxed and natural.

Remember two other important "don'ts" while stretching. First, don't bounce when you stretch. Bouncing only tightens the muscle, and you're more likely to strain a muscle as a result. Second, don't stretch to the point of pain. At this point you may have already injured a muscle. Stretch slowly and hold for 10 to 20 seconds at the point where you begin to feel the muscle pulling.

GETTING STARTED

- Get your doctor's approval. This is particularly important if you are over age 40, have had diabetes for more than 10 years, or have other physical problems, concerns, or questions about exercise.
- Choose an exercise program made up of activities you enjoy and that fits your lifestyle. Exercise should be enjoyable, not a chore!
- Invest in a good pair of exercise shoes. This is important for everyone who exercises regularly, but especially for people with diabetes. Buy shoes that are comfortable and suited to the type of exercise you will be doing. Be careful to avoid blisters or other foot problems during exercise. Treat them immediately if they occur and get help from your health care team if they do not heal promptly.
- Drink plenty of water before, during, and after exercise. Dehydration (a serious loss of body fluids) is very dangerous and can cause heat stroke.
- Start slowly. Learn how to measure your heart rate during exercise and gradually work up to exercising at 70 to 85% of your maximum.
- Make the exercise an enjoyable and necessary part of your life. It should be practical—suited to your schedule. Exercise at the time of day that feels good to you. People with Type I diabetes usually find that it helps their blood glucose control if they exercise at about the same time each day.
- Test your blood glucose frequently to find out how exercise affects you. Get help from your health care team if you need to adjust your food intake or medication.

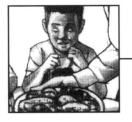

- Warm up and cool down adequately in every exercise session. Hold stretches for 10 seconds and do not bounce or strain. Gradual warm-ups and cool-downs and proper stretching are keys to injury prevention.

- If you want to lose weight, use a combination of a diet designed with your dietitian and exercise of long duration and moderate or even low intensity. Choose more than one type of aerobic exercise and do them on alternate days so you can exercise almost every day.

- Try to increase your day-to-day activity level, changing sedentary routines into mini-exercise sessions. Take the stairs instead of the elevator, walk to the store instead of driving, park a short distance from your destination and walk the rest of the way. Together these behaviors can burn a significant number of calories.

- Make a commitment to exercise and stick with it. An exercise partner can help you stay with it and add to the enjoyment. Just telling others about your exercise program can provide motivation to keep you going.

- You will lose the benefits of exercise very quickly—in a matter of days—if you stop. If you have a layoff period, gradually work back to your previous level of fitness.

- Most importantly, remember to have fun and feel good about yourself. You need to hear "cheering from within." This will be what keeps you going!

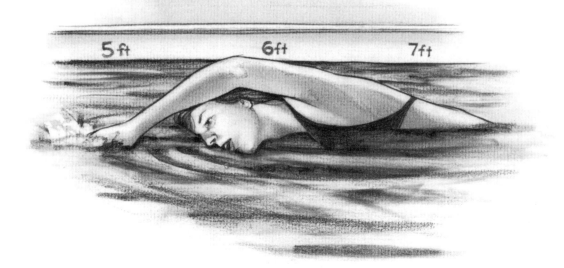

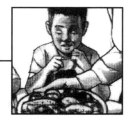

MONITORING YOUR KNOWLEDGE

1. List three benefits of exercise.

_____

_____

_____

2. Name two ways you can tell how hard you are exercising.

_____

_____

3. Name the four parts to an exercise program.

_____

_____

_____

_____

4. What are the three factors of aerobic activity that improve endurance and overall fitness?

_____

_____

_____

Answers on page 117.

CHAPTER 4

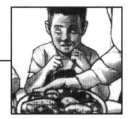

Lucy Mullen, RN, BS, CDE
Judy Ostrom Joynes, MA, RN, CDE

Monitoring:
The Secret to Control

How is it possible to test the amount of glucose (sugar) in the blood?

What do I need to know to test my blood glucose?

Do I need a meter, or is visually reading the testing strip enough?

What is ketone testing, and why is it so important?

Diabetes researchers and health care providers are becoming more and more convinced that testing the level of glucose (sugar) in your blood is one of the most important things you can do to control your diabetes. This is because the results of glucose testing can be used to make important decisions about medication, meal planning, and exercise.

In this chapter we'll explain blood glucose testing and why and how to test urine for ketones if the blood glucose level is high.

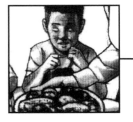

Monitoring blood glucose (testing your blood glucose and keeping track of test results) helps you and your health care team take action to keep your blood glucose levels as close to normal as possible. Studies show that keeping blood glucose levels close to normal seems to be the best way to prevent complications of diabetes. Children seem to follow normal growth and development patterns, the short-term problems of low blood glucose and high blood glucose occur less often, and the long-term problems affecting the small and large blood vessels are minimized.

The information gathered from blood glucose monitoring can be used to help you make changes in your health care plan. Your health care plan includes your insulin schedule, meal plan, and activity plan. By making small changes, you may be better able to control your blood glucose levels (see Chapter 10 for information on how to do this).

TESTING BLOOD GLUCOSE

The oldest method of finding out if there is too much glucose in the blood is by testing the urine. In Chapter 1 we mentioned the ancient technique of placing urine near an anthill to see if the ants would be attracted by the sugar crystals. Another old and crude method was to actually taste the urine to see if it was sweet. Fortunately, much better methods were developed that use strips of chemically treated paper to test the urine. And now, methods have been developed that allow people with diabetes to directly test their blood using plastic strips. The chemically treated pads on the strips can be visually compared to a color chart or read by a machine that shows a very accurate level of glucose.

Before we discuss how to perform these tests, let's review the way glucose gets into the blood and urine. In Chapters 1 and 2 we described how the body digests food, turning much of it into glucose. Glucose then passes through the walls of the intestines into the circulating blood. The glucose travels throughout the body in the bloodstream. When enough insulin is available, the glucose can be taken in by the cells of the body and used for energy. But if no insulin is made by the pancreas (Type I diabetes) or if the insulin is not effective in moving glucose into the cells (Type II diabetes), then glucose builds up in the blood.

The kidneys, which are at the lower back near the spine, remove waste products from the blood by filtering them. This creates urine to carry the

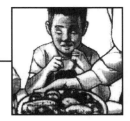

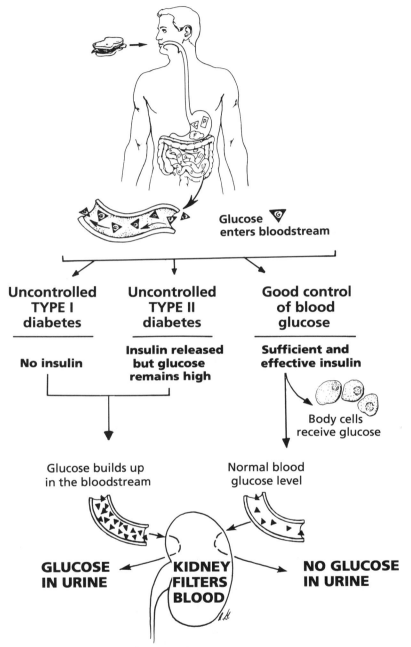

How blood glucose control affects urine glucose levels

waste products out of the body. When blood glucose is in a normal range, almost no glucose is filtered from the blood and removed from the body in the urine. But if the level of glucose in the blood gets too high, the kidneys try to reduce it by washing larger amounts of glucose into the urine. This is why a "positive" urine test for glucose can be taken as a sign of high blood glucose.

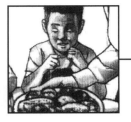

SELF MONITORING OF BLOOD GLUCOSE

Before the 1960s, the only way to directly test the level of glucose in someone's blood was to do an expensive laboratory test. But in the late l960s, methods were developed that allowed people to test blood glucose levels at home. In the late 1970s, these methods became reasonably easy to perform and their cost was reduced enough that they became practical for everyday use. But it wasn't until the early 1980s that these methods came into wide use. Small calculator-like machines called blood glucose meters were developed that used a ray of light to "read" blood glucose test strips. Devices were also developed to help people remove a small drop of blood for each test. Since then, self monitoring of blood glucose has been improved to the point that it's the most reliable method of testing to gather information to achieve and maintain normal blood glucose levels.

BLOOD GLUCOSE MONITORING SUPPLIES

There are a variety of products on the market to be used for self monitoring of blood glucose (see Appendix B for a list). Lancets and holders are used to poke the finger almost painlessly to obtain a small drop of blood for testing. Different types of test strips change color after blood is applied and can be read by visually comparing the color change to a color chart. Different types of instruments called blood glucose meters read these test strips and show the exact blood glucose level. Blood glucose meters are even available that can be used by the blind—they have an electronic voice that reports the glucose level.

Not all of these instruments and products are needed by everyone who wants to do blood glucose monitoring, but just the basic supplies make it a more expensive method than urine testing. And the procedure is slightly more difficult to learn than urine testing. However, even young children can accurately test their blood with proper instruction. Despite the cost and difficulty, the accuracy of blood glucose monitoring is so superior that urine testing for glucose is no longer used.

If you decide to use blood glucose monitoring, first receive proper instruction from your health care team. Your main decision will be whether to use the visual method, the meter method, or a combination of the two.

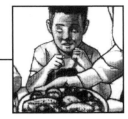

Some people like to leave their meter at home and just carry the bottle of strips to obtain visual readings while at school or work.

Blood-Letting Devices

There are numerous devices available to use to obtain a drop of blood. They are basically the same—a holder that has a spring-driven action, a cap or a platform that determines the depth of the poke, and a disposable lancet (small, short needle). Check with your health care team to see which type works best for you.

Be sure to dispose of the lancets properly. We suggest that you place used lancets in an opaque, puncture-proof container, such as an empty soda pop can. When the container is full, tape it shut and throw it in the garbage.

Visually-Read Blood Testing Strips

If your diabetes is in good control or if you only need a range of blood glucose values to manage your diabetes, you may choose to test with the visual method. To do this, a drop of blood is applied to a chemically treated pad on a strip. The glucose in the blood mixes with the chemical and results in a color change on the pad. The reacted pad is compared to a numbered color chart on the vial of strips.

The color chart does not give specific number readings in mg/dl. It shows ranges, such as 80-120 mg/dl or 120-180 mg/dl. By comparing the color of your test pad with the closest color chart square, you can estimate about where in the range your blood glucose level falls.

Some people prefer to have a specific number reading that tells them their blood glucose level in mg/dl. The same strips that can be visually read can also be used in some blood glucose meters to obtain an accurate mg/dl reading.

Keep in mind that each brand of strips has a different time action and method of blood removal. Know the name of the product you use. If you need to change products, read the directions to make sure you're doing the test correctly.

Meters/Sensors

Blood glucose meters are changing daily. Today many different kinds are available: small, large, fast, slow, strip-requiring, and strip-less. Each is designed to make blood glucose monitoring easier for you. Although there are many kinds of meters, there are actually only three different types: reflectance meters, electrochemistry meters, and glucose sensors.

Reflectance meters are actually color analyzers. When you drop blood on a chemically treated pad, the glucose in the blood mixes with the

69

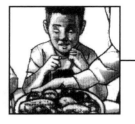

chemical and causes a color change. The more glucose in the blood, the darker the color. A reflectance meter analyzes that color and changes it into a number that reflects the amount of glucose in the blood. For a reflectance meter to work accurately, it must be cleaned regularly and calibrated (adjusted for accuracy) to each container of strips. Check the list in Appendix B for examples of reflectance meters.

Meters based on electrochemistry measure the amount of energy produced when the glucose in the blood mixes with the chemical on the pad. The number corresponds with the results obtained from a reflectance meter. The main thing to remember with this type of meter is to calibrate it. Check the list in Appendix B for examples of electrochemistry meters.

Glucose sensors do not use strips. The blood is placed on a sensor (which needs to be replaced monthly). The meter determines the amount of glucose in the blood through the sensor and, like the reflectance meter, changes it into a number that reflects the amount of glucose in the blood. This type of meter needs to be cleaned and calibrated daily. Check the list in Appendix B for examples of glucose sensors.

All meters and sensors need to be checked periodically with control solutions to make sure they're working correctly. Each control solution has a measured amount of glucose. The amount of glucose in the solution is found on the package insert or strip container. If you perform a test with the control solution and the results match the amount of glucose in the solution, you can assume your meter is working properly, that your strips are okay, and that your technique is correct.

Some reflectance meter companies also issue check strips or check paddles, which are plastic strips of a certain color. Since reflectance meters read color, if the meter always reads the color of the paddle the same or within a small range, you'll know the meter is working correctly.

Each meter should be checked before performing a test, or at least daily. It is also important to clean your meter and then test it with control solutions:

- weekly
- when a new container of strips is opened
- when the batteries are replaced
- whenever you feel your meter is not giving you true information.

If a meter comes with a check paddle, this test should be performed daily.

If you're having a blood glucose test done at a laboratory, you may want to see if your meter matches the laboratory results. Take your meter to the lab and do the test on the meter within 5 minutes of the blood draw. To ensure accuracy, your meter and the laboratory results should be within 15% of each other. Keep in mind that the laboratory blood test will generally be higher by 10 to 15%.

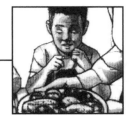

HOW TO TEST BLOOD GLUCOSE

Visual Method

To test blood glucose, get a drop of blood from the sides of the fingertips, ear lobes, or toes. Rotate these sites. (Do not use your toes if your doctor has told you that you have poor circulation or loss of sensitivity in your feet or if you've had diabetes for 10 years or longer.)

1. Prepare the site by washing with soap and warm water. The warm water will increase the blood flow to the area. Dry the area thoroughly. Any moisture or sugar from food left on the site may make the blood glucose reading inaccurate. It's best not to use alcohol to clean the skin. If not completely dry, the alcohol can change the blood glucose reading and cause discomfort as well as cause your skin to become dry and cracked.

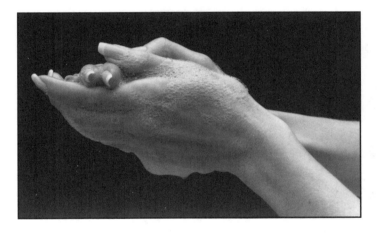

2. Puncture the skin with the blood-letting device.

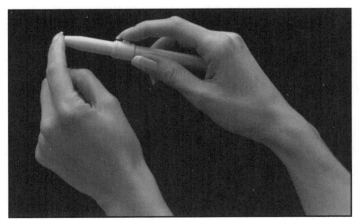

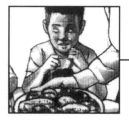

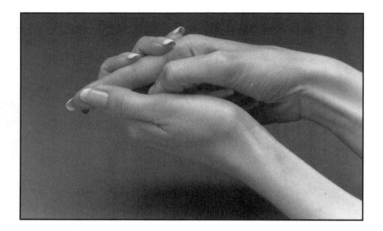

3. Gently massage the area to bring a large drop of blood to the puncture site. When a large drop accumulates, allow it to hang from the site.

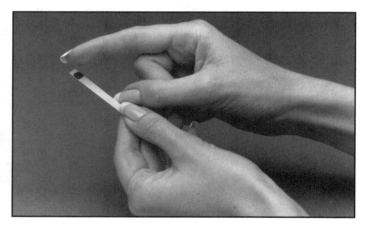

4. Place the large hanging drop of blood on the test pad. Be sure to cover the entire pad with blood. Follow the product's instructions. With some products the blood must be dropped on the pad and with others it can be smeared.

5. Wait the amount of time specified by the instructions to allow a chemical reaction between the glucose and the pad. If the proper time is not used, the results will not be accurate.

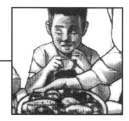

6. Wipe or blot blood from the pad according to product instructions.

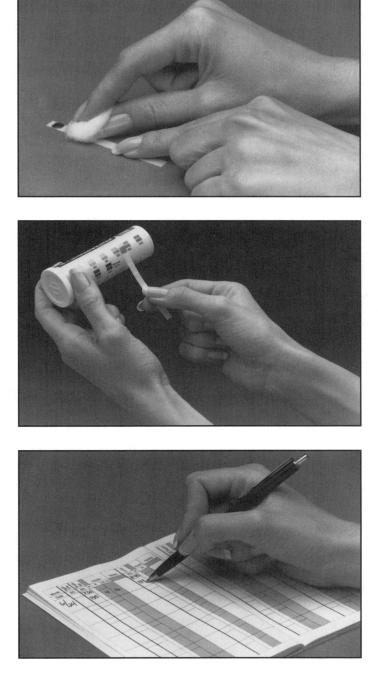

7. Wait another specified time according to instructions.

8. Compare color of pad with color chart on test strip bottle.

9. Write your blood glucose level in your record book.

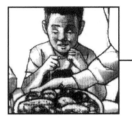

Meter Method

There are many different types of meters and each has its own procedure, so it's difficult to state specific steps to perform the test. Important steps to remember include:

1. Wash site with warm water and soap, and dry thoroughly.

2. Puncture site.

3. Place drop of blood on pad or sensor so that the entire surface is covered.

4. Time the reaction according to directions.

5. Remove blood, if necessary, according to the product directions.

6. Ensure strip placement is correct.

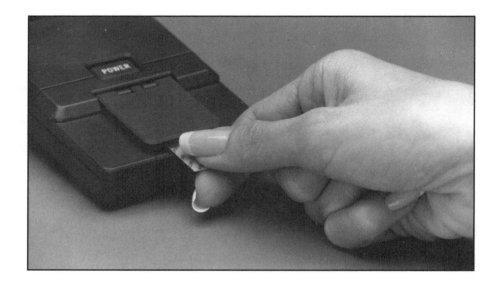

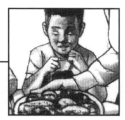

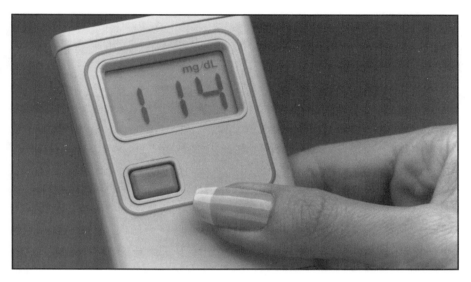

7. Wait for number readout to appear on display.

8. Write your blood glucose level in your record book.

9. Before using a blood glucose meter, check with your health care team to ensure proper testing technique.

WHEN TO TEST

Many people with diabetes now monitor their blood glucose as many as six times a day. It's helpful to test before meals and evening snack, before and after exercise, before you drive, whenever you feel symptoms of low or high blood glucose, or whenever you need to be reassured that you are in control of your diabetes.

The times of day testing is done vary from person to person. However, it's important that you test within an hour of the same times from day to day. This will be discussed further in Chapter 10. Your health care team will make recommendations based on whether you are taking insulin, how often, and how stable your blood glucose level is. General guidelines for testing times include:

- If you are taking insulin to help control Type I or Type II diabetes, it's most helpful to test your blood before breakfast, lunch, dinner, and evening snack.

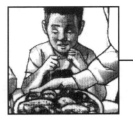

- If you have Type II diabetes and are not taking insulin, and if your blood glucose level stays close to or within the normal range, it may only be necessary to test two or three days per week. Test before breakfast, before your main meal, and 1 1/2 hours after finishing your main meal.

URINE TESTING FOR GLUCOSE

Urine tests show the blood glucose level during the time urine has been building up in the bladder (a sac-like organ that stores urine produced by the kidneys). The advantages of urine testing are that it's easy to learn and not very expensive. The basic disadvantage is that the results don't give a very good reading of the actual blood glucose level at the time of the test. This severely limits the usefulness of urine testing in making decisions about medication, food intake, and exercise—all things that will affect your blood glucose control.

One reason for the lack of accuracy with urine testing is that the method assumes the kidneys will begin removing extra glucose as soon as the blood glucose level exceeds normal range. The trouble is, not everyone's kidneys work that way. Some people can have a positive test when their blood glucose is within the normal range and others can have a negative test when their blood glucose is elevated.

TESTING URINE FOR KETONES

Another test you must know how to perform involves checking the urine for ketones. Ketones are formed in large quantities when the body uses too much fat for energy. When the body uses glucose as its main energy source, the glucose is totally burned up by the cells. But when there is not enough insulin, the body switches over to burning an excessive amount of fat. When the body burns fat as an energy source, it leaves an acid by-product called ketones.

The ketones left behind when the body burns fat can make you very sick if they accumulate in the blood. The kidneys try to remove the ketones just as they remove extra glucose from the blood. But if the body burns large amounts of fat for energy, the kidneys cannot remove enough ketones from the blood. The body cells are then bathed in blood that has too high of an acid level because of the ketones. The sickness caused by having too many ketones in the blood is called ketoacidosis. Ketoacidosis can be a very

76

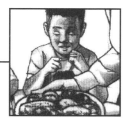

serious sickness, causing stomach pain, nausea, vomiting, dehydration, unconsciousness, and even death if it's not treated promptly and correctly. (Ketoacidosis is explained more completely in Chapter 11).

It's important to test your blood glucose routinely, because it will tell if you should check for ketones in your urine. ***If your blood glucose is 240 mg/dl or higher, you should check a urine sample for ketones.***

General instructions:

1. Dip a ketone test strip in a urine specimen, or pass the chemically treated pad at the end of the strip through a stream of urine.

2. Remove the strip and time the reaction according to directions on the product.

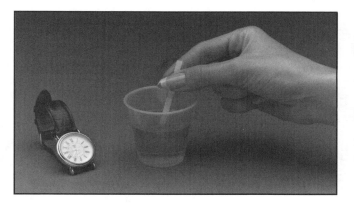

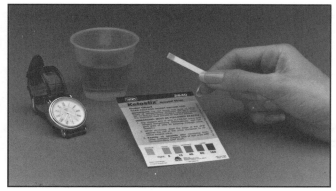

3. The pad will change colors if ketones are present. Compare test strip to the color chart on the package.

4. Record the result.

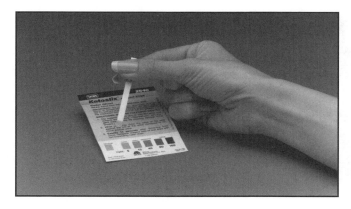

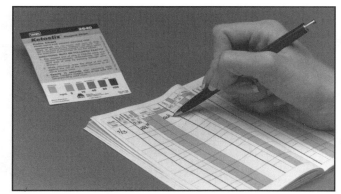

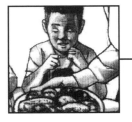

If ketones are present, they are measured as trace, small, moderate, or large. Discuss with your health care team the steps you are to follow if your blood glucose level is elevated and your ketone test is positive. A positive ketone test is like a flashing red light signaling that your diabetes is getting out of control. You may need to make adjustments in your insulin. Call your health care team for advice on how much to adjust your insulin and how often.

So far we have discussed routine tests you can do to help achieve and maintain normal blood glucose. Another valuable test your health care provider can do to gain a more complete picture of your diabetes control is called a glycosylated hemoglobin, or hemoglobin A_1c, test. It can be used with your daily testing records to make decisions about possible changes in your diabetes management.

GLUCOSE MOLECULES

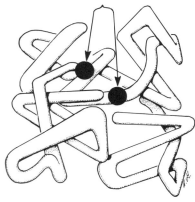

GLYCOSYLATED HEMOGLOBIN

Glucose molecules attach to hemoglobin

GLYCOSYLATED HEMOGLOBIN (HEMOGLOBIN A1C) TEST

Glycosylated hemoglobin means "glucose attached to hemoglobin" (hemoglobin is the part of the red blood cells that carries oxygen to body cells). Hemoglobin A1c is the specific type of hemoglobin often measured to find out how much glucose has become attached over six to eight weeks. If blood glucose has been in the normal range of 70 to 140 mg/dl, the glycosylated hemoglobin test will be within the normal range. If blood glucose levels have been elevated, more glucose will attach itself to the hemoglobin, resulting in an elevated glycosylated hemoglobin reading. This value will be shown as a percentage. To know what your glycosylated hemoglobin number means, you need to know which test your doctor uses and what the normal ranges are for that test. Normally, values vary from laboratory to laboratory depending on the method used for performing the test. Glycosylated hemoglobin tests are usually done once every three to four months.

BLOOD GLUCOSE MONITORING GOALS

The chart on the next page gives you normal and ideal blood glucose goals for people with diabetes. However, each person has individualized target blood glucose ranges based on:

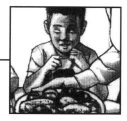

- age
- level of control
- frequency and severity of hypoglycemia
- ability to recognize early warning signs of reactions
- lifestyle
- other medical conditions
- other medications you may be taking
- pregnancy

Keep in mind many people are not able to achieve normal blood glucose goals. Work with your health care team to determine a target blood glucose range appropriate for you. Acceptable blood glucose ranges are often 140 mg/dl in the morning or before a meal and under 200 mg/dl 1 1/2 hours after finishing a meal. Remember, it's very important that you know your target ranges.

BLOOD GLUCOSE RANGES

	Fasting and Before Meals	**1 1/2 Hours After Finishing Meal**
Persons Without Diabetes	70–115 mg/dl	less than 140 mg/dl
Ideal Ranges for Persons With Diabetes	70–120 mg/dl	less than 140 to 160 mg/dl
Acceptable Ranges for Persons With Diabetes	70–140 mg/dl	less than 180 to 200 mg/dl
Pregnant Women With Previous Diabetes	65–95 mg/dl	less than 120 mg/dl

PATTERN CONTROL

It's important to record and use your blood glucose monitoring results to help you achieve as near normal blood glucose as possible. At first, you'll want to use your test results and notes of any changes in food intake or exercise to discuss your diabetes control with your health care team. But as you learn more about how to manage your diabetes, you'll probably want to make minor changes in your health care plan without having to visit or call your health care team.

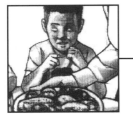

Pattern control is a method used successfully by many people to make changes in insulin doses or food to maintain the best possible blood glucose control. This skill takes time and practice to learn and requires working closely with your health care team. It involves using blood glucose monitoring results over several days to decide if adjustments are needed in insulin or food. Pattern control is not something that can be learned just by reading about it. It must be practiced, and in the beginning your decisions must be discussed with your health care team.

To use pattern control, you should be familiar with the time actions of your insulin or insulins. This information, along with your blood glucose monitoring results and food and exercise records, will help you decide which insulin could be increased or decreased slightly to achieve better control of blood glucose at a specific time of day. Your routine may change during vacations or on holidays or weekends, so it's important to test your blood glucose more frequently to determine if a change is needed in your insulin dose. Chapter 10 covers pattern control in more detail.

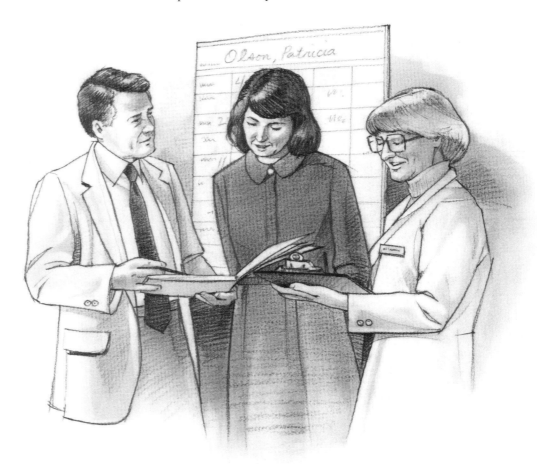

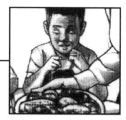

SUMMARY

To summarize, if you take insulin, test blood glucose:

- before meals
- before bedtime snack
- before driving a vehicle and during long trips
- when feeling symptoms of an insulin reaction
- when feeling like blood glucose is high
- when feeling ill

Test urine ketones if blood glucose is 240 mg/dl or higher.

If you do not take insulin, test blood glucose two to three times a day, two to three days a week:

- before you eat in the morning
- before your main meal
- 1 1/2 hours after your main meal

Test more often when you are ill. At those times you may need insulin for a short time to help control blood glucose

Knowing what to do to manage your diabetes is very important. But it's equally important to perform tasks correctly. Work with your health care team to build your skills and review them regularly. Not only will they become easier to perform, but your diabetes control will be improved as your skills improve.

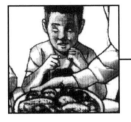

MONITORING YOUR KNOWLEDGE

1. Name two methods you can use to test your blood for glucose (sugar).

_____

_____

2. Name the testing material you use for measuring your blood glucose.

_____

3. List the days and at what times of the day you are to test your blood glucose.

_____

_____

_____

_____

4. What would you do if your blood glucose level was over 240 mg/dl?

_____

5. What is the name of the test done to measure how well your diabetes has been controlled over the past couple of months?

_____

Answers on pages 117 and 118.

CHAPTER 5

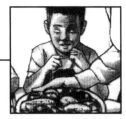

Judy Ostrom Joynes, MA, RN, CDE
Lucy Mullen, RN, BS, CDE

Insulin:
A Message to the Cells

What is insulin?

How is injected insulin different from the insulin the body makes?

What is the correct way to inject insulin?

Insulin is one of many hormones in the body that helps cells do their work. Hormones are chemicals made in the body to control specific body processes. When you have diabetes, your body either doesn't produce enough insulin or doesn't use what it has properly. In order for your body to perform the same tasks it did before developing diabetes, you need to inject insulin. In this chapter, you'll learn about insulin and the skills you'll need to use it properly.

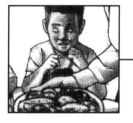

I nsulin is a protein made up of 51 building blocks called amino acids. These are divided into two connected chains, an A chain and a B chain (see illustration). Insulin is produced in the beta cells of the islets of Langerhans in the pancreas. The pancreas also makes, stores, and releases many other hormones, digestive juices, and enzymes.

The production of insulin in the pancreas starts with the formation of a larger hormone called proinsulin. Proinsulin contains the A and B chains of insulin connected to an additional set of amino acids called the connecting peptide, or C-peptide. When proinsulin is broken down in the pancreas, it releases one molecule of insulin and the C-peptide separately into the bloodstream.

Insulin helps transfer glucose from the blood into the body cells to be used as energy for the cells—and therefore the body—to function. Insulin helps store glucose in the form of glycogen in the liver and muscles, which prevents the body from relying on body protein and too much fat for energy. Insulin also helps the body store fat and repair tissue. This prevents muscle breakdown, excessive weight loss, and the buildup of ketones in the blood.

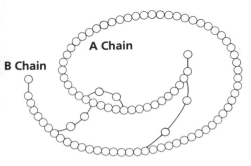

PROINSULIN

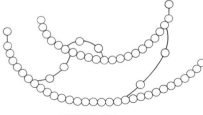

INSULIN

Proinsulin released from the pancreas is changed to insulin

C-peptide splits off, leaving a molecule of insulin containing the A and B chains

THE DIFFERENCE BETWEEN INJECTED INSULIN AND INSULIN THE BODY MAKES

Injected insulin has four major differences from insulin made in the human body:

1. *Source,* or where the insulin came from.
2. *Action time,* or when and how long it is effective.
3. *Concentration,* or how much insulin is in a given amount of liquid.
4. *Purity,* or how many non-insulin hormone parts it contains.

Source

When insulin was discovered in 1921, it became possible to inject insulin into people who would otherwise die of Type I diabetes. This insulin was obtained from the pancreases of cows and pigs. For insulin to work, it must be injected. Insulin is a protein, so if it's taken by mouth the digestive system will destroy it before it can get into the blood.

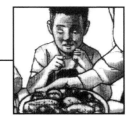

Presently there are several main sources of insulin: beef, pork, and two types of human insulin made in laboratories. A mixture of beef and pork insulins is also manufactured. Pork insulin is more similar in structure to that made by the human pancreas than is beef insulin. In general, insulin most like that made in the human pancreas is less likely to cause problems.

It appears that the ideal form of insulin for injection would be identical to insulin made by the human body. Eli Lilly and Company has been successful in actually creating human insulin, called Humulin. This was done using a laboratory process called recombinant DNA, in which the genes of bacteria are "instructed" to make human insulin molecules. DNA is the basic blueprint of all living things. It carries genetic information from one generation to the next. Recombinant means the formation of new combinations of genes.

The Novo-Nordisk company has developed a process by which the insulin obtained from pigs can be chemically changed so that it's identical in structure to human insulin. This product is called Novolin. Both Humulin and Novolin are now available in the United States.

Action Time

When insulin is released by the pancreas into the bloodstream it's immediately active, or available for use by the cells. This is not so when insulin is injected into the fatty tissue under the skin.

Injected insulin has three action times: short-acting, intermediate-acting, and long-acting. The different action times are a result of the use of zinc or protein in the insulin mixture, which causes the insulin to be absorbed more slowly from the injection site into the blood.

Short-acting insulins, such as Regular, start to work one-half hour to one hour after injection, work most effectively two to four hours later, and last only six to eight hours. Intermediate-acting insulins, such as NPH or Lente, begin to work about two hours after injection, are most effective eight to 12 hours later, and last about 24 hours. Long-acting insulin, such as animal Ultralente, lasts 32 to 36 hours. It's usually given to provide a small, steady release of insulin much like that continuously released by the pancreas of a person without diabetes. Short-acting insulin is used with it to cover increases in blood glucose caused by food intake.

Each insulin action time has a general pattern of when the insulin will become active (onset), when it will be working hardest (peak), and how long it will continue to be active (duration). The following chart shows the general action patterns of the different types of insulin.

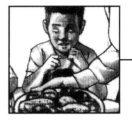

INSULIN ACTION CURVES

Insulin	Onset (hours)	Peak (hours)	Duration (hours)	Maximum Duration (hours)
Animal				
Regular	1/2–2	2–4	4–6	6–8
NPH	4–6	8–14	16–20	20–24
Lente	4–6	8–14	16–20	20–24
Ultralente	8–14	Minimal	24–36	24–36
Human				
Regular	1/2–1	2–3	3–6	4–6
NPH	2–4	4–10	10–16	14–18
Lente	3–4	4–12	12–18	16–20
Ultralente	6–10	?	18–20	20–30

Concentration

Two basic concentrations of insulins are used for daily injections: U-100 and U-40. U-100 means there are 100 units of insulin in each cubic centimeter (cc) of liquid. Therefore, a 10-cc bottle of U-100 insulin contains 1,000 units of insulin. U-40 is a less concentrated form of insulin. It has 40 units of insulin per cc. A 10-cc bottle of U-40 insulin contains 400 units of insulin. U-100 is the concentration most commonly used in the United States, but U-40 is more common in many other countries.

Purity

Over the years, insulin products have been made increasingly pure (free of proinsulin and other hormone parts) through the use of electrical and chemical laboratory techniques. All insulins sold today are greatly improved in purity, but some are very highly purified and are sometimes helpful if problems result from using other insulins.

There are several non-insulin ingredients in a bottle of insulin. These include the diluting solution, a preservative to prevent bacteria from growing, some protein or zinc to lengthen action time, and ingredients used to adjust the acidity of the insulin solution.

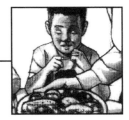

KNOW YOUR INSULIN

Since you don't need a prescription to buy insulin (in most states), you need to know what to ask for. Be sure you know:

- what kind of insulin you use (Regular, NPH, Lente, UltraLente, etc)
- the manufacturer (Lilly or Novo-Nordisk)
- the source (human, animal)
- the concentration (U-100 or U-40)

Look at the insulin bottle. All of this information is on the label. If you can't remember it all, bring your old bottle to your pharmacist, or write the information on a card and keep it in your purse or billfold. You also need to know your dosage, or how much insulin you use and when you take it.

It's very important to use the insulin your physician prescribes for you. If you change manufacturers or sources on your own, you may build up antibodies to the insulin. This means the insulin will not work as well for you. If you change type or concentration, you won't be getting the proper amount when you need it. Remember, insulin is time-released, so take it at the same time (or at least within an hour of the same time) each day.

Besides knowing your insulin, you need to know which syringe to purchase. You'll need the proper syringe to match your insulin concentration. For instance, if you're taking U-100 insulin, you must use U-100 syringes. Today you'll find many different syringes to choose from. There are several manufacturers (B.D., Monoject, Terumo, etc) and calibrations of syringes (100-unit, 50-unit, 30-unit). It's important to know which calibration you are using. If you're using U-100 syringes, usually each line on the syringe equals 2 units of insulin. On the 50-, 30-, and some 100-unit syringes, each line equals 1 unit of insulin. Make sure you know the calibration by counting the lines between the given numbers.

(below, left) Different manufacturers and types of insulin

Everything you need to know about your insulin is listed on the label and box

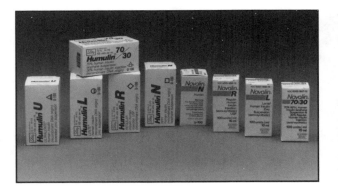

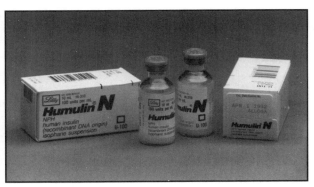

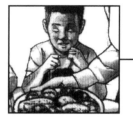

INJECTION AIDS

It's important to know that many aids are available to enhance your ability to inject insulin. Some simply hold the syringe and have a spring action that injects the needle through the skin. Others hold the syringe and inject the needle and the insulin, and still others don't have needles. These are jet injection devices that force insulin through the skin by air pressure. Also available is a catheter-like device that's placed under the skin for two to three days. You can inject insulin into the catheter rather than the skin. Pen-like syringes that hold cartridges of insulin and can inject small amounts of insulin quickly and inconspicuously can also be purchased. If you are having difficulty injecting insulin in the conventional manner, check with your health care team to see if any aids will meet your needs.

STORING INSULIN

Now that you know what you need, you must know how to care for your supplies. Insulin stored at room temperature must be used within one month. Keep it out of direct sunlight and away from heat and cold. If the amount is going to last longer than one month, it's necessary to refrigerate it. Before injecting, remove the insulin from the refrigerator. Draw the insulin into the syringe, warm it in your hands until it reaches room temperature, and inject it. If opened insulin is in the refrigerator for more than three months, discard it. Unopened insulin stored in the refrigerator is effective through the expiration date.

Once you have the right insulin and syringe, you can get ready to draw up your insulin. Pick up the syringe and practice working it. It consists of a needle, a measuring gauge, and a plunger. The plunger moves back and forth to allow you to measure the correct amount of insulin. You are ready!

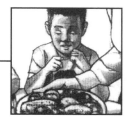

PREPARING ONE TYPE OF INSULIN

If your doctor has prescribed a single type of insulin:

1. Wash your hands.

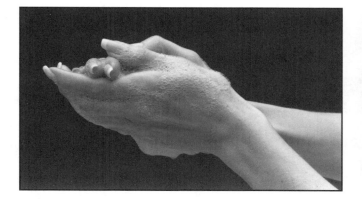

2. Roll the bottle of insulin between your hands to mix the contents.

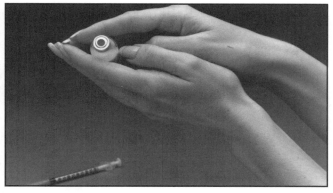

3. Remove the protective covering from the needle.

4. Pull down on the plunger and measure an amount of air in the syringe that is equal to your insulin dose.

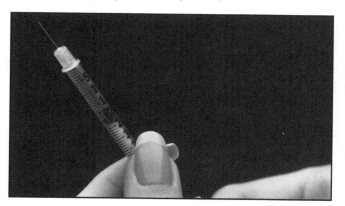

5. With the bottle in the upright position, inject the needle into the rubber stopper. Push down on the plunger and air will flow into the bottle. This air makes it possible to draw insulin out of the bottle.

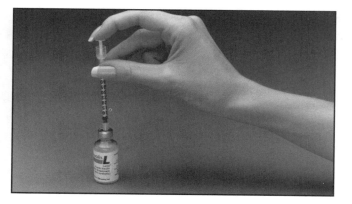

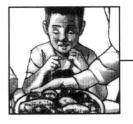

6. Now turn the bottle upside down on top of the needle. Make sure the tip of the needle is covered with insulin.

7. Pull down the plunger, allowing the insulin to enter the syringe.

8. Push the plunger back up. The insulin will return to the bottle.

9. Repeat steps 7 and 8. You are removing air bubbles from the insulin in the syringe to make sure you inject the correct amount.

10. Pull the plunger down to the required amount of insulin. Look to see that there are no·air bubbles in the syringe.

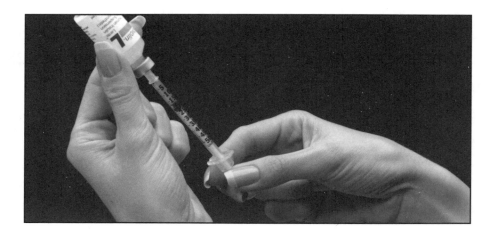

11. Remove the syringe from the bottle.

12. Place the syringe on a flat surface without letting the needle touch anything. The needle is sterile and you want to keep it that way.

13. Go to page 95 for instructions on how to inject insulin.

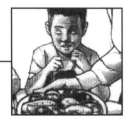

MIXING TWO TYPES OF INSULIN

You can mix two types of insulin in one syringe so you only have to inject once. Make sure you have the correct insulins and know your prescribed dose for each one. To prevent errors, mark the short-acting (Regular) insulin bottle by winding a rubber band around it.

1. Wash your hands.

2. Roll the intermediate- or long-acting insulin between the palms of your hands to mix the contents.

3. Remove the protective covering from the needle.

4. Inject air into both bottles of insulin so you'll be able to draw out the insulin. Pull down on the plunger and measure an amount of air in the syringe that is equal to your dose of intermediate- or long-acting insulin. With the bottle of intermediate- or long-acting insulin in an upright position, inject the needle into the rubber stopper. Push down on the plunger and air will flow into the bottle. Remove the syringe.

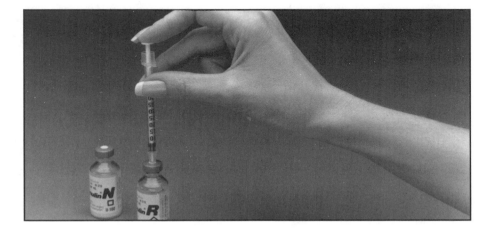

5. Draw up the amount of air equal to your dose of short-acting insulin and inject into the upright bottle.

6. Turn the bottle of short-acting insulin upside down on top of the needle. Make sure the tip of the needle is covered with insulin.

91

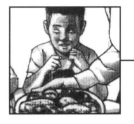

7. Pull the plunger halfway down the syringe, allowing insulin to flow into the syringe.

8. Push the plunger upward and the insulin will flow back into the bottle.

9. Repeat steps 7 and 8 to make sure there are no air bubbles in the insulin in the syringe.

10. Pull the plunger down to the required amount of short-acting insulin. Check to see that there are no air bubbles, then remove the syringe, which now contains your dose of short-acting insulin.

11. Insert the needle of the syringe into the upside down bottle of intermediate- or long-acting insulin. (Remember, air has already been placed inside this bottle.)

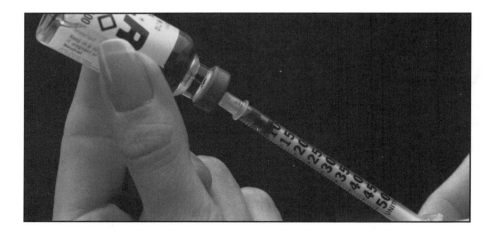

12. Pull the plunger down to the required amount of intermediate- or long-acting insulin. Remember to add the units of short-acting insulin to the units of intermediate- or long-acting insulin to arrive at the total number of units for this step. If you accidentally go beyond the total number, discard the contents and start over.

13. Remove the needle from the bottle and place it on a flat surface where it will not touch anything.

You are now ready to inject the mixed doses of insulin.

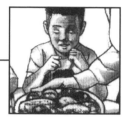

CHOOSING AND PREPARING THE INJECTION SITE

Many different areas (sites) on the body can be used for injecting your insulin (see photographs). You'll be injecting the needle into the fatty tissue, which is called subcutaneous tissue. Any place where there is fatty tissue can be used, such as the back of the arms, the top and outside area of the thighs, the stomach (except for a 1-inch area around the belly button), and the buttocks. Insulin is absorbed most quickly from the stomach, followed by the arms, legs, and buttocks. Absorption may also be speeded slightly if the muscles at the injection site are exercised immediately after injection or if you take a hot bath. While each of these factors may change blood glucose levels only a small amount, together they may have some effect as you strive for more normal blood glucose levels. One suggestion might be to give injections at a particular time of day in one area of the body.

Some persons develop skin problems if the same small area is used repeatedly for injections. Two problems may develop. 1) The skin at the site may begin to break down (atrophy), causing an unsightly depression in the skin, or 2) The skin at the site may become scarred or swollen (hypertrophy). These problems can also change the absorption time of insulin. To avoid these problems, develop a system for rotating and keeping track of your injection sites.

Abdomen

Below shoulder blades

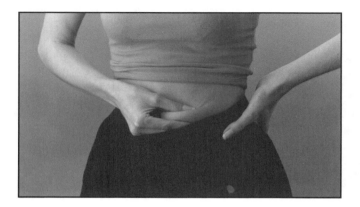
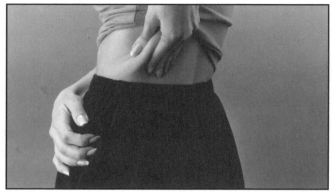

93

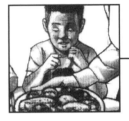

Hip

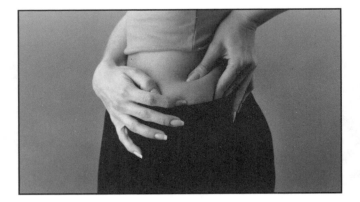

Buttocks

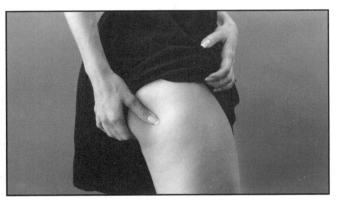

Arm

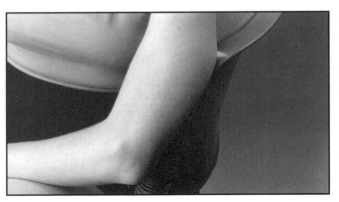

Thighs

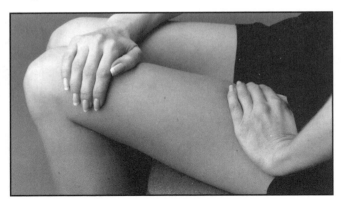

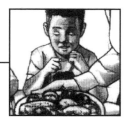

INJECTING INSULIN

1. The site you have selected should be clean.

2. With one hand, pinch the skin together to keep the tissue from moving.

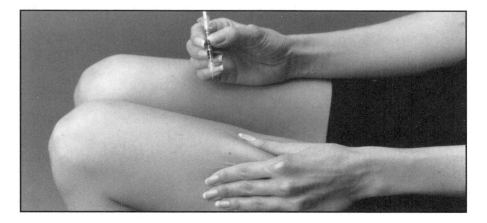

3. With your other hand, pick up the syringe, holding it like a dart.

4. With a dart-like motion, insert the needle into the pinched skin at a 45 to 90 degree angle (see photos). Remember, you want to inject into the subcutaneous fatty tissue. If you have a normal amount of fatty tissue, use a 90 degree angle. For very small children or extremely thin adults, a 45 degree angle may be necessary.

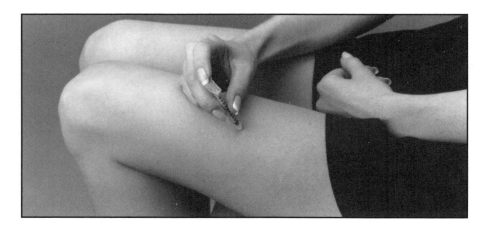

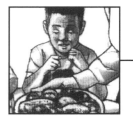

5. Once the needle is inserted, push down the plunger to inject the insulin.

6. Withdraw the needle from the skin, covering the injection site with your finger to prevent insulin from leaking out of the tissue.

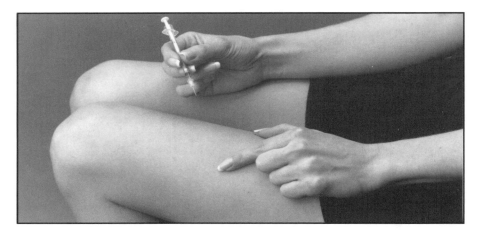

7. Place the cover back on the needle and discard the syringe.

8. Write down in your record book the amount of insulin injected, the time, and the site used.

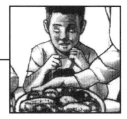

SYRINGE REUSE AND DISPOSAL

Studies have shown that using syringes more than once did not increase the rate of infections. However, proper syringe disposal is important in preventing injury to others by needle pokes as well as cross-contamination from reuse of needles. One option is to purchase a needle clipper. Before disposal, use it to clip the needle off the barrel of the syringe. The needle clipper will hold several years worth of used needles. When it's full, discard it and purchase another. The plastic syringes can be thrown in the garbage. This still becomes an ecological problem because it takes years for plastic to disintegrate. If you have strong feelings about this, you may want to use a glass syringe and sterilize it.

Another means of syringe disposal is to place the entire syringe, with needle attached, into a puncture-resistant metal container. You can purchase these through medical supply companies. Aluminum soda pop cans also work well. The opening is large enough to fit syringes through and small enough to keep them in. Caution: Because you can't see the contents, make sure the cans are clearly labeled and kept out of reach of children. Fill the container, tape it shut, and dispose of it in your garbage.

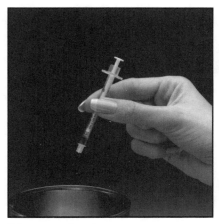

Dispose of syringe

RECORD KEEPING

No one can assess how you're managing your diabetes unless there is a record of your test results and amount of medication taken. Many record books are available for this purpose. Each day write down the amount of medication taken, when taken, where injected, and the test results.

SUMMARY

Very basic but critical steps in gaining control of your blood glucose levels include:

- correctly preparing and injecting insulin
- being consistent in the time of day you inject insulin
- understanding time actions of insulins

If these steps are done incorrectly, it can lead to problems with diabetes management.

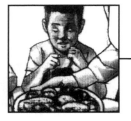

MONITORING YOUR KNOWLEDGE

1. Name three sources of insulin.

_____

_____

_____

2. Name the three action times of injected insulin.

_____

_____

_____

3. What is the most commonly used concentration of insulin in the United States?

_____

4. State the type, manufacturer, source, and concentration of your insulin.

_____

_____

5. Name the supplies you need to inject insulin.

_____

_____

6. Describe how insulin should be stored.

_____

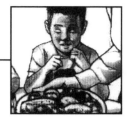

7. Name the steps you need to take to inject insulin.

_____

_____

_____

_____

_____

_____

_____

_____

_____

_____

_____

8. State your prescribed dose and schedule for taking insulin.

_____

_____

_____

Answers on pages 118 and 119.

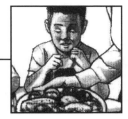

CHAPTER 6

Randi S. Birk, MA, LP

Emotional Adjustment:
The Key to Living Well

"Thank goodness diabetes is controllable!"
But...

"Why me?"

"Why my child?"

When diabetes enters your life, your world is suddenly changed to include new and very special concerns, considerations, and challenges. It's difficult to make lifestyle changes, but it's often harder to adjust emotionally to those changes. This chapter will discuss some common feelings about diabetes and suggest ways of making these feelings part of a healthy adjustment to living with diabetes. The result will be a happy and productive lifestyle for your whole family.

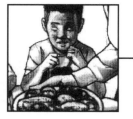

If you recently learned that you or someone close to you has diabetes, you may be feeling somewhat overwhelmed and frightened—perhaps even numb! You may have hoped this was a bad dream from which you would awaken. As reality sinks in, you will probably experience a variety of emotions that range from anger to relief.

As you and your family struggle to cope with diabetes, you will enter an adjustment process. Many emotions will surface, often repeatedly. Identifying and accepting these emotions help the process along.

ADJUSTING EMOTIONALLY

When we think of adjustment, many words come to mind. Webster's dictionary uses words such as settle, resolve, and adapt. Others have described adjustment as change, acceptance, and coping. There is no one correct definition. However, in looking at "adjustment to diabetes," the ultimate goal is to *live well with diabetes*.

We can identify two aspects of living well with diabetes—"living well" and "diabetes." Both are extremely important and clearly affect one another. Ideally, persons with diabetes can achieve a balance between having an active, full, productive life and managing their diabetes. However, at times that balance may be tipped to one side or the other. For example, a person might resist making the lifestyle changes that are necessary for good diabetes management. While he or she may temporarily be living fully, diabetes management suffers. On the other hand, a person may be so concerned about diabetes that unnecessary limits are placed on active living. In neither of these situations is the person really *living well* with diabetes. Eventually this will affect both diabetes management and the rest of the person's life.

How you adjust emotionally helps determine how well you balance diabetes management and living fully. In some ways, adjustment, like insulin, can be viewed as a "key." Just as insulin is the key that allows the cells in our bodies to use food for energy, emotional adjustment is the key that helps you use medical technology and information to manage diabetes and live fully. Because adjustment is so important, this chapter discusses the process and the feelings that may be involved. And remember, the whole family and other loved ones will experience this adjustment and the emotions described—not just the person with diabetes.

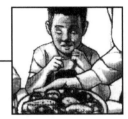

DENIAL (DISBELIEF)

"This isn't really happening."

"I don't have to change. Diabetes isn't forever."

"It's not that serious."

"I don't have to feel anything about my diabetes."

One of the first things many people experience is disbelief: "This can't be happening to me!" When you suddenly learn you have diabetes, you may have frightening and confusing thoughts and feelings. There are many unknowns about diabetes and the future. Until you experienced it personally, you probably had very little accurate information about diabetes. This lack of knowledge can affect your feelings about the disease.

It's natural to avoid unpleasant and scary feelings and to deny the reality of having diabetes. This can be healthy and protective at first. It insulates you from all the scary, confusing feelings that would be overwhelming if you let them in all at once. It "buys time" for you to get used to your situation and the required changes until you're ready and able to deal with them.

We use denial in everyday living. By believing that the accidents, natural disasters, assaults, and other bad things we read or hear about daily won't happen to us, we can go about the business of living fully without constant worry. This is healthy and useful. But sometimes denial becomes unhealthy and affects how we take care of ourselves. For example, when we smoke or drink too much, overeat, or don't wear seat belts, we somehow believe we are specially protected from lung cancer, liver disease, heart problems, or accidents. Similarly, if you continue to deny your diabetes, or feel changes are not necessary for good diabetes management, you won't care for yourself properly. Not only will your future health be at risk, but you won't feel good and you will lack energy.

The loved ones of a person with diabetes also have fears that can be overwhelming. Sometimes they deny the diabetes or their feelings about it. If this continues, it can give the person with diabetes the message that his or her diabetes is not real or serious and that proper management is not necessary.

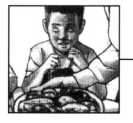

FEAR

"What will this mean for my life?"

"What's going to happen?"

As denial grows weaker, reality becomes increasingly clear. You or your loved one has diabetes, and you need to make some changes. But what does it all mean? Will you/they still be able to live a full life? Although you probably now have a few more facts about diabetes than before it was diagnosed, it's all still quite new. It's difficult to put aside the false and negative stories you may have heard or read, or perhaps even past experiences with a family member whose diabetes was poorly controlled.

Diabetes is serious. It requires change and that's scary. It's common to feel a loss of control over your body during the time right after diagnosis. Your body, which you trusted without question, has betrayed you by failing to function as it should. Being in the hospital at this time can add to the fear. And you don't yet have the information you need to regain control of your body and your life. You might feel anything from mild nervousness to downright terror, and the intensity of your fear may change from time to time.

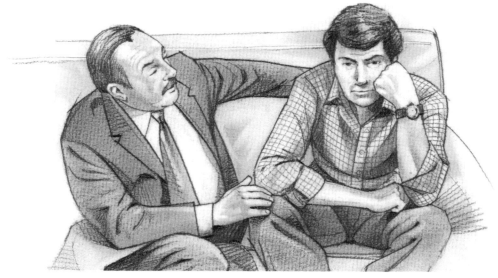

But just as denial was useful at first, fear also has a purpose. Fear, along with the discomfort of being out of control, can motivate you to seek the answers you need to live well with diabetes. Limited and appropriate fear, which is really just respect for consequences or danger, motivates us to

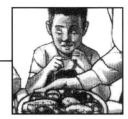

proceed carefully in life. However, too much fear over a long period can also lead to a feeling of hopelessness. And when you have no hope, you have no reason to care for yourself, feeling "it doesn't matter anyway."

When family members or others feel overly fearful about their loved one's diabetes, they sometimes react by becoming overprotective. They may unnecessarily restrict otherwise safe activities or situations. They may also become overly demanding about following a diabetes management plan. Over time, this can cause the person with diabetes to actually accept less responsibility for his or her management. It can also lead to rebellion against those rigid demands and the loved one who is making them.

ANGER

"Why me?" "Why my child?"
"Why do I have to do all this stuff?"
"It isn't fair!"
Everyone who has diabetes or loves someone who has diabetes feels anger at one time or another. It's natural to feel angry when changes happen in our lives that are unwanted, unexpected, undeserved, and beyond our control. Diabetes is all those things. It demands that you make changes in your life and requires extra attention and energy for day-to-day management.

It's healthy and normal to feel angry once in a while. In daily living, our anger often gives us the energy we need to deal with or remove ourselves from an unpleasant situation. Since you can't remove yourself from having diabetes, your anger will affect how you deal with it. It can help you gain energy to meet the challenge of diabetes management. It's very important to recognize your anger and accept that it's all right to be angry for a while.

People vary in how often they get angry, how long they stay angry, and how they direct their anger. This also varies within a person from time to time. As with other emotions, anger can become unhealthy if it is felt too strongly, for too long, or is directed in a harmful manner. For example, sometimes anger at diabetes is misdirected at family members, causing them to be treated unkindly. Sometimes anger continues for so long or is so strong that it interferes with daily diabetes management, causing personal harm.

Loved ones also feel anger as a normal part of their adjustment process. But again, when it's felt too strongly, for too long, or directed at the person with diabetes instead of at the diabetes, it can hurt that person's ability to live well with diabetes.

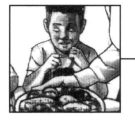

GUILT

"What did I do to deserve this?"

"If I just hadn't eaten so much sugar..."

"The diabetes must have come from my side of the family."

Guilt is an emotion we feel when we think we are responsible for something bad happening. You may have this feeling because of a misunderstanding of diabetes. For example, some people mistakenly think diabetes is caused by eating too much sugar or is inherited from just one parent. They might feel guilty if they always had a sweet tooth and then developed diabetes, or if a parent had diabetes and now their child does. If you believe people "get what they deserve," you might wonder what you have done to deserve diabetes.

Some guilt is healthy and useful. We all need to have a conscience in order to live responsibly in society. Feelings of guilt can serve as a sign that we have slipped in the goals we set for ourselves, such as to follow a meal plan, quit smoking, or test blood glucose (sugar) regularly. The intensity of our guilt and how we respond to it is important. If you feel somewhat guilty about "cheating" on your diet and accept that you're human and made a mistake and will try to do better, your guilt has proved to be healthy and appropriate. However, if you feel too guilty, you may be telling yourself you are "bad" or "a failure." These messages are likely to make you miserable and depressed, giving you little motivation to correct the mistake and improve your diet or work toward other goals.

Parents feel responsible for their children's well-being and may therefore feel guilty because they couldn't prevent the child's diabetes or can't get him or her to maintain better control. This kind of guilt is based on ideas that are untrue or unclear and, therefore, not realistic or helpful. Since the reasons for these feelings of guilt may be beyond our control or are in the past, the guilt accomplishes nothing but frustration, self-criticism, and depression.

When family members feel guilty about a loved one's diabetes, they may treat that person differently to try to make up for it. Parents, spouses, or other family members sometimes feel guilty and react by becoming overindulgent. They may set few limits, lower their expectations for positive, appropriate, responsible behavior, and otherwise try to make up for the loved one's misfortune. This can have very unhealthy consequences.

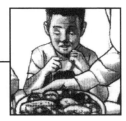

DEPRESSION

"I feel so sad."

"I just don't feel like doing anything."

"I feel so alone, no one understands."

After you've tried a number of ways to cope with diabetes—avoidance or denial, fear, seeking information, anger—and you realize diabetes will not go away, you may feel depressed, sad, defeated, or resigned.

Depression is a normal response to being unable to change a situation we don't like. Diabetes and the changes it requires are forever, and you can't make them go away. It's understandable and healthy for you to feel depressed for a while. In fact, recognizing and accepting your sad feelings are important to your adjustment to diabetes. During the time you are sad, you often make the necessary change in your self-image to include diabetes. This is a very important part of adjustment. It helps you focus on your new limits and the changes you must make. You learn to accept your new life, like many others before you.

We've all had to accept some limitations in life and at times have felt sad or depressed because of them. For example, you may have wanted to be athletic, artistic, tall, beautiful, or rich. By accepting our limits, we are able to move on and make realistic choices about life and make the most of our strengths.

Of course, depression can become unhealthy if it lasts for a long time or is very severe. People who are severely depressed often lack energy, have little appetite, and experience changes in their sleeping patterns. They may feel isolated, and this may cause them to avoid others, which adds to their feelings of isolation. In addition, people who are very depressed usually feel hopeless. They may not take care of themselves, since it doesn't appear to matter what they do.

When family members feel depressed about their loved one's diabetes for a long time, they can convey a message of hopelessness. This can affect how the person cares for himself or herself.

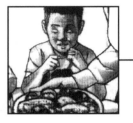

HOW DO YOU FEEL ABOUT DIABETES?

Here are some clues:

- Do you believe you can avoid your diabetes treatment plan without consequences?
- Do you hope your diabetes will somehow go away if you ignore it?
- Do you believe you are no different now than you were before you developed diabetes and that you don't need to change?

If so, you may be feeling disbelief, denying that you truly have diabetes and that it's permanent, serious, and going to take time to adjust to.

- Are you absolutely rigid about your meal plan and injection times?
- Do you feel diabetes has so many possible complications that your situation is hopeless?
- Do you resist allowing your child with diabetes to sleep overnight at a friend's house or go to camp?

If so, you may be feeling fear.

- Do you feel life is terribly unfair?
- Do you find yourself irritable with family members, friends, or health care team members for no apparent reason?
- Do you refuse to follow the recommendations of your medical team?

Perhaps you are angry.

- Do you want to do things for your child to somehow make up for his or her diabetes?
- Do you expect less of your family member with diabetes because he or she already has enough to deal with?
- Do you feel like a failure when even one blood glucose test is high?

Then you may be experiencing guilt.

- Do you feel sad and tired all the time?
- Do you avoid other people because no one seems to understand you anymore?
- Have you stopped enjoying activities you used to think were fun?

If so, you may be depressed.

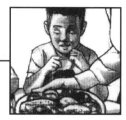

DEALING WITH EMOTIONS AND FEELINGS

Denial, fear, anger, guilt, depression—these are just some of the feelings you may have about diabetes. They are not unique to people or families with diabetes. Everyone feels these emotions from time to time. These emotions are in themselves neither good nor bad, healthy nor harmful. Each one can be helpful and useful as you strive to live well with diabetes, but each also can become unhealthy and interfere with your life. Understanding how that might happen can help you avoid or recognize problems if they develop.

DETERMINING IF AN EMOTION IS HEALTHY OR UNHEALTHY

An emotion becomes unhealthy when it upsets the balance you're striving for—that is, living well with diabetes. For example, people who for a long time deny they have diabetes, or that it is serious or forever, will manage their diabetes poorly. An equally unhealthy imbalance will result if a person is extremely fearful and unnecessarily restricts his or her activities.

Two factors largely determine whether an emotion will interfere in your life: its intensity (how strongly you feel it), and its duration (how long you feel it). Feeling is not an all-or-nothing process. For example, you don't feel guilty about everything or about nothing, but rather experience guilt within a range between those extremes. And you will likely feel different amounts of an emotion at different times. You might feel very depressed at one point, mildly sad at another, and not at all depressed on a third occasion. When you experience an emotion to an extreme degree, for example intense fear, your ability to maintain the balance of living fully and managing diabetes is reduced.

How long you experience an emotion is also important. It's very normal and healthy for people to be angry when they learn that they or a loved one has diabetes. However, continuing to feel anger about the disease several years later is clearly unhealthy because it will interfere with the long-term management of diabetes.

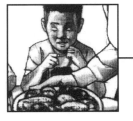

Is there a limit on how long a person can feel an emotion before it becomes unhealthy, or an amount beyond which an emotion is too strong? No. Just as there isn't one right insulin dosage or caloric intake for everyone, there isn't one right length of time or intensity to feel emotions. Each person will respond differently, and it's important to recognize and accept those differences. However, as with food and insulin, extremes may be a problem.

RECOGNIZING WHEN EMOTIONS BECOME A PROBLEM

If you're aware of the balance you want to maintain in your life, then you can be aware when that balance is tipped. If your diabetes is out of control or if there is a problem area within the rest of your life—conflict within your family, difficulties in school or at work, problems with friends, or limitations in your activities—it's time to ask yourself some questions.

Why are you experiencing this difficulty? If your diabetes is out of control, have you experienced a change in medication, food, or activities that is temporarily affecting your blood glucose, or is this a long-term problem? Problems in the rest of your life will not always be related to your diabetes. For example, you may simply be having difficulty with a school subject or dislike your new boss. However, there are also times when your feelings about diabetes will affect how you interact with family members, friends, and employers and which activities you choose to participate in or limit.

What can you do once you determine that some of your feelings have become an obstacle to living well with diabetes? Identifying that there is a problem is a healthy, positive first step. Next you must try to identify what you are feeling.

Often when you know what you are feeling, you can change how you express this feeling. For example, once you realize you are really angry at your diabetes and not your spouse, you can work toward expressing anger in a way that won't hurt you or others. You might release this anger through sports or exercise, or talk it out with family members, friends, or clergy. If you recognize that it is fear that stops you from letting your child become independent or guilt that keeps you from setting limits, you might be able to take a deep breath and let go—a little at a time—or feel better about setting some realistic expectations.

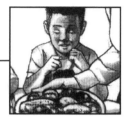

These changes may not be easy and they won't happen overnight. You can change what you feel and how you express your emotions. Sometimes you might need help. It's often more difficult to struggle with feelings alone. Support from others can be critical. You need to accept and actively seek emotional support from family, friends, and your health care team. Some people find it very rewarding to join a support group made up of others experiencing similar feelings or challenges. Contact your local diabetes chapter or your health care team for information about support groups in your area.

If you have identified a problem related to your feelings about diabetes and have realized it's something with which you need help, it's time to seek professional help. Counselors, social workers, and psychologists are skilled professionals who can help you identify your feelings and work toward a more healthy expression of those feelings. This could be a key to successfully coping with diabetes in yourself or your family. The earlier this action is taken, the easier it will be to work out a solution.

ACCEPTANCE

"I don't always like watching how much food I eat, but I understand how important that is to me."

"I have diabetes, so I guess I am going to have to make some changes."

Hopefully—sometimes sooner, sometimes later—you'll come to the point where you "accept" diabetes. That doesn't mean you like having

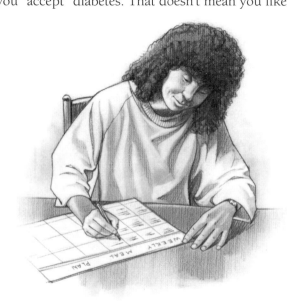

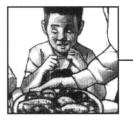

diabetes, want it, or feel happy that you or a family member has it. It only means you fully admit to yourself and others that you or a loved one has diabetes. You admit that it's part of you or them. At that point, you're able to choose to make the necessary changes good diabetes management requires. But at the same time you avoid setting unnecessary limits or restrictions. You've achieved that balance described earlier and are "living well with diabetes." It's desirable for everyone to be able to accept the limitations or challenges he or she is given in life. With this acceptance, you can then focus not on your limitations but rather on your strengths.

IS ACCEPTANCE THE SAME FOR EVERYONE?

While most people experience many of the feelings we have described; each person is unique, and his or her emotional responses will also be unique. The adjustment process is not a neat, orderly, predictable process that everyone moves through in the same way. We do not proceed from one feeling to another and then magically arrive at acceptance and live happily ever after.

IS ACCEPTANCE FOREVER?

Not exactly. Just as a smooth pond occasionally and temporarily experiences rippling, there will be occasional "ripples" in your acceptance. There will be times, perhaps, when the long-term, or "forever," aspect of diabetes temporarily becomes too much. Or when an important decision or life event causes you to be faced again with some of the old fears, anger, or sadness about your diabetes. It's not unusual to return every once in a while to some of the feelings you experienced during your initial adjustment. Sometimes you might repeat the whole process, again returning to acceptance.

With acceptance come other feelings, such as pride. You can feel proud that you're coping well, taking excellent care of yourself, and meeting your challenges. You feel in control of your diabetes and your life. You are the driver rather than the helpless bystander. And you can feel hope, not necessarily that a cure for diabetes will be found tomorrow, but that the growing knowledge and understanding of the disease will help you live fully and well with diabetes.

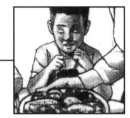

MONITORING YOUR KNOWLEDGE

1. What is the ultimate goal in adjusting to diabetes?

_____

2. What is one of the first feelings many people experience when they learn they have diabetes?

_____

3. Name four other common feelings people may experience when they learn they have diabetes.

_____

_____

_____

_____

4. How do you know if your feelings are healthy or unhealthy?

_____

5. What must you do to achieve a balance between *living well and diabetes?*

_____

Answers on page119.

ANSWERS

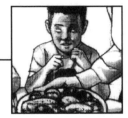

Monitoring Your Knowledge

CHAPTER 1

1. Diabetes is a *serious disease that affects the way your body uses food. Food is changed into glucose, which is carried to your body's cells by the bloodstream. Insulin (a hormone made in the pancreas) allows glucose to enter the cells where it is changed into energy or stored for later use. In diabetes, your body either doesn't make enough insulin or can't use insulin correctly. As a result, glucose builds up in the bloodstream. High blood-glucose levels are one of the main symptoms of diabetes. Today diabetes cannot be cured, but it can be controlled.*

2. The name of the hormone that lowers blood glucose is *insulin.*

3. The blood glucose level in people who do not have diabetes rarely falls below *70 mg/dl* or goes higher than *140 mg/dl.*

4. The two main types of diabetes are:
- *insulin-dependent diabetes mellitus (IDDM), or Type I diabetes*
- *noninsulin-dependent diabetes mellitus (NIDDM), or Type II diabetes.*

5. Differences between Type I and Type II diabetes include (list three):
- *Age of onset. Type I usually begins in children or young adults, whereas Type II usually occurs in adults over age 40.*
- *Persons with Type I diabetes are usually lean at diagnosis, whereas persons with Type II diabetes are frequently obese.*
- *Symptoms at onset of Type I seem to appear suddenly, while the symptoms of Type II diabetes are more gradual and may not be obvious.*
- *Persons with Type I diabetes require insulin by injection. Persons with Type II diabetes may require insulin to control their blood glucose levels but are not dependent on insulin injections for life.*
- *Persons with Type I diabetes experience the short-term complications of diabetes: insulin reactions and ketoacidosis. Persons with Type II diabetes are unlikely to experience these problems unless they take injected insulin.*

6. Treatment for Type I diabetes consists of *insulin injections, meal planning, exercise, and blood glucose monitoring.* Treatment of Type II diabetes consists of *meal planning, exercise, blood glucose monitoring, and sometimes diabetes pills (oral hypoglycemic agents) or insulin injections.*

7. The type of diabetes that develops during pregnancy is called *gestational diabetes mellitus.*

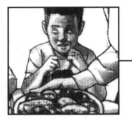

ANSWERS

■ CHAPTER 2

1. There are four reasons why it's important to watch what you eat if you have diabetes (list two):

- ■ *to help keep your blood glucose level as close to normal as possible*
- ■ *to help achieve healthy levels of blood cholesterol and triglycerides*
- ■ *to help you reach and stay at a reasonable body weight*
- ■ *to help you plan healthful meals that meet all your nutritional needs*

2. The nutrients found in food that require insulin to be used correctly by the body are: *carbohydrates, protein, and fat.*

3. The six exchange lists are: *1) starch/bread, 2) meat and meat substitutes, 3) vegetable, 4) fruit, 5) milk, and 6) fat.*

4. Free foods contribute *less than 20 calories per serving.*

5. A meal plan tells you *how many exchanges you can select for each meal and at snack times.*

6. Factors that determine how many calories you need include:

- ■ *your age*
- ■ *your height, current and desirable weight, and frame size*
- ■ *your activity level*

7. The two types of fiber found in foods are:

- ■ *water-insoluble fibers (generally found in brans, whole grains, and some vegetables)*
- ■ *water-soluble fibers (generally found in legumes, oats, barley, some fruits and vegetables)*

8. The different types of fat found in foods are (list three):

- ■ *saturated fatty acids (generally found in animal foods, such as meats, whole milk, dairy products, butter, lard, coconut, palm, or palm kernel oil, hardened shortenings)*
- ■ *unsaturated fatty acids (generally found in oils, such as safflower, sunflower, corn, and soybean)*
- ■ *monounsaturated fatty acids (found in olive oil, canola oil, peanut oil, olives, peanuts, most nuts and seeds)*
- ■ *omega 3 fatty acids or fish oils (found in fatty fish and fish from cold water)*

ANSWERS

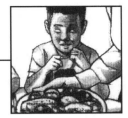

CHAPTER 3

1. Benefits from exercise include (list three):
- *improved fitness (flexibility, muscle strength and endurance, and heart and lung efficiency)*
- *weight control*
- *lower blood glucose levels*
- *reduced risk factors for heart disease*
- *lower blood pressure*

2. Two ways to tell how hard you are exercising are:
- *heart or pulse rate, which tells you how many times your heart is beating; and*
- *perceived exertion, by which you rate how hard you "perceive," or feel, you are exercising and how tired you are.*

3. The four parts to an exercise program are:
- *warm-up*
- *training or aerobic exercise*
- *muscle strengthening*
- *cool-down*

4. Three components of an exercise program that build endurance and overall fitness are:
- *intensity, or how hard you should work*
- *duration, or how long you should exercise*
- *frequency, or how often you should exercise.*

CHAPTER 4

1. Two methods you can use to test your blood for glucose are:
- *using visually-read blood testing strips, or*
- *using a blood glucose meter or sensor.*

2. I test my blood glucose by using a _____.

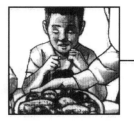

ANSWERS

3. I test at the following times during the day:

————————, ————————, ————————,

————————, ————————, ————————,

and on the following days:

————————, ————————, ————————,

————————, ————————, ————————,

————————, ————————, ————————.

4. If your blood glucose is 240 mg/dl or higher, ***you should check a urine sample for ketones.***

5. The ***glycosylated hemoglobin test*** measures how much glucose has become attached to hemoglobin over the past six to eight weeks.

CHAPTER 5

1. Sources of insulin are (list three): ***beef, pork, mixtures of beef and pork, human insulin made in laboratories.***

2. The three action times of injected insulin are: ***short-acting, intermediate-acting, and long-acting.***

3. The most commonly used concentration of insulin in the United States is ***U-100.***

4. The kind of insulin I take is ———————————————.

It is manufactured by ———————————————.

The source of the insulin is ———————————————.

The concentration is ———————————————.

5. To inject insulin you need ***insulin and insulin syringes.***

6. Insulin you are using can be stored ***at room temperature, but must be used within one month. It should be kept out of direct sunlight and from heat and cold. If it will last longer than one month it should be refrigerated. Unopened insulin should be refrigerated.***

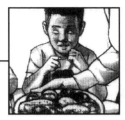

7. Steps for injecting insulin are:
  - *clean the site*
  - *pinch the skin together*
  - *pick up the syringe, hold it like a dart*
  - *insert needle straight into the pinched skin*
  - *push down plunger*
  - *withdraw needle, cover site with your finger*
  - *place cover back on needle and discard syringe in the appropriate container*

8. take the following dose or doses of insulin at the following times:

Time	Dose	Time	Dose	Time	Dose
____	____	____	____	____	____

Time	Dose	Time	Dose	Time	Dose
____	____	____	____	____	____

CHAPTER 6

1. The ultimate goal of adjusting to diabetes is to *live well with diabetes.*

2. The first feeling that you may experience when you learn you have diabetes is *disbelief.*

3. Other common feelings you may have are:
  - *fear*
  - *anger*
  - *guilt*
  - *depression*

4. An emotion becomes unhealthy when it *upsets the balance* you are striving for—that is, living well with diabetes.

5. To achieve a balance between living well and diabetes, you need to *reach a point of acceptance.* This doesn't mean that you like having diabetes, want it, or feel happy that you or a family member has it. With acceptance, you can choose to make the necessary changes good diabetes management requires.

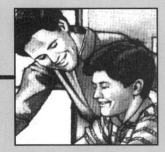

Living Well

Controlling Diabetes With Insulin

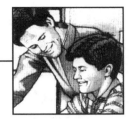

CHAPTER 7

Martha L. Spencer, MD

Your Health Care Plan:
Individualized for Your Lifestyle

How do you know if you have Type I diabetes?

What is a health care plan?

What should you expect your doctor to do during your routine visits?

What is intensive insulin therapy?

How can diabetes education help you?

Insulin-dependent (Type I) diabetes is a disease that can be controlled, but even so, it has an enormous effect on you and your family. Each person reacts differently to the physical and emotional stresses of diabetes and must be treated individually. The exciting challenge you face is to work with your health care team to find out just how healthy you really can be!

This chapter explains how you can work with your health care team to plan your diabetes management. It also explains the importance of regularly updating that plan and frequently checking for early signs of long-term complications.

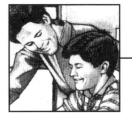

About 10 to 15% of all persons with diabetes have Type I diabetes. It usually occurs in children and in adults less than 40 years old, although it can develop at any age. About one of every 600 children in the United States has Type I diabetes. In persons with Type I diabetes, little or no insulin is produced by the pancreas, so insulin must be injected.

Although excellent insulins are currently available, the insulin we inject is not supplied to the body in the precise way the pancreas does. This means that meals, exercise, and injections of insulin must be carefully planned and carried out each day. Since it's rare that any two persons do the same activities, eat the same foods, and require the same amounts of insulin each day, it's not surprising that each person must have an individual diabetes health care plan. These detailed plans must be developed by both you and your health care team.

Failure to carry out your health care plan can lead to wide swings in blood glucose levels. Over time, this can contribute to the many complications of diabetes. You can help prevent these swings be monitoring blood glucose, following a meal plan consistently, and making changes in the amount and kind of insulin you take and the time you take it.

HOW IT STARTS

The symptoms of Type I diabetes (such as thirst, frequent urination, tiredness, and weight loss despite eating large amounts of food) usually appear suddenly. Children may start wetting the bed. Often a urinary infection is suspected. The total time between onset of symptoms and diagnosis may be only a few days or weeks. Occasionally, onset of symptoms will be more gradual, with small amounts of glucose found in the urine during a routine examination.

Type I diabetes is diagnosed when two blood glucose tests are over 200 mg/dl. Further testing rarely needs to be done. Some people, especially young children, may have stomach pain and vomiting as a result of the onset of diabetes. These people need immediate treatment and may require hospitalization. Their blood glucose level is usually very high, and large amounts of ketones are present in the urine. This means there is not enough insulin for the body to use glucose effectively for energy. The body must rely on fat for energy, which results in too many ketones in the blood (ketoacidosis). Ketoacidosis needs to be treated immediately. If not, it can lead to death.

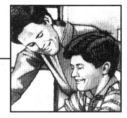

TREATMENT

Once Type I diabetes is detected, it's important to begin treatment as soon as possible. In the past, everyone diagnosed with Type I diabetes was hospitalized. Now, specialized health care teams in diabetes clinics can start insulin therapy and teach people how to manage their diabetes during a series of clinic (outpatient) visits. When outpatient health care is available and the diabetes has been detected before a person becomes seriously ill with ketoacidosis, hospitalization is not necessary.

During these first clinic visits (or days in the hospital), you'll learn:

- what diabetes is
- how to inject insulin
- how to test blood glucose and urine ketones
- how to plan meals
- how to recognize and treat symptoms of low and high blood glucose

Ongoing treatment of diabetes is a complex process that requires a special management plan for each person. When diabetes is detected, you should have a complete physical examination, nutrition history, and assessment of activity level. It's also necessary to identify sources of stress that could affect blood glucose, as well as sources of emotional support for you and your family. With this information, a meal plan and insulin schedule can be designed according to your activity level and time schedules.

THE HEALTH CARE PLAN

Together, the meal plan, activity plan, and insulin schedule are called the *health care plan.* The diabetes health care plan must be individualized to your lifestyle. Ideally, each person with diabetes should work with an experienced diabetes health care team, which may consist of a nurse educator, dietitian, counselor or social worker, and doctor. In smaller communities, some of these team members may not be available. Where services are limited, your doctor may wish to work with a diabetes center near your area. Most important is that all aspects of a person's life are considered in determining the health care plan.

Because diabetes is so serious, the major goal of the health care plan is to keep the body functioning as close to normal as possible. In people who

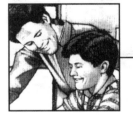

do not have diabetes, blood glucose levels are between 70 and 115 mg/dl before meals and below 140 mg/dl after meals. In people with diabetes, the goal is to keep blood glucose levels between 70 and 140 mg/dl before meals and below 200 mg/dl 1 1/2 hours after ending a meal. Blood glucose levels under 70 mg/dl are not safe for a person with diabetes because the insulin you inject cannot be turned off.

Other important goals of the health care plan include maintaining normal blood fat (lipid) levels; maintaining normal weight, growth, and development in children; maintaining a reasonable weight in adults; and preventing ketoacidosis and serious insulin reactions.

Achieving and maintaining these goals are challenges that require lifestyle changes for the whole family. It's important that you and your family learn all you can about diabetes, assume major responsibility in daily diabetes management, and work with your health care team.

Sharing responsibility with your health care team includes being seen regularly for routine health care and reevaluation of your health care plan. You must learn when, how, and whom to contact when you have questions or problems. Your health care team is not there just to treat you when you are sick. Their focus is on helping you stay well and *live well*.

MEAL PLANNING AND EXERCISE

Meal planning is one of the most important parts of diabetes control. The rest of your health care plan is based on a relatively consistent food intake. For children, the meal plan is designed for normal growth and development. For adults, it is designed to help maintain a reasonable weight.

A meal plan usually consists of three meals and one to three snacks a day. The number of snacks and timing of meals are designed to fit your lifestyle. Once a meal plan has been designed, it's important that meals and snacks be eaten at about the same time each day. See Chapter 8 for details on meal planning.

Activity, or exercise, is another important part of the health care plan. People with Type I diabetes are encouraged to make exercise part of their lifestyle. Most people who exercise feel better, take better care of themselves, and take an active interest in living a healthful life.

In children it's hard to predict when activity will take place. Unpredictable activity, inability to recognize symptoms of low blood glucose, and variability in appetite all contribute to children having wider swings in blood glucose than are seen in most adults. Chapter 9 includes guidelines and information to help you design a safe and effective exercise program.

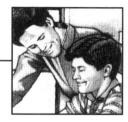

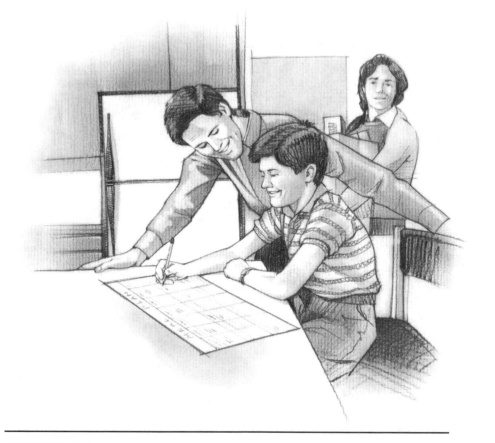

INSULIN

In Type I diabetes, the pancreas cannot make its own insulin. Since insulin is necessary for you to stay alive, it must be replaced. Insulin taken by mouth is destroyed by stomach acids, so it must be injected under the skin.

There are three basic types of insulin—short-acting, intermediate-acting, and long-acting. They differ in how quickly they begin to work (onset), when they have their greatest effect (peak), and how long they work (duration). Depending on a person's insulin needs, these insulins are taken either alone or in combination. The many different types of insulin serve to better copy the way the pancreas works.

Insulin should be taken within an hour of the same time from one day to the next. For example, if you normally take your insulin at 7 AM on weekdays, the injection should be taken no later than 8 AM on weekends. Your injection should be taken approximately one-half hour before you begin eating your meal. This way the Regular insulin has started to be absorbed into the bloodstream, and its blood glucose-lowering effect will occur at about the same time the food you are eating is being changed into glucose and released into the bloodstream. You can see that taking your

127

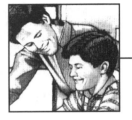

insulin injection right before a meal would not be ideal. For some people, absorption of insulin may differ from the norm. Some may have fast absorption and need to take their insulin 15 to 20 minutes before a meal, whereas others may have slow absorption and need to take their injection up to 45 minutes before a meal. You may already know the best time interval for you. If you don't, it's best to start with the one-half hour period.

A combination of short-acting and intermediate-acting insulin is often recommended to be given twice a day, with the first injection 30 minutes before breakfast and the second 30 minutes before supper. Although this varies from person to person, about two-thirds of the total daily insulin is usually given in the morning and one-third in the afternoon or before supper. Intermediate-acting and long-acting insulins should be given at about the same time each day.

If your doctor has asked you to mix two different types of insulin for injection, it's especially important that you receive instruction in how to prepare and measure the doses to receive the correct amount of each insulin.

What usually happens with Type I diabetes is that at the beginning, the pancreas is making very little insulin. Often, the pancreas' ability to make insulin may temporarily recover, causing a rapid decrease in the need for injected insulin. This may occur two weeks to six months after the onset of diabetes and is called the "honeymoon period." It may last weeks or even months. During this time a single injection of intermediate-acting insulin may meet the person's needs, and sometimes no insulin is needed.

Many insulin schedules, in addition to those already mentioned, may be used to obtain the blood glucose goals you and your health care team have identified. Your doctor will usually prescribe the simplest insulin schedule and progress to a more complex insulin schedule if and when the need arises. There is no one right insulin dose or schedule. Each must be individualized and adjusted when necessary. Insulin requirements do change, particularly in children because of growth, illness, and seasonal changes in activity.

INTENSIVE INSULIN THERAPY

Intensive insulin therapy involves injecting more than one kind of insulin more than twice a day or using an insulin pump to improve diabetes control. It's usually used when maximum control of diabetes is desired. Some people believe it provides a more flexible lifestyle, although the best control is still achieved when meals and activity are kept fairly consistent.

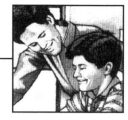

In general, meal times should not vary by more than an hour and meal sizes should remain consistent so it will be easier to judge insulin requirements. An evening snack is important to prevent low blood glucose during the early morning hours.

Persons wanting to use intensive therapy must be highly motivated and knowledgeable about nutrition, exercise, insulin action and adjustments, and physical and emotional stress. And they must learn how all of these things affect blood glucose levels. They must test blood glucose at least four times a day to make sure blood glucose goals are being achieved and to determine insulin doses. This is even more important for people using insulin pumps. For more information on intensified insulin therapy, see Chapter 24 or the International Diabetes Center's workbook, *Intensified Insulin Management for You.*

THE INSULIN PUMP

An insulin pump is a battery-powered microcomputer a little larger than a deck of cards. The pump is worn on the outside of the body. Inside the pump is a syringe, or reservoir, that is filled with insulin every two to three days. Insulin is delivered to the body through a small plastic tube attached to a needle inserted into the skin and taped in place. The needle and tubing are replaced when the pump is refilled with insulin. Only short-acting (Regular) insulin is used in a pump. Instructions to deliver different amounts of insulin at different times of the day can be entered through a keyboard on the pump. Insulin pumps are being developed that can monitor blood glucose levels and deliver insulin appropriately.

MONITORING

The best way to determine how successfully you are balancing food, insulin, and activity is to measure your blood glucose. The most valuable information is obtained if blood tests are done before each meal and at bedtime. Other times to test are when blood glucose is low (especially when you suspect low blood glucose levels at night), when you are ill, or when there is a change in your schedule. However, testing in itself does not improve blood glucose control. Test results must be recorded. You and your

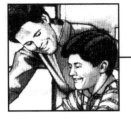

health care team must use these records to help you learn how activity, food, insulin, and stress are related. Adjustments in your health care plan are based on these results.

Besides blood glucose testing, it's important to know how to test for ketones in the urine. This must be done whenever your blood glucose is 240 mg/dl or higher or if you're feeling ill. The presence of ketones in the urine, along with high blood glucose, means there is not enough insulin to allow the body to continue to use glucose for energy. The body has switched over to using too much fat for energy. This can be caused by too little insulin, too much food, or an unusual amount of stress. A blood glucose test of 240 mg/dl or higher and a positive ketone test are a warning that some changes need to be made immediately to prevent ketoacidosis. This will be discussed in Chapter 11.

WHAT SHOULD BE DONE DURING ROUTINE HEALTH CARE VISITS

Through routine visits to your health care team, you can work together to evaluate your blood glucose control and make changes as needed. You should visit your health care team every three to four months. If your diabetes is not in good control, more frequent visits may be necessary.

During each routine visit, your doctor will order a glycosylated hemoglobin test from the laboratory. This test provides very valuable information, because it shows what your average blood glucose level has been over the previous six to eight weeks. The glycosylated hemoglobin level for people without diabetes who have been tested in our laboratory is 4.6 to 5.8%. Each laboratory has its own normal level. Your result must be interpreted according to your laboratory's normal value. Your doctor will do this and discuss the result with you. The test results, along with your daily blood glucose records, allow you and your health care team to evaluate how your health care plan is working. If the levels are higher than expected, your insulin, meal plan, or exercise pattern needs to be adjusted.

Glycosylated hemoglobin measurements do have some limitations. As with any laboratory test, they must be done very carefully to provide accurate results. The test does not reveal if you have had problems with low blood glucose, and is not helpful in pinpointing what you need to change to improve your average blood glucose level. This is why it's important to

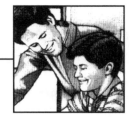

test and to record accurate daily blood glucose readings and work with your health care team to make changes if necessary.

Blood glucose control is not the only factor that will be checked in routine visits. Each year you should have a complete physical examination. Any changes that are occurring may need more extensive evaluation. Your blood pressure will be checked, sometimes two or three times to obtain a reliable result. Your doctor will check your eyes, feet, heart sounds, pulses, organs, and the condition of the skin at your injection sites. Ask questions about what is being checked and discuss with your doctor how signs of long-term complications can be detected. If you have had diabetes more than five years and are over 12 years of age, your eyes should be examined by an ophthalmologist (eye doctor) annually. The ophthalmologist will use eye drops to enlarge (dilate) the opening to your eye. Then he or she will look at the back of the eye for any changes diabetes may have caused. For complete information on diabetes and the eye, see Chapter 19.

Your blood cholesterol and triglyceride levels (under 180-200 milligrams is desirable for cholesterol and under 150 milligrams for triglycerides) should be checked annually. If a child's cholesterol is initially normal, it only needs to be checked every two years. Other blood and urine tests are done annually to check for signs of kidney problems. Good blood glucose control and early detection of long-term complications can best be achieved by these preventive measures.

YOUR RESPONSIBILITIES

It's important that you participate in your health care visits. To do this you need to follow the health care team's recommendations for monitoring, record the results, and bring the meter and record book to each clinic visit. Each person with diabetes is different. It's up to you to collect the information to help yourself and your health care team.

If your blood glucose levels aren't in line (low or high) with your goals, make adjustments or call your health care team. Don't wait until your next clinic visit. The chart below outlines what you and your health care team need to do. That way you can work together to achieve the best diabetes control possible.

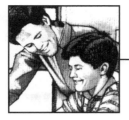

HEALTH CARE RESPONSIBILITIES

	You	**Your Health Care Team**
Clinic Visits	Bring record book Bring meter Ask questions Help in decision-making process	Look at record book Compare current status with past medical status Perform yearly physical exam Provide continued education update Provide yearly meter check Order glycosylated hemoglobin test and, when needed, blood cholesterol and triglyceride tests
Hypoglycemia	Be consistent with times of insulin and needs Test more often with schedule changes Adjust health care plan or call for help when schedule changes Pay attention to blood glucose under 70 mg/dl and adjust health care plan	Work with you to set reasonable blood glucose goals Provide information on preventing severe reactions Respond to phone calls
Hyperglycemia	Follow sick day plan when ill Test blood glucose more often and test urine for ketones when blood glucose is over 240 mg/dl or when you're ill Call when ketones are moderate or large, when vomiting, or if ill more than 24 hours	Educate on sick day plan Respond to phone calls

EDUCATION

Diabetes education allows you to work with your health care team and is one of the most important tools you have. The learning process is most successful when approached in three basic stages: survival skills, in-depth education, and ongoing education.

When you are first diagnosed you need "survival skills," which include learning:

- the kind and amount of insulin to take and how to inject it
- the kind of foods you need to eat and when to eat them
- how to test and record blood glucose and urine ketones

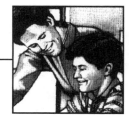

- how to recognize, prevent and treat low and high blood glucose
- where to buy your diabetes supplies, how you'll pay for them, and how to store them

This a lot of information to learn when you're still in shock over hearing that you have a disease that will be with you for the rest of your life. Any attempts to learn more about diabetes at this time usually fail.

Once you've had a chance to adjust emotionally and are familiar with the routine of managing your diabetes, it helps to learn all about diabetes and how you can live well with it. This may take several months. At this time, you'll be able to apply what you learn to your own experiences, which will help you remember the information. This is a good time to attend an in-depth education program, such as the week-long program offered by the International Diabetes Center or its Affiliates around the country. A good program will help you and your family work as a part of the health care team. You'll be able to help reevaluate your health care plan and make any adjustments needed to improve your diabetes control and/or quality of life.

You will always need to keep updating your knowledge of diabetes. Researchers and doctors are discovering new and better treatment methods every year, so it's important to remain informed about this progress. Your local affiliate of the American Diabetes Association can tell you about programs in your area. Your own health care team can also answer many of your questions and concerns.

Since your diabetes will be changing constantly, you need to learn how to modify your health care plan to allow for these changes. Seasonal activity, work schedules, health problems, life changes, and many other things can affect diabetes and require changes in your health care plan. Your health care team can help you make changes in your insulin schedule, meal plan, or activity schedule to allow you to control your diabetes without needlessly restricting your lifestyle. The more you learn about diabetes, the more you'll be in control of it, rather than it being in control of you.

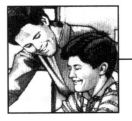

SUMMARY

Studies have shown that the success of the diabetes health care plan is affected by several things:

- how serious you are about controlling your diabetes
- how well the health care plan is made, understood, and followed
- how well the health care plan is adapted to your lifestyle
- how you adjust emotionally to diabetes
- how much support you receive from family members and others

People with diabetes must not be thought of as "diabetics" who must live restricted lives. They should be thought of as persons who happen to have diabetes, a disease that fortunately can be made part of a very healthy, productive, and full life.

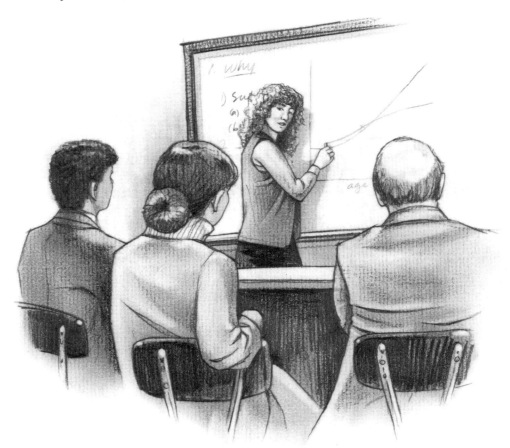

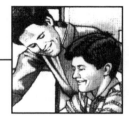

MONITORING YOUR KNOWLEDGE

1. To achieve good control of your diabetes, who is the most important team member?

_____

2. Why do you need a special treatment plan?

_____

3. Name four of your responsibilities related to blood glucose monitoring.

_____

_____

_____

_____

4. Name three responsibilities of your health care team.

_____

_____

_____

5. How can diabetes education help you?

_____

Answers on page 191.

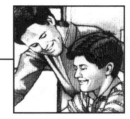

CHAPTER 8

Marion J. Franz, MS, RD, CDE
Diane Reader, RD, CDE
Gay Castle, RD, CDE

Nutrition:
The Key Is Consistency

Why is an individualized meal plan necessary?

Why is consistency so important?

What's the best way to handle delayed meals?

Meal planning is an important part of the health care plan for Type I diabetes. But even though paying attention to what you eat can help control blood glucose and blood fat levels, it's a mistake to think you are eating just to control your diabetes. A well-designed meal plan provides all the nutrients necessary for a healthful lifestyle, with enough variety to be enjoyable and enough flexibility to allow for your personal likes and dislikes. A meal plan is not a "diabetic diet," it's a way of eating that is recommended for everyone, whether you have diabetes or not.

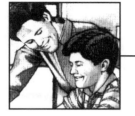

The general nutritional recommendations for persons with diabetes focus on "wellness" and help everyone eat better. They do not provide specific guidelines related to diabetes management. For this you must have an individualized *meal plan*. Your meal plan will be designed to meet your diabetes needs as well as your caloric and nutrient needs based on your age, height and weight, activity level, lifestyle, and food preferences.

A meal plan can best be developed by working with a registered dietitian (a health professional with the letters "RD" after her or his name). An RD will explain what is important in meal planning and then teach you how to do it. By learning more about nutrition and your meal plan you can add variety to your meals and flexibility to your lifestyle. You will also be better able to solve the problems and situations you encounter in your daily eating habits.

Your nutrition needs may change as a result of changes in weight, activity, lifestyle, or growth, and it's important to have them reflected in your meal plan. Changes can be made in your meal plan to reflect a healthier lifestyle, or simply to make things more convenient for you. Your meal plan should be reviewed at least two to four times a year. This will ensure that it's meeting your needs and that you feel comfortable with it. Children's meal plans ideally should be reviewed every three months but certainly no less than twice a year (before and after the school year).

THE IMPORTANCE OF CONSISTENCY

Once your meal plan has been established and you feel you can follow it regularly, your insulin needs can be adjusted to your food intake and regular activity. This is why it's so important to be consistent in following your meal plan. By eating about the same amount of food at the same times each day and by doing regular blood glucose testing before meals and at bedtime, you or your health care team can make adjustments in your insulin therapy. This is the best way to keep blood glucose levels as close to the normal range as possible.

Remember, in persons who don't have diabetes, the body matches the amount of insulin it produces to the amount of food eaten. This is what you and your health care team are trying to duplicate by balancing your food intake, activity, and insulin. If a person without diabetes eats more food one day than the next, the body makes more insulin as needed. In a person with diabetes the body can't do this, so blood glucose has to be kept

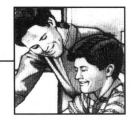

in line by a consistent balance of food, activity, and insulin. Routine meal times and day-to-day consistency in the number of calories eaten will help make blood glucose control easier.

DESIGNING YOUR MEAL PLAN

Your meal plan will include the number of exchanges you should eat and at what times you should eat them, based on the timing of your injections and the type of insulin you take. This means you probably need three meals and at least two to three snacks each day. Snacks are very important for matching the time action of insulin. An injection of a short-acting and intermediate-acting insulin before breakfast often makes a morning snack necessary, especially for children. The time action of intermediate-acting insulin makes an afternoon snack necessary; sometimes children do better with two afternoon snacks. An evening snack is important to balance the insulins acting throughout the night.

Blood glucose monitoring can help you find out how different foods affect your blood glucose so you can make appropriate decisions about how to use them in your meal plan. As you learn more about your meal plan and gain practice in adjusting food, insulin, and activity based on blood glucose tests, you will find yourself getting more flexible about meal planning. Blood glucose monitoring is also used to make adjustments in insulin. However, don't react to one high blood glucose by skipping snacks or cutting back on meals. Wait for patterns to develop, and then make appropriate changes in insulin or food. See Chapter 10 for more information on pattern control.

Exercise and normal activity levels, such as the types and times of your usual activity (work, school, home) as well as exercise, sports practices, and competition, also affect how your meal plan is designed. It's helpful if your activity patterns can also be consistent. Not only is it easier to work your needs into the meal plan, but your body will adapt to a regular training pattern. This, in turn, can help blood glucose control.

You may need to increase your food intake after, and perhaps before, activity or exercise that you don't do regularly. The best way to decide how much food you need is to monitor blood glucose levels before and after exercise. For guidelines on how to adjust food based on blood glucose levels, see the table on page 157.

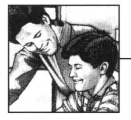

HANDLING SCHEDULE CHANGES

We've discussed how important consistency is in the timing of insulin injections and meals. A schedule or daily routine is a basic tool in diabetes management to help control blood glucose levels. However, there are always times when situations come up, such as delayed and changed meal times and holidays, that call for changes in your usual schedule or daily routine. You need to know how to handle these situations in a safe manner in order to stay within your diabetes management plan.

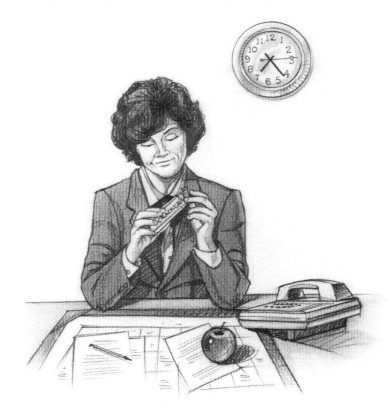

The easiest schedule change to deal with is one that's planned. However, even a very organized and structured person can face an unexpected problem. Therefore, the first rule is to be prepared! That means you must carry some food with you as you work, travel, shop, exercise, and drive. A fruit or starch exchange, such as a box of raisins, package of crackers, or plain granola bars is often convenient.

140

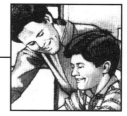

Let's examine some common scheduling problems. Remember, these are very general guidelines. If you have questions about your care, don't hesitate to contact your health care team.

DELAYED MEALS

Sometimes you may find it necessary to delay meals because of work or social commitments. What's the best way to handle this? If a meal is delayed by one hour, have a fruit or starch exchange (15 grams of carbohydrate) at the scheduled meal time. This is particularly important if you take your insulin injection at the usual time. (However, you can delay your insulin for up to an hour. In that case you would take your insulin and have your meal as usual.) The following diagram shows how to delay your supper an hour:

Usual Schedule	Delayed Meal Schedule
5:30 PM: Insulin (Regular or Regular and intermediate-acting)	5:30 PM: Insulin (usual dose)
	6 PM: 1 fruit (1/2 cup orange juice)
	7 PM: Supper (subtract 1 fruit)
6 PM: Supper	10 PM: Evening snack
10 PM: Evening snack	

If the meal is delayed for longer than 1 1/2 hours, you have several options. The first option is to move the evening snack to the meal time and have the meal later. (This option is especially important if you are taking only one injection of insulin in the morning.) For example, if you will be eating supper out at 8:30 and your supper hour is usually 6:00, use the following suggestion:

Usual Schedule	Delayed Meal Schedule
5:30 PM: Insulin (Regular or Regular and intermediate-acting)	5:30 PM: Insulin (usual dose)
	6 PM: Evening snack
	8:30 PM: Supper
6 PM: Supper	*(check blood glucose before going*
10 PM: Evening snack	*to bed to see if an additional snack*
	is needed)

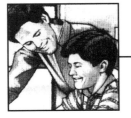
If you take two injections of insulin, another option may be better. If supper is not delayed more than 1 1/2 hours, you can wait, take your insulin before the meal, and then have the snack at bedtime. Delaying the second injection too long, however, may cause an overlap of intermediate-acting insulin action the next morning. To prevent this, you can use the third option (below). Take your intermediate-acting insulin at the usual time and take the regular insulin before your meal:

Usual Schedule	Delayed Meal Schedule
5:30 PM: Insulin (Regular and intermediate-acting) 6 PM: Supper 10 PM: Evening snack	5:30 PM: Insulin (intermediate-acting) 6 PM: 1/2 Evening snack 8 PM: Insulin (Regular) 8:30 PM: Supper (also rest of snack) *(check blood glucose before going to bed to see if an additional snack is needed)*

Of course, if you have an intermediate-acting insulin before bed you can continue to do that and simply have the regular insulin before supper. If supper is delayed too long it may be a good idea to have a fruit or a starch exchange from your evening snack around 6 PM.

Making any of the above changes will probably affect your blood glucose tests because you may be testing closer to the larger meal than you normally do. But because you will know why your glucose level is higher, you won't need to make any changes in your insulin dosages. The next day return to your usual schedule, and your blood glucose level should again return to normal.

An important word of caution: If you find your bedtime blood glucose level is higher than usual, do NOT take extra regular insulin at that time. By the time insulin is at its peak of action the elevated blood glucose from the meal will have decreased. The time to take extra Regular insulin is before a meal, not after. However, the difficulty in doing this is knowing how much extra Regular insulin to take. In general, remember that it should be very small amounts, one or two units. The best advice is to check with your health care team. They can advise you on the best way to handle situations such as the above.

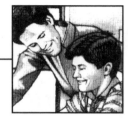

HOLIDAY MEALS

Some holiday and special occasions create very different meal times. By following some simple guidelines, people with Type I diabetes can also make changes in the meal plan to adapt to holiday eating schedules. For example, if the family chooses to have the holiday meal at 2 or 3 PM and you are scheduled to eat at noon and 6 PM, what can you do to enjoy the holiday festivities with your family and friends? Begin by having the exchanges of your afternoon snack at noon. Then, at 2 or 3 PM have the exchanges of your lunch meal plan. If you are really being honest about it, this holiday meal will probably use up part of your supper meal plan as well. Do save a portion of the evening meal plan exchanges to eat at the routine supper hour.

So if you keep your morning insulin schedule the same, use the following suggested schedule:

Usual Schedule		Holiday Schedule	
7:30 AM:	Insulin	7:30 AM:	Insulin
8 AM:	Breakfast	8 AM:	Breakfast
10 AM:	Morning snack	10 AM:	Morning snack
Noon:	Lunch	Noon:	Light lunch (afternoon snack exchanges)
3 PM:	Afternoon snack	2 PM:	Dinner (lunch and part of supper exchanges)
5:30 PM:	Insulin	5:30 PM:	Insulin
6 PM:	Supper	6 PM:	Snack (rest of supper exchanges)
10 PM:	Evening snack	10 PM:	Evening snack

Making the changes just shown will probably throw your blood glucose tests off for the day because you may be testing closer to meal times than you normally do. But by knowing what has affected the blood glucose tests, you don't need to make any changes in the insulin program. Keep in mind that dividing your meal plan into different size meals and snacks won't get you in trouble as long as your total carbohydrate and calorie intake for the day (preferably for each four to six hour period) remains the same. For persons taking insulin, delaying meals WILL cause problems! One of the

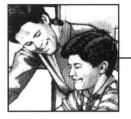

factors that determines how much insulin is needed in a day is the total number of calories eaten, and this should remain constant. Remember that making these changes should be reserved for very special occasions.

WEEKENDS AND BRUNCHES

It's tempting to sleep in on Saturday and Sunday mornings or on your day off. However, doing this can play havoc with your insulin schedule. Therefore, try to keep on your usual Monday to Friday schedule. If you need more sleep, it's best to get up, take your usual insulin injection, eat breakfast, and go back to bed and sleep.

If a brunch is planned, follow your usual morning routine and eat a small breakfast, have brunch in place of your morning snack, and eat your morning snack at your usual lunchtime:

Usual Schedule		Brunch Schedule	
7 AM:	Insulin	7 AM:	Insulin
7:30 AM:	Breakfast	7:30 AM:	Small breakfast (1–2 starch/breads)
9:30 AM:	Morning snack	9–10 AM:	Brunch (rest of breakfast and lunch exchanges)
Noon:	Lunch	12–1 PM:	Morning snack
3 PM:	Afternoon snack	3 PM:	Afternoon snack

INTENSIFIED INSULIN THERAPY

The basis of meal planning for intensified insulin therapy continues to be a meal plan using the exchange system. However, with intensified insulin therapy small adjustments are made in Regular insulin for anticipated changes in meals. Decisions as to how to make these adjustments are based on carbohydrate counting. The easiest way to begin judging how much extra insulin may be needed for extra carbohydrate is to use the following guidelines: add 1 unit Regular insulin to the usual Regular insulin dose for each extra 15 grams of carbohydrate added to a meal.

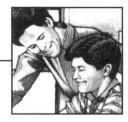

Two precautions should be kept in mind: First, varying meal sizes too often can worsen control of diabetes. The more consistent the content and timing of meals, the easier it is to maintain consistent blood glucose values. Because there is no magic formula for deciding how much extra insulin is needed to cover every food, trial and error must be used. Second, experimenting with new foods and eating larger meals and snacks tend to cause weight gain.

Although use of multiple injections may provide somewhat increased flexibility of meal times, meals must still be reasonably routine in their timing. Multiple injections are most successful when meals are eaten within an hour of the usual schedule.

It's important to also remember to not adjust insulin based on blood glucose levels taken one or two hours after eating a meal. Regular insulin should only be added to the insulin injection taken before a meal. After insulin adjustments are made, it's important to look at post-meal blood glucose values to assess how well the adjustment worked. For additional information on intensified insulin therapy, see the International Diabetes Center's workbook, *Intensified Insulin Management for You.*

SUMMARY

Meal planning by the person with diabetes depends on a certain amount of self-control as well as adequate information. With this combination, you too can enjoy an active social life and even "have a ball."

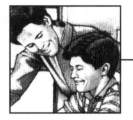
MONITORING YOUR KNOWLEDGE

1. List three things that determine what your meal plan will be.

_____

_____

_____

2. What is the most important lifestyle factor for persons who take injected insulin?

_____

3. To delay meals an hour, you need to eat about how many grams of carbohydrate?

_____

Answers on page 192.

CHAPTER 9

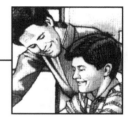

Marion J. Franz, MS, RD, CDE
Jane Norstrom, MA

Exercise:
Clues for Safe Participation

Will exercise help me control my diabetes?

What do I need to know to exercise safely?

Will I have to make adjustments to my insulin and food whenever I exercise?

Diabetes should not be used as an excuse to avoid exercise. Although research shows that regular exercise may not improve blood glucose control in Type I diabetes, it has many benefits that can't be tested or measured. Exercise improves self-image, increases your ability to do work, enhances your sense of well-being, and enriches and adds "quality" to your life.

If you have Type I diabetes, you should exercise to improve overall fitness. You are also encouraged to get involved in other recreational and, if you wish, competitive activities. This chapter has information that will help you begin or continue to exercise safely so you can enjoy the same benefits of exercise other people do. And for most people, the benefits far exceed the risks.

147

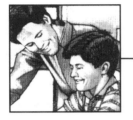

When it comes to exercise for people with Type I diabetes, there may be some extra benefits. For one thing, exercise can add to the blood glucose-lowering effects of injected insulin. This means people who exercise regularly usually have lower insulin requirements than those who don't exercise. A smaller amount of insulin is needed for muscle cells to use glucose during exercise than at rest. This effect lasts for 24 to 48 hours after exercise. Muscle and liver glycogen (stored carbohydrate) is used for fuel during exercise and must be replenished afterward. As a result, exercise improves the use and storage of glucose and decreases the amount of insulin required.

Exercise also helps you achieve a "low-risk" profile for heart disease. A low-risk profile means it's important for you to be lean, have normal blood pressure, not smoke, and have low blood cholesterol values. Normal blood pressure is particularly important because high blood pressure can increase the severity of long-term problems that occur with diabetes, such as eye and kidney problems. Regular exercise decreases blood pressure. Regular exercise can also assist with weight control. It increases the number of calories you use and it can help to keep food intake at more appropriate levels.

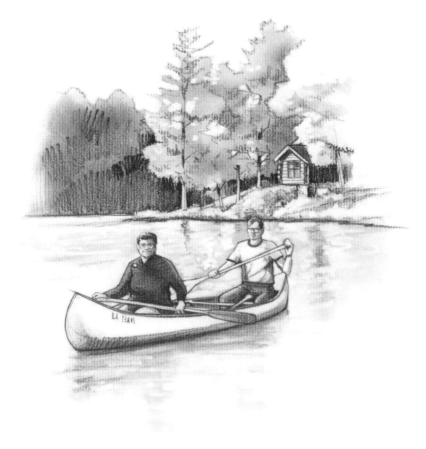

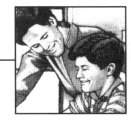

Overall improved blood glucose control, however, has not been found to be a benefit of exercise for persons with Type I diabetes. Researchers have studied how exercise affects glycosylated hemoglobin (which shows your average blood glucose level during a certain length of time), but none of them has been able to prove that exercise helped to improved glycosylated hemoglobin values. In fact, it was found that exercise often made blood glucose levels harder to control.

One problem with exercise is that persons with diabetes tend to overeat when exercising. They may be over cautious and fear hypoglycemia, or they may believe the exercise will reduce any high blood glucose level that results from overeating. Whatever the reason, exercise should not be viewed as an opportunity to indulge in foods that are usually avoided, such as candy bars, desserts, and regular soda pop. Lack of overall improved blood glucose control surprised the researchers, because blood glucose levels had dropped during the exercise sessions. It was concluded that without changing food and insulin, physical training alone usually doesn't improve overall blood glucose control.

Blood glucose monitoring is your most effective tool for correctly deciding when and how much to increase food or how to reduce insulin. You will be your own best teacher when making decisions about blood glucose control during exercise.

GETTING STARTED

Before starting any exercise program, be sure your diabetes is under good control. It's important to start slowly and gradually build up endurance.

When you begin an exercise program, the exercise may cause blood glucose levels to change unpredictably. People who exercise regularly usually have fewer blood glucose control problems than those who are just beginning to exercise or who exercise only occasionally.

The key to safe exercise is to monitor your blood glucose before and after exercise. If you'll be exercising for a long period you should also monitor blood glucose during exercise. Keep a record of the test results, time of exercise, what you ate, and what type of exercise you did and for how long. Discuss your records with your health care team. Together you can develop guidelines for adjusting food intake and insulin.

A good general "rule of thumb" regarding exercise concerns blood glucose levels, food intake, and insulin adjustment.

If your blood glucose is less than 100 mg/dl before exercise, eat a pre-exercise snack. See the following chart for snack ideas.

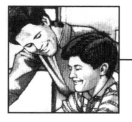

If it's 100 to 150 mg/dl, go ahead and exercise and, if necessary, eat a snack afterwards.

If your blood glucose is greater than 250 mg/dl, check urine for ketones. If ketones are positive, improve control by adjusting insulin. Don't exercise until ketones are negative.

PRE- AND POST-EXERCISE SNACKS

Food	Amount	Carbohydrate Content	Exchanges
Bagel or English muffin	1/2	14 gms	1 starch/bread
Graham cracker squares	3	15 gms	1 starch/bread
Snack crackers	4–5	15 gms	1 starch/bread
Muffin	1	17 gms	1 starch/bread, 1 fat
Pretzels	6 3-ring	14 gms	1 starch/bread
Soup (not cream)	1 cup	15 gms	1 starch/bread
Yogurt (plain or sweetened with NutraSweet®)	1 cup	16 gms	1 milk
Apple	1 medium	22 gms	1 1/2 fruit
Banana	1 small	22 gms	1 1/2 fruit
Dried fruit	1/4 cup	10 gms	1 fruit
Orange	1 medium	18 gms	1 fruit
Raisins	2 Tbsp	15 gms	1 fruit
Fruit juice	1/2 cup	15 gms	1 fruit

Before starting any exercise program you need to be aware of the risks of hypoglycemia and from hyperglycemia.

HYPOGLYCEMIA

Exercise can increase the risk for hypoglycemia, especially if it isn't done regularly or if it's done for long periods. Hypoglycemia can occur during exercise, usually when you exercise for longer than an hour. It can also

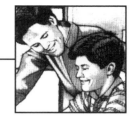

occur up to 30 hours after vigorous or prolonged exercise or exercise that is done sporadically. In a study of 300 adolescents with Type I diabetes, hypoglycemia was more common four to ten hours after exercise than during exercise or even one to two hours after exercise.

How does this happen? Insulin prevents the liver from releasing glucose. In persons who do not have diabetes, insulin levels automatically decrease with exercise. This prompts the liver to release more glucose to keep blood glucose levels in the normal range, even though exercising muscles can use 20 times more glucose than non-exercising muscles.

However, if you have Type I diabetes, your body cannot decrease its level of circulating insulin when you begin to exercise. Your level of circulating insulin will depend on how much you took by injection. When insulin in the blood doesn't decrease, the liver doesn't release glucose. As a result, your body uses what glucose is available, but no extra glucose is released to meet the added needs of the exercising muscle. This can result in hypoglycemia.

After exercising, your blood glucose can continue to drop for two reasons. First, your body cells require less insulin to use or store glucose after exercising. Second, your body has to replace the stored carbohydrate (glycogen) you used during exercise.

Hypoglycemia can be prevented by increasing food eaten after and/or before exercise or by reducing the dose of insulin acting during the time of activity. See page 157 for general guidelines on how to begin doing this.

Monitor your blood glucose levels at one- or two-hour intervals, especially after strenuous exercise. This will help you assess how you respond to exercise and make the necessary adjustments in insulin and food intake. It's often more important to eat a small snack after exercising than before. And just as important, don't assume you've exercised safely and don't disregard making appropriate food or insulin adjustments after exercise is completed.

HYPERGLYCEMIA

Although low blood glucose as a result of exercise is usually the major concern, exercise can at times raise blood glucose levels. One factor that determines the effect exercise has on blood glucose levels is the availability of insulin to muscle cells. One of insulin's primary roles is to allow muscle cells to use glucose. With exercise, less insulin is needed for this to happen, but you do need some insulin. Therefore, if you begin exercising with an

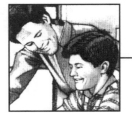

insulin deficiency—such as occurs with uncontrolled diabetes—blood glucose levels and ketones can rise.

How does this happen? When blood glucose is high (generally greater than 250 to 300 mg/dl) because of poor control, it means not enough insulin is available. You need adequate amounts of insulin available to help the muscle cells use the glucose needed during exercise. Activity is not a replacement for insulin. If blood glucose levels are high, the exercising muscles still need glucose and will send a message to the liver to release stored carbohydrate (glycogen). This will stimulate release of glucose. But because not enough insulin is available, the glucose won't be able to leave the blood stream to the cells, causing blood glucose to rise even further during exercise. Meanwhile, the exercising muscles still need a source of energy. Since the extra glucose can't be used, the body responds by releasing fat to be used instead. However, the amount of fat released is more than the exercising muscles can use, which can lead to an increase in blood ketone levels.

Hyperglycemia is of particular concern when diabetes has been poorly controlled over several days or more. If you start with a blood glucose level greater than 250 to 300 mg/dl, you may find that exercise doesn't decrease it. However, with mild to moderate hyperglycemia (blood glucose levels under 250 to 300 mg/dl), moderate exercise almost always results in a desirable reduction of blood glucose levels.

Exercise of high intensity can also cause blood glucose levels to be higher after exercise than before. This can happen even if blood glucose levels are in the normal range before beginning the exercise. High intensity exercise is so strenuous that you become short of breath and have to stop because of exhaustion. Generally, this type of exercise can only be done for short periods. Examples would be pedaling a bicycle very rapidly, sprinting, climbing stairs quickly, and weight lifting.

TIMING OF EXERCISE

The time of the day you choose to exercise may also be important. For instance, "morning people" may choose to exercise before breakfast. This is usually a good time to exercise because blood glucose levels tend to be higher during the early morning hours. However, the opposite may be true and some people may have lower blood glucose levels before breakfast. So, if you choose to exercise before breakfast, we suggest you do a blood glucose test first. If the level is 100 mg/dl or higher, eat or drink 10 to 15 grams of

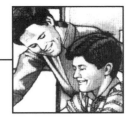

carbohydrate, then exercise. If blood glucose is lower than 100 mg/dl, add another 10 to 15 grams of carbohydrate, wait 10 to 15 minutes, and test again. If it is then above 100 mg/dl, go ahead and exercise. After exercise do another blood glucose test, take your morning insulin, eat breakfast, and get on with the day.

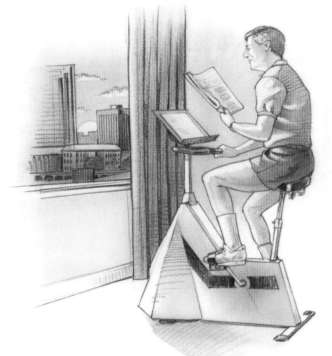

Another good time to exercise may be after breakfast (or other meals), since blood glucose levels tend to be the highest during these times. This may be inconvenient because of work or school. But if you can work it out, eat your usual breakfast or meal, exercise, and then have your usual snack. You may find you don't need any extra food.

If you prefer exercising after work or later in the afternoon, do a blood glucose test and follow the recommendations for food adjustment on page 157. Eat the snack before exercising.

If you want to exercise in the evening, take your evening insulin (if you're on two injections of insulin), and eat dinner. Wait an hour or so to give your food time to digest. (This isn't really necessary, but many persons find they exercise better if they wait awhile after eating.) Then exercise. Test your blood glucose before your evening snack. You may need to add some extra food to that snack, depending on the type and amount of exercise you

153

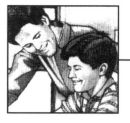

performed and the level of your blood glucose. Again, follow the recommendations on page 157. If you exercise later in the afternoon or evening, don't go to bed without a snack. Remember that blood glucose levels can continue to drop for hours after exercise.

GENERAL GUIDELINES FOR SAFE EXERCISE

Ideally, you would exercise at about the same time each day and at the same level of intensity. For practical reasons, this is rarely possible. You may need to make adjustments, especially in food intake, depending on the time of day you are exercising. Exercise may initially cause blood glucose levels to change unpredictably. Your level of fitness also can affect glucose stability—if you already exercise regularly you will have fewer diabetes control problems than if you are just beginning to exercise or exercise only occasionally.

Listed below are general precautions you need to take when planning an exercise program:

1. Be sure you are in good control of your diabetes. Remember, the effect of exercise will depend on whether enough insulin is available to allow the muscle cells to use glucose for energy. If your blood glucose is over 250 to 300 mg/dl and ketones are present, it may be better to delay exercise until your diabetes is under better control.

2. Test your blood glucose before and after the exercise session. If you exercise for a long time, test during the exercise as well. Blood glucose testing is essential to record your response to exercise and to plan for safe exercise sessions. Carefully finding out how exercise affects your blood glucose levels will decrease the risk of having an insulin reaction.

3. Be aware of the peak times of injected insulin and the excessive lowering of blood glucose levels that exercise may produce at these times. Regular insulin peaks in three to four hours. NPH or Lente peaks in eight to ten hours. An ideal time to exercise is after a meal, especially after breakfast, since blood glucose levels tend to be the highest during the morning hours. If you do exercise when insulin is peaking, be sure to plan for appropriate increases in

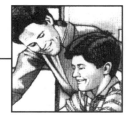

carbohydrate before or after exercise.

4. Blood glucose can continue to decrease for up to 30 hours after exercise, especially after vigorous or prolonged exercise or exercise that is not done regularly. Blood glucose often drops between four and ten hours after exercise. Reports have shown that hypoglycemia during exercise, or even one to two hours after exercise, is not as common as hypoglycemia later. Replacing stored carbohydrate used during exercise can take many hours. By monitoring blood glucose levels at two-hour intervals after strenuous exercise, you can assess how you respond to the blood glucose-lowering effects of exercise.

5. You may need to increase your food intake to accommodate activity or exercise. In your meal plan you will plan for regular periods of activity. Well-trained persons who regularly exercise usually need less additional food than individuals who exercise only occasionally. Care should be taken to not eat too much food before exercise. Guidelines for increasing food should be based on blood glucose levels before and after exercise and on how close to regularly scheduled meals and snacks exercise occurs. If blood glucose is below 100 mg/dl, eat a snack before exercising. In general 10 to 15 grams of carbohydrate—one fruit or starch exchange—should be eaten before an hour of moderate exercise, such as tennis, swimming, jogging, cycling, or gardening. For more strenuous activity of a one- to two-hour duration, such as football, hockey, racquetball, basketball, strenuous cycling or swimming, or shoveling heavy snow, 30 to 50 grams of carbohydrate—one-half a meat sandwich with one milk or fruit exchange—may be needed. Mild exercise, such as walking a half mile, will probably not require any extra food.

   The effect of exercise on blood glucose levels varies greatly. Everyone exercises at different intensities and uses insulin and food differently. The guidelines given in the table on page 157 are only suggestions. They can help you plan food for exercise and make food changes based on your blood glucose level. But, it's still important that you monitor your blood glucose level and adapt these guidelines to your own needs.

   Along with food intake, exercisers must remember the need for increased fluid intake. Cool water, sports drinks, or diluted fruit juices are good choices. Persons whose diabetes is poorly controlled are particularly prone to dehydration when exercising on warm days.

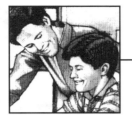
6. Injection sites are not a major concern, unless the injection is done in a part of your body you will be exercising immediately. If it's been more than 40 minutes between the injection of Regular insulin and the start of exercise, more than half of the injected insulin will be mobilized from the injection site. Likewise, absorption of intermediate-acting insulin remains unaffected when exercise is begun 1 1/2 hours after an injection. If you exercise immediately after an insulin injection, inject into an area not involved in the exercise, such as the abdomen.

7. Be sure to carry identification and a source of readily available carbohydrate with you when you exercise.

ADJUSTING INSULIN FOR EXTENDED EXERCISE

When you exercise strenuously over an extended period, such as all morning, all afternoon, or all day, it may be difficult to avoid low blood glucose by just increasing food intake. In such cases, you can reduce the dose of the insulin that will be acting during the time of activity. In effect, the exercise will take the place of the missing insulin and, together with food intake, will keep blood glucose in the normal range. Use the following guideline to adjust your insulin.

Decrease insulin acting during the exercise time by 10% of the total insulin dose. For example:

Insulin dose: 10 Regular, 20 NPH before breakfast
                  3 Regular, 5 NPH before supper
Total: 13   +   25   =   38 units

10% of 38 (38 x .10) is 3.8 units, which can be rounded to 4 units.

In this case, you would decrease insulin by 4 units for exercise. For instance, fast-acting insulin acts during the morning hours. For cross-country skiing all morning, you would decrease the morning Regular insulin by 10% of the total insulin dose. The morning insulin would then be 6 Regular (10 minus 4) and 20 NPH.

Intermediate-acting insulin taken before breakfast acts during the afternoon hours. For canoeing all afternoon, the morning insulin would be 10 Regular and 16 NPH (20 minus 4).

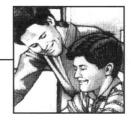

MAKING FOOD ADJUSTMENTS FOR EXERCISE: GENERAL GUIDELINES

Type of Exercise and Examples	If Blood Glucose Is:	Increase Food Intake By:	Suggestions of Food to Use
Exercise of short duration and of low to moderate intensity (walking a half mile or leisurely bicycling for less than 30 minutes)	less than 100 mg/dl	10 to 15 gms of carbohydrate per hour	1 fruit or 1 starch/bread exchange
	100 mg/dl or above	not necessary to increase food	
Exercise of moderate intensity (one hour of tennis, swimming, jogging, leisurely bicycling, golfing, etc)	less than 100 mg/dl	25 to 50 gms of carbohydrate before exercise, then 10 to 15 gms per hour of exercise	1/2 meat sandwich with a milk or fruit exchange
	100 to 180 mg/dl	10 to 15 gms of carbohydrate	1 fruit or 1 starch/ bread exchange
	180 to 300 mg/dl	not necessary to increase food	
	300 mg/dl or above	don't begin exercise until blood glucose is under better control	
Strenuous activity or exercise (about one to two hours of football, hockey, racquetball, or basketball games; strenuous bicycling or swimming; shoveling heavy snow)	less than 100 mg/dl	50 gms of carbohydrate, monitor blood glucose carefully	1 meat sandwich (2 slices of bread) with a milk and fruit exchange
	100 to 180 mg/dl	25 to 50 gms of carbohydrate, depending on intensity and duration	1/2 meat sandwich with a milk or fruit exchange
	180 to 300 mg/dl	10 to 15 gms of carbohydrate	1 fruit or 1 starch/ bread exchange
	300 mg/dl or above	don't begin exercise until blood glucose is under better control	

Reprinted, with permission, from *Diabetes Actively Staying Healthy (DASH): Your Game Plan for Diabetes and Exercise,* by Marion J. Franz, MS, RD and Jane Norstrom, MA. Minneapolis: International Diabetes Center, 1990.

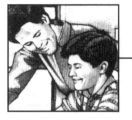

For activity lasting the entire day, such as downhill skiing, the Regular and NPH insulins would each be decreased by 10%. This means the morning insulin would be 6 Regular (10 minus 4) and 16 NPH (20 minus 4). On such days you may also need to decrease your insulin at suppertime.

Blood glucose testing before and after physical activity allows you to make adjustments in these general recommendations. Furthermore, be aware of specific warning signs of approaching hypoglycemia, especially after activity. Test your blood glucose when you notice such symptoms to make sure they are signs of low blood glucose. Also make sure that others are aware of your diabetes and know what to do if you need help.

RISKS AND PRECAUTIONS

Before you start an exercise program, you may need a detailed medical evaluation. This is especially important if you're over age 40 and have had diabetes for more than 10 years.

Strenuous exercise can make eye, kidney, and nerve problems worse. Because exercise can cause blood pressure to rise, it can put persons with eye problems at increased risk. Therefore, strenuous exercise, especially if it involves abrupt changes in head motion, should be avoided because it could cause hemorrhage or bleeding within the eye. Lifting heavy weights also should be avoided if eye hemorrhage or bleeding has occurred.

Kidney changes also can occur. Some protein is usually excreted in the urine during exercise, with or without diabetes. But for some reason, persons with diabetes seem to excrete more protein than normal when they exercise. We don't know yet if this is a serious problem.

If you have any nerve problems (neuropathy), avoid activities that might cause joint or bone injury. You also need to check your feet regularly for injuries and be sure you wear well-fitting shoes and socks.

For persons with known heart disease, it's important that "stress testing" be done before beginning an exercise program. If you're in this category, have an experienced exercise physiologist or physical therapist trained in this type of exercise planning prepare an exercise prescription. Chest pain, irregular heartbeat, dizziness, unusual fatigue, visual disturbance, or nausea should alert you to stop exercising and check with your doctor.

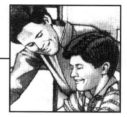

SUMMARY

Exercise should be a necessary yet enjoyable. Remember these main points:

- Blood glucose monitoring is essential for recording your response to exercise and planning safe exercise sessions.

- It's important that your diabetes is in good control. If your blood glucose is more than 250 mg/dl and ketones are present, exercise can worsen control. Exercise of high intensity can also cause hyperglycemia.

- If possible, exercise after your usual meals or snacks to improve blood glucose response to food.

- When you don't exercise after a meal, care must be taken not to eat too much extra food before exercising. However, if your blood glucose is less than 100 mg/dl, eat a snack first.

- Consider delaying extra food intake until after exercise. Hypoglycemia can occur for up to 30 hours after exercise, especially after vigorous or prolonged activity or exercise that is done sporadically. A sandwich along with a glass of milk may be needed to prevent overnight hypoglycemia.

The blood glucose responses to exercise depend on many variables—nutrition, training level, metabolic control, intensity, duration, and time of day you exercise. You are strongly encouraged to exercise whenever you find it convenient for a number of reasons—to maintain physical fitness, for recreation, and to get the same benefits from exercise that people without diabetes do.

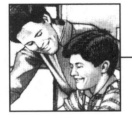

MONITORING YOUR KNOWLEDGE

1. The key to safe exercise is _____

2. Hypoglycemia can occur for up to how many hours after exercise?

_____

3. What can cause hyperglycemia after exercising?

_____

4. In general, how much carbohydrate is needed for an hour of moderate exercise?

_____

Answers on page 192.

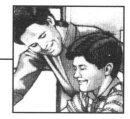

CHAPTER 10

Judy Ostrom Joynes, MA, RN, CDE

Pattern Control:
Monitoring Your Way to Better Blood Glucose Control

Which insulin do you adjust if your blood glucose reading is too high? What if it's too low?

Do you know how much to change your insulin?

How do you find out what causes high blood glucose values in the morning?

For many years it was believed the best treatment for diabetes was to manage complications as they developed. Now we know more can be done. It's the day-by-day, hour-by-hour management that makes the difference in the length and quality of life of persons with diabetes.

Pattern control is a way to carefully control blood glucose levels by using results of blood glucose monitoring to make changes in insulin, food intake, and exercise. If done properly, these changes can help people achieve and maintain blood glucose levels as near normal as possible and, as a result, the best possible diabetes control. This chapter explains how pattern control works and what you'll need to know to make it work for you.

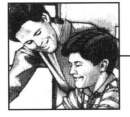

Using the information collected through routine blood glucose monitoring can help you prevent the sudden, severe problems of low blood glucose (hypoglycemia) as well as high blood glucose (hyperglycemia) and ketoacidosis. It can also help prevent the intermediate problems associated with growth and development in children and with pregnancy in women. With optimal blood glucose control, children with diabetes follow the same growth and development patterns as those without diabetes. When blood glucose is carefully controlled before and during pregnancy, outcomes for both mother and baby equal those in women without diabetes.

There is also strong evidence that careful control of blood glucose prevents development of long-term complications, such as eye, nerve, kidney, and large blood vessel problems. For the last several years, the National Institutes of Health (NIH) has funded a national research study that will hopefully provide more information on how diabetes control affects the development of some long-term problems. In the meantime, many diabetes experts believe that control will make a difference in preventing the development of long-term problems.

MONITORING AND RECORDING

Pattern control is based on blood glucose monitoring, and it can benefit anyone with diabetes. It can be especially helpful to:

- persons on insulin therapy or using insulin pumps
- women with gestational diabetes
- persons with kidney problems or on kidney dialysis
- children under age five
- persons who have nighttime hypoglycemia
- athletes in training
- persons who use meal planning in combination with oral medications

By recording results of blood glucose monitoring, you can map out changes in glucose levels throughout the day. This allows you to see how insulin, exercise, and different foods affect your blood glucose levels. In many ways, blood glucose monitoring puts you in control of diabetes, instead of diabetes controlling you.

Some people may have learned blood glucose monitoring from reading books, watching a videotape, or hearing from a friend down the street.

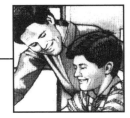

However, monitoring is expensive and time-consuming, so it's best to be sure it's done accurately and with the correct information. Local hospitals and diabetes associations usually have diabetes educators who are skilled in teaching proper technique. For more information on blood glucose monitoring, meters, and testing procedures, see Chapter 4.

ENSURING GOOD CONTROL

Inaccurate results from blood glucose testing cause people to make inaccurate insulin adjustments. This increases problems with their diabetes. That's why it's important to learn correct blood glucose testing techniques. Your testing technique should be checked at least once a year by a qualified health professional. If a problem with technique is suspected, have your blood glucose results checked with your doctor's laboratory.

Once you have mastered the monitoring technique, the next step is identifying blood glucose goals. For newly diagnosed persons, the goals are often higher than for those who are fairly well-versed in managing their diabetes. Ideally, these goals would be 70 to 120 mg/dl before meals, although levels to 140 mg/dl would be acceptable. After meals, blood glucose levels should not exceed 200 mg/dl, but the ideal level is 160 mg/dl or less. As you get better at diabetes management, the goals should be placed more in line with these ideal levels.

HOW OFTEN TO MONITOR

Several things determine how often you should test your blood glucose:

- type of diabetes
- level of control desired
- frequency of insulin injections or use of an insulin pump
- financial limitations

Generally speaking, people who take insulin, whether they have Type I or Type II diabetes, should test four times a day—before each meal and at bedtime. As their skills improve, each test will take about two minutes, or a total of eight minutes each day. If you look at it that way, monitoring really doesn't take much time.

Some people may have to test more frequently. If you've had high morning blood glucose levels or sleep disturbances, you may be asked to

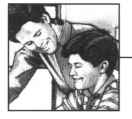

test at 3 AM. Suspected low blood glucose may also require additional testing. Often people think their blood glucose is low and then check with their meters only to find it's perfectly normal. Stress and other factors totally unrelated to blood glucose can cause symptoms similar to those brought on by hypoglycemia, so people are often asked to test during these times as well. You will also have to test more often during illness or when there is a change in routine or in insulin dose, type, or timing.

People who manage their Type II diabetes with meal planning alone or with meal planning combined with diabetes pills take a slightly different approach to blood glucose monitoring. We recommend the following.

Test a minimum of two to three days per week. (Test on one or two weekdays and one weekend day.)

Test two to three times per day on the days you test—before eating breakfast, before your main meal, and occasionally 1 1/2 hours after finishing your main meal. (Blood glucose levels are at their highest one to two hours after a meal.)

INTERPRETING THE RESULTS

Knowing how to correctly read blood glucose records is important if you are to properly manage your diabetes. Of the various record books available, the better ones have places for recording morning, noon, supper, and evening insulin, the time tests were done, and the results. These record books also remind you to check for ketones if blood glucose is high. There should be a place for notes to keep track of anything that might have influenced your glucose levels on a particular day, such as exercise, changes in food intake, illness, stress, or hormonal changes.

Memory meters that electronically store blood glucose results are convenient, but you should still record the values and insulin doses in a record book at the end of the day. The way memory meters store information does not allow you to look at blood glucose values in patterns so you can use them to make insulin adjustments.

People often evaluate their blood glucose control by looking at how the levels varied throughout the day. The first example shows that three of the four tests for Monday were in the target blood glucose range of 70 to 140 mg/dl. Each of the next two days show the same thing, making it look as if target goals were achieved most of the time.

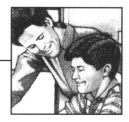

	Breakfast	Lunch	Supper	Evening Snack
Monday	84	171	114	97
Tuesday	78	222	104	135
Wednesday	90	201	117	103
Thursday	86			

A daily rise and fall can give you some information, but you can get more information by looking for consistent patterns in blood glucose levels over at least three days at the same time.

	Breakfast	Lunch	Supper	Evening Snack
Monday	84	171	114	97
Tuesday	78	222	104	135
Wednesday	90	201	117	103
Thursday	86			

It's apparent that all three lunchtime levels are higher than the target range. Regular insulin taken before breakfast peaks, or has its strongest blood glucose-lowering effect, two to four hours after injection, or before lunch.

The pattern in the previous example shows that the breakfast Regular insulin should be increased, but people often think they need to add an injection of Regular at lunch instead. If they do this, the extra Regular insulin will reach its peak at about the same time as the intermediate-acting NPH insulin taken at breakfast. This could possibly cause problems with hypoglycemia later in the day.

The next example shows a pattern of high blood glucose levels at supper.

	Breakfast	Lunch	Supper	Evening Snack
Monday	84	114	171	97
Tuesday	78	104	222	135
Wednesday	90	117	201	103
Thursday	86			

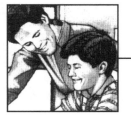

NPH or Lente insulin taken before breakfast has its strongest blood glucose-lowering effect late in the afternoon, or before supper. The pattern above shows that the breakfast NPH should be increased.

Regular insulin taken before supper peaks before the evening snack. The high glucose levels recorded in the following example show that the supper Regular insulin should be increased.

	Breakfast	Lunch	Supper	Evening Snack
Monday	84	97	114	171
Tuesday	78	135	104	222
Wednesday	90	103	117	201
Thursday	86			

Fasting (breakfast) glucose levels are controlled by NPH or Lente insulin taken before supper. In the following example, the breakfast glucose levels are elevated.

	Breakfast	Lunch	Supper	Evening Snack
Monday	84	97	114	78
Tuesday	171	135	104	90
Wednesday	222	103	117	86
Thursday	201			

When breakfast glucose levels are high, it's important to judge why. It could be caused by a continuous rise in blood glucose during the night. It could be caused by *rebounding* (going from low to high) after nighttime hypoglycemia. Rebounding is explained in detail in Chapter 11. Or, it could be caused by the dawn phenomenon (which suggests that blood glucose levels usually increase during the early morning hours). The best way to determine why breakfast blood glucose levels are high is to do a 3 AM blood glucose test. Look at the following chart.

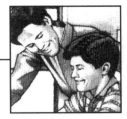

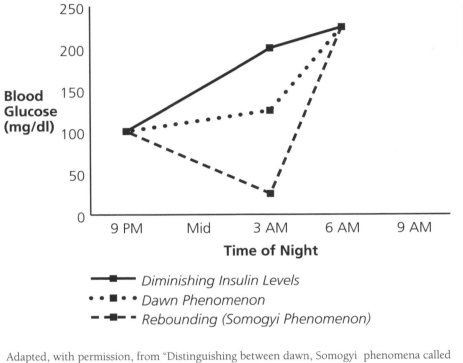

Blood Glucose (mg/dl)

Time of Night

— ■ — Diminishing Insulin Levels
• • ■ • • Dawn Phenomenon
– – ■ – – Rebounding (Somogyi Phenomenon)

Adapted, with permission, from "Distinguishing between dawn, Somogyi phenomena called critical for proper patient management." *Diabetes Outlook* (published by the Pfizer Laboratories and Roerig Division, Pfizer, Inc) 1987;22:3.

The top line in the chart shows decreasing insulin levels and increasing glucose levels. This is one of the most common patterns. It's seen when a person isn't receiving enough insulin during the nighttime hours. If the liver doesn't get enough insulin during the night, it will start to secrete stored glucose. This causes blood glucose to rise steadily through the night. You can detect this pattern by testing blood glucose at 3 AM. If it's high, you need more insulin activity during the nighttime hours. If you're taking NPH insulin only at breakfast, this pattern shows a need for a second injection of NPH at supper. If you are already taking an injection of NPH at supper, it may need to be increased.

The second line on the chart shows the dawn phenomenon. In many persons, blood glucose is often normal until 3 AM but starts to rise in the early morning hours. This increase is thought to be related to a morning peak of hormones, which works against insulin and causes the liver to release stored glucose. If you detect this pattern, moving your NPH injection from supper to evening snack may be of help. If you already take NPH at evening snack, this pattern shows that you need to increase the dose.

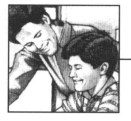

The third line on the chart shows rebounding (sometimes called the Somogyi phenomenon). Intermediate-acting insulin taken before supper may sometimes cause hypoglycemia around 3 AM. When your body senses this low blood glucose, the liver tries to restore glucose levels to normal but often releases too much stored glucose. This causes blood glucose to be high at breakfast. If you detect this pattern, you need to decrease your supper or evening snack NPH.

INSULIN DOSE ADJUSTMENT

When you adjust your usual insulin doses, either up or down, keep a few things in mind. First, adjust only one insulin at a time. Second, adjust it no more than 1 to 2 units at a time. And third, adjust it no more often than every three to four days.

PRACTICE EXAMPLES

Let's practice looking at the effects of different insulins with the following six examples. In all cases, assume that food and exercise have remained constant. As you consider these examples, remember the target range for blood glucose is 70 to 140 mg/dl before meals and at evening snack.

Example 1

Month / Date	Night-Time BG	Break-fast BG	K	R	N/L/UL	Notes	Lunch BG	K	R	Insul. Notes
May		7:30			N		11:45			
1		112	12	22			202			
		7:00					12:12			
2		98	12	22			192			
		7:15					12:15			
3		70	12	22			225			

Supper BG	K	R	N/L/UL	Notes	Evening Snack BG	K	R	N/L/UL	Comments
5:30			N		10:00				
98	9	14			89				
5:45					9:30				
104	9	14			72				
6:00					9:45				
117	9	14			95				

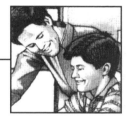

Which blood glucose values are not within the target range? Which insulin affects those blood glucose values? What changes should be made and why?

Answer (Example 1)

In detecting a pattern, you can see that the breakfast blood glucose values are all within the target range (70 to 140 mg/dl). Lunch blood glucose values are elevated for three days. Supper and evening snack blood glucose values are normal. Therefore, it would be correct to increase the breakfast Regular insulin by 1 to 2 units. This should lower the lunch blood glucose value.

Example 2

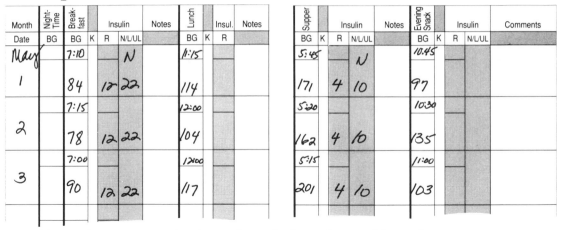

Month	Night-Time	Break-fast		Insulin		Notes	Lunch		Insul.	Notes	Supper		Insulin		Notes	Evening Snack		Insulin		Comments
Date	BG	BG	K	R	N/L/UL		BG	K	R		BG	K	R	N/L/UL		BG	K	R	N/L/UL	
May 1		7:10			N		11:15				5:45			N		10:45				
		84	12	22			114				171	4	10			97				
2		7:15					12:00				5:20					10:30				
		78	12	22			104				162	4	10			135				
3		7:00					12:00				5:15					11:00				
		90	12	22			117				201	4	10			103				

Would you change any insulin dose? If so, which insulin would you change and why?

Answer (Example 2)

In this example, hyperglycemia is occurring before supper. The correct approach would be to increase the breakfast NPH insulin by 1 to 2 units. This should lower the blood glucose level before supper.

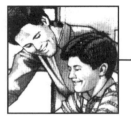

Example 3

Month	Night-Time	Break-fast	Insulin			Notes	Lunch		Insul.	Notes
Date	BG	BG	K	R	N/L/UL		BG	K	R	
May 1		7:15			N		12:00			
		120	8	16			77			
2		7:30					12:15			
		189	8	16			119			
3		7:15					12:10			
		95	8	16			87			
4		7:00								
		88								

Supper		Insulin			Notes	Evening Snack		Insulin			Comments
BG	K	R	N/L/UL			BG	K	R	N/L/UL		
5:20			N			10:30					
103	6	14				164					
5:30						10:30					
82	6	14				199					
5:45						10:20					
76	6	14				214					

Would you change any insulin doses? If so, which insulin would you change and why?

Answer (Example 3)

Although the breakfast blood glucose readings have one value higher than the target range, there is no pattern of high blood glucose values at breakfast. Therefore, it's not necessary to change the supper NPH dose. Lunch and supper blood glucose values are normal. Since the evening snack values are consistently high, it would be correct to increase the Regular at supper by 1 to 2 units.

Example 4a

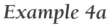

Month	Night-Time	Break-fast	Insulin			Notes	Lunch		Insul.	Notes
Date	BG	BG	K	R	N/L/UL		BG	K	R	
May 1		7:15			N		11:45			
		251	8	16			119			
2		7:20					12:15			
		168	8	16			112			
3		7:10					11:50			
		189	8	16			79			

Supper		Insulin			Notes	Evening Snack		Insulin			Comments
BG	K	R	N/L/UL			BG	K	R	N/L/UL		
5:30			N			10:30					
105	12	24				86					
5:35						11:00					
84	12	24				76					
5:30						10:45					
114	12	24				82					

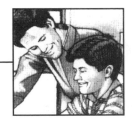

Would you change any insulin doses? If so, which insulin would you change and why?

Answer (Example 4a)

It's easy to detect that the breakfast blood glucose values are higher than the target values of 70 to 140 mg/dl. The insulin that would affect the breakfast blood glucose value is the intermediate-acting NPH taken at supper. However, before you automatically increase the supper NPH, you need to determine what is happening in the middle of the night. That's why we have you measure 3 AM blood glucose values.

Example 4b

Month Date	Night-Time BG	Break-fast BG	Insulin K	R	N/L/UL	Notes	Lunch BG	K	Insul. R	Notes
May 4		7:15 / 162		8	N / 16		12:00 / 112			
5	3AM / 60	7:00 / 181		8	16		12:15 / 108			
6	3AM / 56	7:10 / 176		8	16		11:45 / 99			

Supper BG	K	Insulin R	N/L/UL	Notes	Evening Snack BG	K	Insulin R	N/L/UL	Comments
5:45 / 84		12	N / 24		10:45 / 96				
5:30 / 118		12	24		11:00 / 83				
6:00 / 86									

You did two 3 AM blood glucose tests with results of 60 and 56 mg/dl. Based on this pattern of blood glucose values, what changes would you make?

Answer (Example 4b)

Month Date	Night-Time BG	Break-fast BG	Insulin K	R	N/L/UL	Notes	Lunch BG	K	Insul. R	Notes
May 6	3AM / 56	7:10 / 176		8	N / 16		11:55 / 99			
7	3AM / 120	7:15 / 120		8	16		12:20 / 102			
8	3AM / 134	7:20 / 110		8	16		12:00 / 88			

Supper BG	K	Insulin R	N/L/UL	Notes	Evening Snack BG	K	Insulin R	N/L/UL	Comments
6:00 / 86		12	N / 22		10:30 / 96				
5:15 / 98		12	22		10:30 / 73				
5:20 / 112									

171

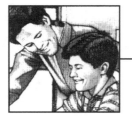

If your answer is that you are seeing a rebound effect, you are correct. Start by lowering the NPH insulin 2 units at supper and check its effect for two or three days.

Example 4c

Month	Night-Time	Break-fast	Insulin			Notes	Lunch		Insul.	Notes
Date	BG	BG	K	R	N/L/UL		BG	K	R	
May 4		7:15			N		12:00			
		162	8	16			112			
5	3AM 144	7:00 181	8	16			108			
6	3AM 164	7:10 176	8	16			11:55 99			

Supper	Insulin			Notes	Evening Snack	Insulin			Comments
BG	K	R	N/L/UL		BG	K	R	N/L/UL	
5:45 84	12	24	N		10:45 96				
5:30 118	12	24			11:00 83				
6:00 86									

What if the 3 AM blood glucose levels were 144 and 164 mg/dl. What action would you take?

Answer (Example 4c)

The high 3 AM blood glucose levels tell you there is not enough insulin during the night. Start by increasing your supper NPH by 2 units. Watch your blood glucose values for two days and do at least another 3 AM blood glucose test. If your 3 AM and breakfast blood glucose levels are still high, increase the supper NPH insulin by another 2 units.

High breakfast blood glucose can be a problem to control on the conventional two-shot insulin program. Increasing or decreasing the NPH insulin at supper doesn't always correct the problem. If you move the supper NPH to evening snack, the peak action of the NPH will be shifted so that 3 AM hypoglycemia can be avoided and more insulin may be present in the post-3 AM period.

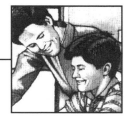

Example 5

Month	Night-Time	Break-fast	Insulin			Notes	Lunch		Insul.	Notes
Date	BG	BG	K	R	N/L/UL		BG	K	R	
May		7:30			N		12:15			
1		166	3	20			114			
		7:45					12:10			
2		241	3	20			89			
	3AM	7:30					12:30			
3	110	236	3	20			102			

Supper		Insulin			Notes	Evening Snack		Insulin			Comments
BG	K	R	N/L/UL			BG	K	R	N/L/UL		
5:30			N			10:30					
78	5	10				117					
5:45						10:15					
103	5	10				107					
5:30						10:10					
106	5	10				93					

Would you add a third insulin injection to this program? If so, how would you change the insulins?

Answer (Example 5)

The 3 AM blood glucose level is normal, but the breakfast blood glucose level is high. If you shift the supper NPH to evening snack, the NPH will peak closer to breakfast, which should correct this problem. The dose of Regular insulin before supper is not changed because it's needed to cover supper. When you change the dose of NPH to evening snack, it may be best to cut back the size of the dose at first. If necessary, the dose can be increased. The 3 AM and breakfast blood glucose levels will help guide you in reaching the right dose.

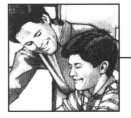
Example 6

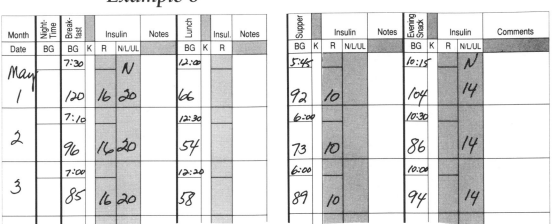

Month	Night-Time	Break-fast	Insulin			Notes	Lunch		Insul.	Notes
Date	BG	BG	K	R	N/L/UL		BG	K	R	
May 1		7:30			N		12:00			
		120	16	20			66			
2		7:10					12:30			
		96	16	20			54			
3		7:00					12:20			
		85	16	20			58			

Supper	Insulin			Notes	Evening Snack	Insulin			Comments
BG	K	R	N/L/UL		BG	K	R	N/L/UL	
5:45					10:15			N	
92	10				104			14	
6:00					10:30				
73	10				86			14	
6:00					10:00				
89	10				94			14	

Would you change any insulin doses? If so, which insulin would you change and why?

Answer (Example 6)

In this example, hypoglycemia is occurring at lunch. The correct change would be to decrease the breakfast Regular insulin by 1 or 2 units (assuming that activity level and food intake remain the same).

POST-MEAL BLOOD GLUCOSE LEVELS

When do you test post-meal blood glucose levels? Generally, we try to achieve pre-meal blood glucose levels in the target range. In most people this usually brings post-meal blood glucose levels into reasonable range. However, if your glycosylated hemoglobin (HbA1c) doesn't match your pre-meal glucose levels, it may be important to evaluate the post-meal values. To do this, test your blood glucose 1 1/2 hours after you finish eating your meal or about two hours from the time you started eating. Members of your health care team will help you interpret these results.

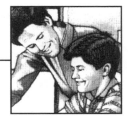

SUMMARY

Diabetes is the sort of disease that requires careful management and a good working relationship with your health care team. Pattern control can help you gain better control of your diabetes, as demonstrated by the examples in this chapter. Pattern control consists of looking for a pattern of blood glucose values over two to three days and making changes in your insulin program to correct for patterns of high or low blood glucose. Remember, when making pattern control changes, adjust only the insulin that affects the abnormal blood glucose values. The chart below provides a quick review of insulin action and refers you to the corresponding patterns in this chapter.

Insulin	Blood Glucose Test Showing Insulin Action	Corresponding Pattern
Breakfast Regular	Noon	Example 1 Example 6
Breakfast NPH/Lente	Supper	Example 2
Supper Regular	Evening Snack	Example 3
Supper NPH/Lente	3 AM and Breakfast	Example 4a Example 4b Example 4c
Evening Snack NPH/Lente	3 AM and Breakfast	Example 5

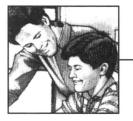

MONITORING YOUR KNOWLEDGE

Suppose someone is taking Regular and NPH insulin at breakfast and supper:

1. Which insulin affects noon blood glucose levels?

    _____

2. Which insulin affects supper blood glucose levels?

    _____

3. Which insulin affects bedtime blood glucose levels?

    _____

4. Which insulin affects morning blood glucose levels?

    _____

5. Give three reasons why a morning blood glucose level might be too high.

    _____

    _____

    _____

6. Why might NPH insulin be moved from supper to evening snack?

    _____

Answers on page 193.

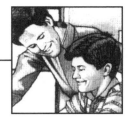

CHAPTER 11

Martha L. Spencer, MD

Immediate Complications:

The Ups and Downs of Blood Glucose

What is the difference between hypoglycemia and hyperglycemia?

What are their causes and how do you prevent them?

When and how should you test for a low or high blood glucose level?

The overall goal in managing diabetes is to maintain blood glucose levels no lower than 70 mg/dl at any time and no higher than 200 mg/dl 1 1/2 hours after a meal. This is thought to be the best way to avoid complications of diabetes.

Diabetes complications are divided into three groups based on how long it takes them to develop: immediate or acute, intermediate, and long-term. This chapter discusses how to prevent, recognize, and treat low blood glucose (hypoglycemia), which causes insulin reactions, and high blood glucose (hyperglycemia), which can lead to ketoacidosis. These are the acute, or immediate, problems faced by people with Type I diabetes.

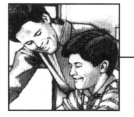

It's difficult for a person with diabetes to duplicate the blood glucose adjustments made by a healthy pancreas. Balancing food, insulin, and activity is a challenge. Even when these factors are balanced, unusual emotional or physical stress can result in wider than normal swings of blood glucose.

Immediate complications, namely insulin reactions and ketoacidosis can develop in minutes, hours, or days. Intermediate complications, which can develop in months or a few years, include failure to grow normally (Chapter 31) and problems during pregnancy (Chapter 22). Long-term complications take years, even decades, to develop. These include small blood vessel problems, which cause eye and kidney disease, and large blood vessel problems, which cause heart disease and stroke. Another long-term complication is damage to nerves, which can lead to a loss of sensitivity and function in some parts of the body. Long-term complications are discussed in Section IV.

LOW BLOOD GLUCOSE, OR HYPOGLYCEMIA

Insulin reaction, reaction, insulin shock, hypoglycemia—all of these terms refer to the body's response to blood glucose below 70 mg/dl. Hypoglycemia can be caused by one or a combination of three things: too much insulin, too little food, or an increase in activity. It can happen suddenly, usually just before mealtimes, during or after exercise, and at times when insulin is having its greatest effect.

When blood glucose gets too low, the body tries to protect itself by releasing a hormone called adrenalin, or epinephrine, which is the same hormone released during stressful situations. This can cause you to feel anxious, shaky, sweaty, dizzy, or suddenly hungry. You, and even others who do not have diabetes, may have these feelings during a stressful situation. It's important to test your blood glucose, if possible, to find out if you're having an insulin reaction or just responding normally to stress. If the test reads below 70 mg/dl, treat the reaction by following the instructions in the next paragraphs.

If blood glucose continues to be low, the brain sends out warning signals. You may develop a headache, blurred vision, or numbness or tingling of the lips. People around you may notice that you have become pale, clumsy, or confused or are acting differently. If you have any of these

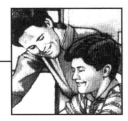

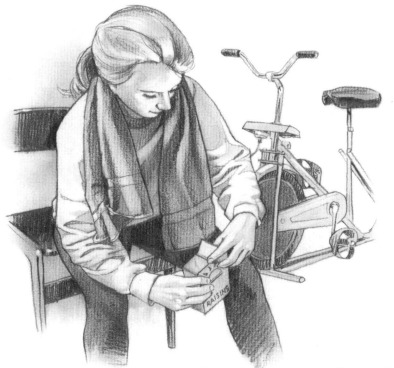

signs, check your blood glucose. If the test reads below 70 mg/dl, treat the symptoms by eating 15 grams of carbohydrate (glucose). If you're unable to test your blood glucose, go ahead and treat the reaction anyway. Suitable foods and amounts are listed below:

- 15 grams of carbohydrate from glucose tablets
- 1 small box (2 tbsp) raisins
- 1/2 cup regular soda pop (not diet)
- 4 or 5 dried fruit pieces
- 2 large sugar cubes
- l Fruit Roll-Up
- 5 small sugar cubes
- 1/2 cup fruit juice
- 6 or 7 LifeSavers
- 1/3 bottle Glutose (or other forms of glucose available at your pharmacy)
- 1 cup milk

Remember that it takes a while for the glucose you've eaten to get into your bloodstream and begin to be used by the body. If you don't feel better in 15 to 20 minutes, eat the same amount of food again. If you continue to feel as if you're having a reaction, check your blood glucose. If it's still below 70, repeat the treatment a third time. If there is no response in 15 to

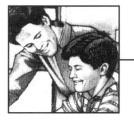

20 minutes, call your health care team. An untreated reaction can lead to severe hypoglycemia. Severe hypoglycemia lasting several hours can result in brain damage and death.

Food used for treating hypoglycemia is considered an addition to your regular meal plan. Do not subtract this food from your next snack or meal. Always carry some form of carbohydrate with you, especially when you're driving. Eat 10 to 15 grams (the amount of carbohydrate in one fruit exchange) of the food at the first sign of an insulin reaction.

The best way to prevent hypoglycemia is to make sure you and your health care team are achieving a good balance of food, insulin, and exercise. The following points are keys to preventing reactions.

- Test routinely and use the results to make changes to avoid low or high blood glucose levels.
- Follow your meal plan.
- Do not delay meals or snacks by more than one-half hour. (This includes breakfast and other meals on weekends and holidays.)
- Monitor blood glucose and, if necessary, eat extra food before and during unscheduled or unusually long exercise.
- Be alert to changes in your daily routines that may affect blood glucose level.
- Measure your insulin carefully.
- Take other medications exactly as prescribed.
- Remember, alcohol can lower blood glucose. Discuss its effects with your health care team. See Chapter 25 for more information.
- Be aware of early warning signs, and always carry some form of carbohydrate so you can treat reactions promptly.

SEVERE HYPOGLYCEMIA (INSULIN REACTION)

If low blood glucose is not treated with some form of glucose, and if stress hormones are not able to raise the blood glucose level, severe hypoglycemia may develop and lead to unconsciousness and seizures. Hypoglycemia is considered severe anytime the person needs help treating it. He or she may become confused, act strangely, have convulsions, and lose consciousness. Severe hypoglycemia lasting several hours can result in brain damage and

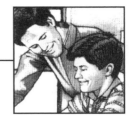

death if not treated. The person may refuse food or be unable to eat if these symptoms develop, and the reaction must be treated by someone who knows how to inject a substance called glucagon.

Glucagon is a hormone produced by a group of cells (alpha cells) in the pancreas. It has the opposite effect of insulin—it raises blood glucose. Glucagon can be used to treat hypoglycemia in semiconscious or unconscious persons, or in persons who refuse or are unable to take food or drink by mouth. Glucagon, like insulin, is a hormone that must be given by injection. When injected, glucagon causes glucose stored in the liver to enter the blood, raising the blood glucose level. Glucagon is a safe medication that should be kept in the home and wherever else a person with diabetes spends large amounts of time.

Glucagon is a prescription medication. Contact your health care team for a prescription and renewals as needed. Before use, glucagon can be stored at room temperature. When properly stored, glucagon is effective for several years. Be sure to periodically check the expiration date on the box so you can replace it before it actually expires.

Periodically review the instructions for injecting glucagon with those who live and work with you. Glucagon comes in two bottles that must be mixed before it can be injected. Store glucagon with a 100-unit syringe taped to the box. The instructions for mixing and giving glucagon are included in the glucagon kit. It should be injected the same way and in the same parts of the body as insulin. There are also glucagon emergency kits made up of diluting fluid already in a syringe and a bottle of powder. This saves one step in mixing. If glucagon is mixed but not used, it will be effective for 48 hours if refrigerated.

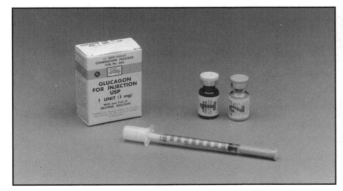

Glucagon comes in two bottles that must be mixed before it can be injected.

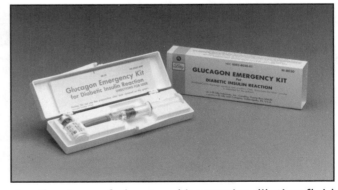

Another type of glucagon kit contains diluting fluid already in a syringe and one bottle of powder

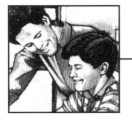
The following instructions are important after someone has been treated with glucagon.

- If no response occurs within 15 to 30 minutes, call for emergency assistance.
- When the person is alert enough to swallow, start offering small amounts of regular soda pop, soda crackers, or dry toast. Be aware that glucagon can cause an upset stomach, nausea, or vomiting.
- If he or she is able to keep these foods down, offer additional food such as milk and a sandwich.
- If the nausea and vomiting continue, follow the sick-day meal plan and contact the health care team.
- When the treatment has raised blood glucose levels above 70 mg/dl, continue to test blood glucose four times a day for the next two days to avoid further episodes. The insulin dose may need to be adjusted if blood glucose tests continue to run low.

Some people have hypoglycemic unawareness, which means severe insulin reactions may occur without any warning signs. It may be necessary to adjust blood glucose goals and to monitor more frequently to prevent these reactions.

Severe hypoglycemia should be avoided if at all possible. If it does occur, review with your health care team the events that led to the severe reaction. Was there something unusual in your lifestyle, food intake, activity patterns, and so on? Consult your health care team for help in making insulin adjustments if necessary. Most severe reactions occur when there has been a change in routine.

REBOUNDING

Frequent blood glucose testing provides information that can be used to avoid wide swings in blood glucose levels. These wide swings can occur because of stress hormones the body releases when the blood glucose level gets too low. The stress hormones can prevent severe hypoglycemia, but they sometimes keep on raising the blood glucose until the level is above the normal range. When high blood glucose levels result from a hormone reaction to hypoglycemia, the effect is called *rebounding*. This was first described by Dr Michael Somogyi and is sometimes called the Somogyi effect.

If you and your doctor are not aware that high blood glucose levels are a result of rebounding, the decision may be made to increase the insulin

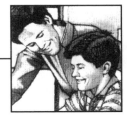

dose. This can result in too high a dose of insulin (over-insulinization), which will only make the problem worse. The insulin causes the blood glucose to drop too low, which causes the liver to release stored glucose. This chain reaction results in a high blood glucose level. The error can be discovered by testing blood glucose every two hours or so during the day and night to try to find out whether the insulin dose actually is causing hypoglycemia. Another clue would be that the response to increasing the insulin dose is higher rather than lower blood glucose levels. The dosage may have to be lowered or spread over several injections throughout the day to avoid the rebounding effect.

Overtreating a reaction can also cause rebounding. Because of the resulting high blood glucose, the person doesn't eat all his or her food and takes extra short-acting insulin. Never increase insulin or decrease the amount of food on the basis of one or two high blood glucose tests unless urine ketones are present. Always wait to see if a pattern develops over several days. Then if you're not sure how to adjust insulin, or if blood glucose is not controlled by your adjustments, discuss the situation with your health care team. See Chapter 10 for a discussion of pattern control.

HIGH BLOOD GLUCOSE (HYPERGLYCEMIA) AND KETOACIDOSIS

High blood glucose can lead to ketoacidosis. Ketoacidosis develops when there is not enough insulin in the blood to allow glucose to be used for energy. The body then must rely on fat for its energy needs. When the body must use too much fat for energy, the fat can't be broken down completely by the liver, and ketones are formed. Besides keeping blood glucose in the normal range, insulin also prevents the uncontrolled breakdown of fat. When fat is burned, ketones may be produced too rapidly and in larger quantities than the body can use. When the body doesn't have the help of adequate amounts of insulin, the ketones build up in the blood and then are filtered into the urine so the body can get rid of them. When present in large amounts in the blood, ketones cause ketoacidosis. If untreated, ketoacidosis can lead to coma and even death.

Large amounts of ketones make you feel nauseated, so you may not be able to eat your usual meal plan. The high blood glucose causes you to lose large amounts of body fluids through excessive urination, and it's hard to drink enough fluids to completely replace the amount lost. This leads to a drying out of body tissues (dehydration), which is very dangerous. If you

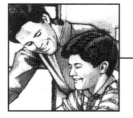

are vomiting or have diarrhea, you can become dehydrated very quickly. This is especially true for small children. Signs of dehydration are dry mouth and sunken eyes.

When blood glucose is over 240 mg/dl for several days, you may experience symptoms of thirst, dry mouth, frequent urination, weight loss, and tiredness. If the high blood glucose persists and the urine becomes positive for ketones, then you may have abdominal pain, nausea, and vomiting. Your face may become flushed and you may have blurred vision. You need immediate medical attention if you become drowsy, start breathing rapidly, or lose consciousness. You may have to be hospitalized.

Ketoacidosis can become very dangerous and cause unconsciousness (diabetic coma) and death if not treated immediately. It can be detected early if you are testing blood glucose regularly. Test urine for ketones if a blood test is 240 mg/dl or higher or if you feel ill, even when you blood glucose level is in the target range. Call your health care team if any of the following warning signs are present:

- moderate to large ketones in the urine along with high blood glucose levels
- severe nausea
- vomiting
- abdominal pain
- rapid breathing

Ketoacidosis usually develops when there is not enough insulin to handle unusual amounts of stress from illness, infection, or extreme and prolonged emotions. If an illness such as the flu or a bad cold prevents you

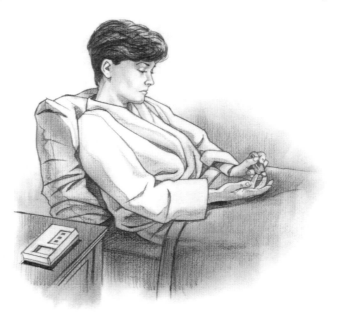

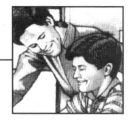

from eating your prescribed meal plan, it is important to follow the sick-day meal plan as described on page 186.

HOW ILLNESS AFFECTS FOOD NEEDS

Another potential problem time for persons on insulin is sick days. Diabetes can get out of control quickly during illness. Fever, dehydration (loss of body fluid), infection, and the stress of illness can all trigger the release of "stress" hormones (glucagon, epinephrine and norepinephrine, cortisol, and growth hormone) that raise blood glucose levels. As a result of this, the body requires additional insulin.

People with Type I diabetes must have insulin throughout illness to prevent ketoacidosis. People with Type II diabetes who take insulin or diabetes pills to help control blood glucose also must continue taking their medication. Even people with Type II diabetes who are not taking insulin or diabetes pills may temporarily need insulin to control blood glucose during times of illness.

During a brief illness you can manage your food and insulin balance by following the guidelines explained on the next page. These guidelines apply to mild, one-day illnesses. If you're ill for longer than one day, call your health care team for additional advice.

GUIDELINES FOR MANAGING A BRIEF ILLNESS

1. When you're ill, it's very important to take your usual dose of insulin. Your need for insulin continues or increases during illness. Never omit your insulin.

2. You should monitor your blood glucose and test urine for ketones at least four times a day—before each meal and at bedtime. This may need to be done more often when you're ill. Even with blood glucose monitoring, you still need to test urine for ketones. If your blood glucose reading is higher than 240 mg/dl, it's especially important to test a urine sample for ketones. The combination of high blood glucose and moderate to large ketones in the urine is a danger signal. Call your health care team if this happens.

185

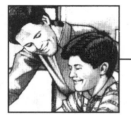

SICK DAY MENU

	Food	Carbohydrate Content
8:00 AM	1 slice toast	15 gm
Spread throughout morning	12 oz sugar-containing soda pop	30 gm
Noon	1 cup soup	15 gm
	6 saltine crackers	15 gm
Spread throughout afternoon	12 oz sugar-containing soda pop	30 gm
6:00 PM	1/2 cup Jello	20 gm
Spread throughout evening	12 oz sugar-containing soda pop	30 gm
		155 gms

3. If you can't eat your regular foods, replace them with carbohydrates in the form of liquids or soft foods (see the examples listed in the chart on page 187). Eat at least 50 grams of carbohydrates every three to four hours, especially if your blood glucose level is 240 mg/dl or less. This will provide some readily available sugar so your body won't have to burn fat for energy, which produces ketones. It will also prevent blood glucose from dropping too rapidly. It's important to eat these foods in small, frequent feedings. The sick day menu shown above will give you an idea of when and what to eat.

If your blood glucose levels are higher than 240 mg/dl, don't be too concerned if you're unable to eat the entire 50 grams of carbohydrate. However, be sure to continue to drink liquids, especially those that don't contain calories, such as water, broth, diet soda pop, and tea.

4. Drink a large glass of calorie-free liquid every hour. During illness body fluids and minerals are lost rapidly and must be replaced to prevent dehydration. This is especially true if you have fever, diarrhea, or vomiting. If you feel nauseated or are vomiting, take small sips of liquid—one or two tablespoons every 15 to 30 minutes—and call your health care team.

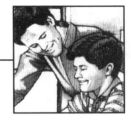

Foods Containing 10 Grams Carbohydrate	Quantity
Carbonated beverages containing sugar (ginger ale, cola)	1/2 cup (4 oz)
Popsicle	1/2 twin bar
Corn syrup or honey	2 tsp
Granulated sugar	2 1/2 tsp (5 small cubes)
Sweetened gelatin (Jello®)	1/4 cup
Coke syrup	1 tbsp (1/2 oz)

Foods Containing 15 Grams Carbohydrate	Quantity
Orange juice, grapefruit juice	1/2 cup
Grape juice	1/3 cup
Ice cream	1/2 cup
Cooked cereal	1/2 cup
Sherbet	1/4 cup
Jello	1/3 cup
Broth-based soups, reconstituted with water	1 cup
Cream soups	1 cup
Carbonated beverages containing sugar (ginger ale, cola)	3/4 cup (6 oz)
Milkshake	1/4 cup
Milk	1 1/2 cups (10 oz)
Eggnog, commercial	1/2 cup
Tapioca pudding	1/3 cup
Custard	1/2 cup
Yogurt, plain	1 cup
Toast	1 slice
Saltine crackers	6

FOODS TO REPLACE MEALS DURING BRIEF ILLNESS

The listed foods are often tolerated by people during periods of illness. To replace 10 or 15 grams of carbohydrate, use any of the listed foods in the amount indicated.

5. Call your health care team if:
   - you can't keep any liquids or carbohydrates down for more than eight hours
   - you're unable to eat regular foods for more than one day
   - you are vomiting or have diarrhea.
   - you begin to breathe rapidly, become drowsy, or lose

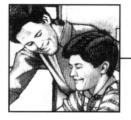

consciousness.

When illness subsides, you can return to your regular meal plan (and regular insulin schedule if your doctor has changed it during the illness). Call or visit your health care team if you think continued insulin adjustments might be necessary.

SUMMARY

Immediate or acute problems faced by persons with Type I diabetes are hypoglycemia, which can lead to insulin reaction, and hyperglycemia, which can lead to ketoacidosis. The best way to prevent these complications from occurring is to keep your blood glucose above 70 mg/dl and below 200 mg/dl 1 1/2 hours after a meal.

Because hypoglycemia and hyperglycemia are dangerous, it's important that you know the causes, the warning signs, and how to treat these conditions appropriately.

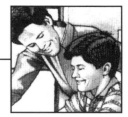

MONITORING YOUR KNOWLEDGE

1. Name three things that can cause hypoglycemia.

_____

_____

_____

2. What should you do to treat blood glucose levels under 70 mg/dl?

_____

3. What does glucagon do?

_____

4. What can high blood glucose levels (hyperglycemia) lead to?

_____

5. List five warning signs that tell you ketoacidosis is developing.

_____

_____

_____

_____

_____

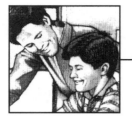

6. List the four main things you must do when you are ill.

_____

_____

_____

_____

Answers on pages 193 and 194.

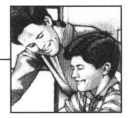

CHAPTER 7

1. *You* are the most important team member when it comes to controlling your diabetes. *Achieving and maintaining health care goals are challenges that require lifestyle changes for you and your whole family. It's important that you and your family learn all you can about diabetes, assume major responsibility in daily diabetes management, and work with your health care team.*

2. You need a special health care plan *because you are unique and your health care plan must be individualized to your lifestyle.*

3. Your responsibilities related to blood glucose monitoring include:

- *doing the test*
- *recording the results*
- *looking at the readings and showing them to your health care team*
- *using the information to help improve diabetes control*

4. Your health care team's responsibilities include (list three):

- *looking at your record book*
- *ordering a glycosylated hemoglobin test from the laboratory at each routine visit*
- *performing a yearly physical exam*
- *checking blood pressure*
- *checking eyes, feet, heart sounds, pulses, organs, and the condition of the skin at injection sites*
- *arranging a yearly exam by an ophthalmologist*
- *ordering a yearly blood cholesterol and triglyceride test*
- *comparing current status with past medical status*
- *providing continued education updates*
- *providing yearly meter check*

5. Diabetes education can help you *work with your health care team and is one of the most important tools you have.*

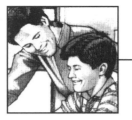

ANSWERS

Monitoring Your Knowledge—Section II

CHAPTER 8

1. Factors that determine your meal plan include:
- *your diabetes needs*
- *calorie and nutrient needs based on your age, height and weight, and activity level*
- *lifestyle*
- *food preferences*

2. The most important lifestyle factor for persons who inject insulin is *to be consistent in following a meal plan. By eating approximately the same amount of food at the same times each day and by doing regular blood glucose testing, you or your health care team can make adjustments in your insulin therapy. This is the best way to keep blood glucose levels as close as possible to the normal range.*

3. To delay meals an hour, you need *about 15 grams of carbohydrate (one fruit or starch exchange) at the scheduled mealtime. This is particularly important if you take your insulin injection at the usual time.*

CHAPTER 9

1. The key to safe exercise is *to monitor blood glucose before and after exercise. If you're exercising for a long time, you should also monitor blood glucose during exercise.*

2. Hypoglycemia can occur up *to 30 hours after vigorous or prolonged exercise or exercise that is done sporadically.* Hypoglycemia can also occur during exercise, especially when you exercise for longer than an hour.

3. Hyperglycemia after exercise *is of concern when diabetes has been poorly controlled over several days or more. If you start exercising with a blood glucose level greater than 250 to 300 mg/dl, especially if ketones are present, you may find that exercise does not decrease your blood glucose levels but instead can cause additional hyperglycemia. Exercise of high intensity can also cause blood glucose levels to be higher after exercise than before. This can happen even if blood glucose levels are in the normal range before starting exercise.*

4. In general, *10 to 15 grams of carbohydrate (one fruit or starch exchange) should be eaten after or before an hour of moderate exercise.*

ANSWERS

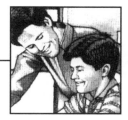

CHAPTER 10

1. *The breakfast Regular insulin* affects noon blood glucose levels.

2. *The breakfast NPH insulin* affects supper blood glucose levels.

3. *The supper Regular insulin* affects bedtime blood glucose levels.

4. *The supper NPH insulin* affects morning blood glucose levels.

5. A morning blood glucose level may be high because:

- *of a continuous rise in blood glucose during the night*
- *of rebounding (going from low to high) after night-time hypoglycemia*
- *of the dawn phenomenon (which suggests that blood glucose levels usually increase during the early morning hours)*

The best way to determine why morning blood glucose levels are high is to do a 3 AM blood glucose test.

6. Supper NPH might be moved to the evening snack *if increasing or decreasing the supper NPH does not correct a problem with morning blood glucose levels. High blood glucose can be a problem to control on the conventional two-shot insulin program. If you move the supper NPH to the evening snack, it will shift the action of the NPH so that 3 AM hypoglycemia can be avoided and more insulin may be present after 3 AM.*

CHAPTER 11

1. Three things that can cause hypoglycemia are:

- *too much insulin*
- *too little food*
- *an increase in activity*

2. To treat blood glucose levels under 70 mg/dl, *eat 15 grams of carbohydrate (glucose). (If you are unable to test your blood glucose, go ahead and treat the symptoms of a reaction anyway.) If you don't feel better in 15 to 20 minutes, eat the same amount of food again. If you continue to feel as if you're having a reaction, check your blood glucose. If it's still below 70 mg/dl, repeat the treatment a third time. If there is no response in 15 to 20 minutes, call your health care team. An untreated reaction can lead to severe hypoglycemia.*

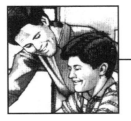

ANSWERS

3. Glucagon, a hormone produced by a group of cells (alpha cells) in the pancreas, *has the opposite effect of insulin—it raises blood glucose levels. Glucagon, like insulin, must be given by injection. When injected, glucagon causes glucose stored in the liver to enter the blood, raising the blood glucose level.*

4. High blood glucose levels (hyperglycemia) can lead to *ketoacidosis.*

5. Warning signs of ketoacidosis are:

- *moderate to large ketones in the urine along with high blood glucose levels*
- *severe nausea*
- *vomiting*
- *abdominal pain*
- *rapid breathing*

6. When you have a brief illness, you should do the following to prevent ketoacidosis:

- *Take your usual dose of insulin. Your need for insulin continues or even increases during illness.*
- *Monitor your blood glucose and test urine for ketones at least four times a day—before each meal and at bedtime. The combination of high blood glucose and moderate to large ketones in the urine is a danger signal. Call your health care team if this happens.*
- *If you can't eat your regular foods, replace them with carbohydrates in the form of liquids or soft foods. Eat at least 50 grams of carbohydrates every three to four hours, especially if your blood glucose level is 240 mg/dl or less.*
- *Drink a large glass of calorie-free liquid every hour. If you're feeling nauseated or are vomiting, take small sips of liquid—one or two tablespoons every 15 to 30 minutes—and call your health care team.*
- *Call your health care team if:*
- *you can't keep any liquids or carbohydrates down for more than eight hours*
- *you're unable to eat regular foods for more than one day*
- *you are vomiting or have diarrhea*
- *you begin to breathe rapidly, become drowsy, or lose consciousness*

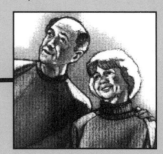

Living Well

Managing Diabetes With Meal Planning, Exercise, and/or Oral Agents

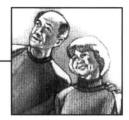

CHAPTER 12

Priscilla M. Hollander, MD

Your Health Care Plan:
"Meal Planning- and Exercise-Dependent" Diabetes

How is Type II diabetes different from Type I diabetes?

Who gets Type II diabetes?

How is Type II diabetes managed?

Diabetes can appear at any age, but diabetes that appears in adulthood (Type II) is quite different from diabetes that appears in childhood (Type I). Type I diabetes is often called insulin-dependent diabetes because insulin injections are necessary. Type II diabetes is often called noninsulin-dependent diabetes, although it would be more helpful if it were called "meal planning-and-exercise-dependent diabetes." This is because nutritional guidance and exercise advice are always the first "medicines" given to people with Type II diabetes. However, if blood glucose (sugar) cannot be controlled with a program of meal planning, exercise, and weight loss (if necessary), diabetes pills (oral agents) or insulin injections may be added to the health care plan.

Many health care professionals, and even many persons with Type II diabetes, have not appreciated the need to care for this form of

197

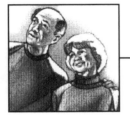

diabetes. We hope this chapter will help you care for your Type II diabetes just as aggressively as if it were Type I diabetes. The methods are a little different, but the goals are the same: a healthy today and many healthy tomorrows.

In the past, Type II diabetes was sometimes called "adult-onset" or even "borderline" diabetes. Such descriptions and the general approach to managing Type II diabetes made it seem like a less serious form of the disease than Type I diabetes. We now know that sudden problems (such as ketoacidosis and hypoglycemia) are unlikely with Type II diabetes, but other serious medical problems can result if it's undiagnosed or poorly treated. For instance, Type II diabetes:

- affects the large blood vessels and increases the chance for heart attack or stroke by two to four times
- affects the small blood vessels and causes problems such as eye disease (retinopathy)
- causes problems with blood circulation that can lead to foot infections and possible amputation
- damages nerves in various parts of the body, which can result in loss of feeling and impaired function in affected areas.

Prevention and treatment of Type II diabetes complications are discussed in Section IV.

THE DIFFERENCE BETWEEN TYPE II AND TYPE I

Type II is by far the most common of the two types of diabetes. It affects 85 to 90% of all Americans known to have diabetes, or more than six million people. An additional seven million people are estimated to have Type II diabetes that has not yet been diagnosed. In the United States, one of five people over age 65 and one of four people over age 85 have Type II diabetes. If this trend continues, by the year 2000 almost 15 million Americans over age 40 will have this disease.

In both Type I and Type II diabetes, people have high blood glucose levels. The difference is in the importance of injected insulin for treatment.

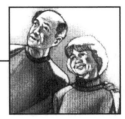

Insulin acts like a key, "unlocking" areas on the outside of the cell wall and allowing glucose to pass into the cell where it can be used or stored for energy. These areas on the cell wall where insulin attaches are called *insulin receptor sites.*

Cells with normal number of insulin receptor sites allow glucose to enter to be used and/or stored for energy

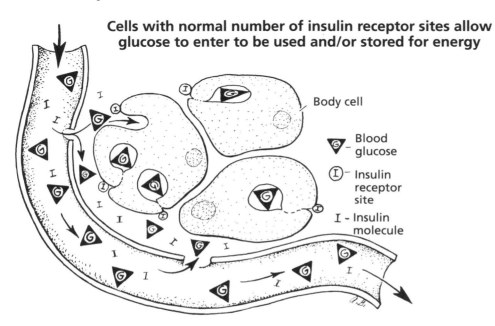

Body cell

Blood glucose

Insulin receptor site

I - Insulin molecule

Cells with decreased number of insulin receptor sites and changes within the cell cause insulin resistance

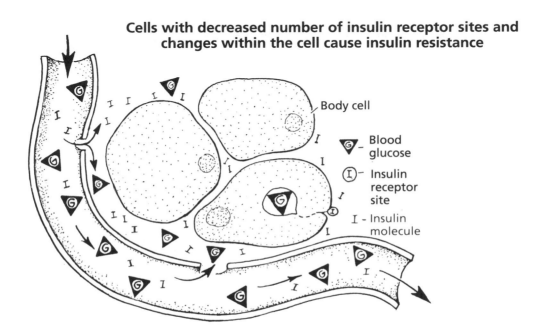

Body cell

Blood glucose

Insulin receptor site

I - Insulin molecule

With Type I diabetes the pancreas produces little or no insulin, making it difficult for glucose to enter body cells. The body must then rely on fat for energy, which produces too many ketones and possible ketoacidosis. Persons with Type I diabetes cannot survive without insulin injections.

With Type II diabetes the pancreas is capable of producing insulin, but the insulin is not effective enough to keep blood glucose at a normal level. Type II diabetes may decrease the number of receptor sites so that the cells become less effective at using insulin. The cells also seem to change the way they use insulin in the process of burning glucose for energy. The decrease in receptor sites and changes within the cells reduce the body's ability to remove glucose from the blood. This problem is called *insulin resistance*.

Although insulin resistance is common in Type II diabetes, it's also seen in other conditions, such as obesity. If this is the case, why don't all obese people have Type II diabetes? For one thing, not all obese people have a tendency to develop diabetes. Their pancreases can produce the extra insulin needed to control blood glucose levels. In fact, obese people have higher levels of insulin in their blood than people who are not obese. These higher insulin levels are necessary to allow their body cells to use glucose normally.

We know Type II diabetes is associated with insulin resistance, but problems with insulin production also occur. The pancreas may be able to produce insulin, but it obviously doesn't produce enough to overcome the insulin resistance. Therefore, blood glucose levels are high, resulting in the diagnosis of Type II diabetes.

FACTORS IN DEVELOPING TYPE II DIABETES

Heredity plays a major role in the development of Type II diabetes. Certain families will have a genetic background that makes them more likely to develop the insulin resistance associated with the disease. Think about your family tree. Most people with Type II diabetes have at least one relative (or several relatives) with Type II diabetes. The pattern of inheritance, however, is difficult to predict. In some families, Type II diabetes can be seen in every generation; in others it may skip a generation. It may affect all siblings in the family or only one or two. For some persons, the history of Type II diabetes would be found not in their first degree relatives but in cousins, aunts, uncles, and grandparents. Type II diabetes may also occasionally appear in persons who have no obvious family history of the disease. Because family history is such an important predictor of Type II diabetes,

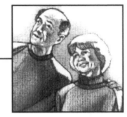

it's important for members of high-risk families to be checked regularly for diabetes, especially after they reach the age of 40.

Because Type II diabetes is inherited, its incidence may be higher in some groups than others. Native Americans have a particularly high incidence of Type II diabetes. (For example, up to 60% of adult Pima Indians have it.) Both Mexican Americans and Black Americans are at higher risk for developing Type II diabetes than the general population.

Obesity is another factor that may be important in the development of Type II diabetes. Since obesity can cause insulin resistance in persons with a genetic tendency to develop diabetes, it may cause diabetes to appear earlier than usual. Studies show that about 60 to 80% of all persons with Type II diabetes are obese.

DIAGNOSIS

Both Type I and Type II diabetes are diagnosed on the basis of elevated blood glucose levels. Normal fasting (before meals) blood glucose levels are between 70 and 115 mg/dl. Diabetes is diagnosed when fasting blood glucose levels are higher than 140 mg/dl on two occasions or when they are below 140 mg/dl but higher than 200 mg/dl two hours after a 75-gm *glucose tolerance test.* (For a glucose tolerance test, a person drinks a liquid that contains glucose. Samples of blood are then drawn every hour for three hours to see how the body deals with glucose over time.)

Symptoms of Type I diabetes usually occur quickly, with fasting blood glucose levels going from normal to 300 to 400 mg/dl in a matter of days or weeks. In Type II diabetes, blood glucose levels may rise very slowly over many months or even years. A person's average blood glucose may be 110 mg/dl one year, 140 mg/dl the next year, and 160 mg/dl the following year. In fact, it may take several years until blood glucose levels get high enough to cause the kidneys to filter glucose into the urine so it can be detected by routine urine tests. Symptoms of diabetes, such as frequent urination and extreme thirst, begin to appear when average blood glucose levels exceed what is called the *renal threshold* (the blood glucose level at which glucose begins to spill into the urine). In most people, the renal threshold is between 180 and 200 mg/dl.

In the past, urine testing or the glucose tolerance test was commonly used to diagnose Type II diabetes. Neither method is as useful as the elevated fasting blood glucose level. Urine testing is inadequate because the urine does not become positive with glucose until glucose has reached the renal threshold. This may take several years in some people with Type II

201

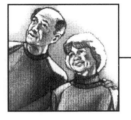

diabetes, so the disease would be undiagnosed for several years. That is why seven million people are believed to have Type II diabetes that has not yet been detected. An oral glucose tolerance test is not always a good way to predict who is going to develop diabetes.

MANAGEMENT OF TYPE II DIABETES

The goals of treatment in Type II diabetes are really quite similar to those for Type I. The first goal is to maintain good blood glucose control. Blood glucose control means keeping blood glucose levels as close to normal (70 to 140 mg/dl before meals; below 180 to 200 mg/dl after meals) as possible. A number of animal and human studies show that elevated levels of blood glucose effect the development and severity of long-term complications of diabetes. The second goal, which is equally important, is to achieve a general sense of well-being.

HEALTH CARE PLAN FOR TYPE II DIABETES

Perhaps a good name for Type II diabetes would be Meal Planning-and-Exercise-Dependent diabetes. This describes the first approach to treating Type II diabetes. Remember, the goal in treatment of Type II diabetes is to keep blood glucose levels normal by making insulin more effective. The focus is on decreasing insulin resistance. Unlike Type I diabetes, in which insulin is almost always necessary for survival, Type II diabetes can be controlled with meal planning, exercise, and weight loss. All three approaches have been successful in decreasing insulin resistance and lowering blood glucose.

At diagnosis, your health care team will help you set up the best individual program for you. Chapter 13 describes meal planning for persons with Type II diabetes, and Chapter 14 describes a good exercise program. This approach to Type II diabetes can work for many people at first. Especially when combined with weight loss, persons may do well on such a program for months to several years. However, if blood glucose levels do not respond to meal planning alone, you may need to add an *oral hypoglycemic agent* (diabetes pill).

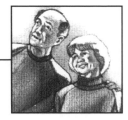

ORAL AGENTS

Since the discovery of insulin, scientists have been trying to find a diabetes medicine that does not have to be injected. Unfortunately, insulin cannot be taken by mouth because it's a protein and, like other proteins, it is digested in the stomach and is not effective. In the 1950s, scientists discovered a group of drugs that improved the body's ability to use insulin. These pills are called oral hypoglycemic agents, or sometimes just *oral agents.* They help increase the effectiveness of the body's insulin. They are not oral insulin and should not be thought of as a substitute for insulin.

Despite more than 30 years of research, scientists are still not completely sure how oral agents lower blood glucose. However, they do know that in order for them to work, your own pancreas must still be producing insulin. Therefore, they are useful only in Type II diabetes and not in Type I diabetes.

Oral agents are believed to work in a number of different ways.

- They may stimulate the pancreas to release more insulin.

- They may help lower glucose at the cell level by increasing the effectiveness of insulin at the cell receptor site, thus decreasing the problem of insulin resistance.

- They may help regulate the liver's metabolism of glucose. Because the liver has stored glucose, it plays an important role in determining blood glucose levels in both Type I and Type II diabetes.

Most diabetes specialists agree that oral agents should be tried if nutritional management is not successful in treating diabetes. Listed below are some guidelines for using oral agents:

1. Only people with Type II diabetes who are over age 40 are given oral agents. Occasionally people in their 30s may be diagnosed with typical Type II diabetes and may respond to oral agent treatment.

2. Oral agents are tried after attempts at meal planning, regular exercise, and weight loss have not been successful in providing reasonable blood glucose control.

3. Use of oral agents is continued if blood glucose levels are reasonably controlled (usually under 120 mg/dl fasting and 180 mg/dl 1 1/2 hours after eating).

4. If high blood glucose levels persist despite a maximum dose of oral agents, insulin treatment may be necessary.

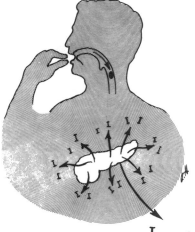

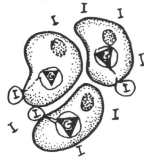

Oral agents increase the effectiveness of the body's insulin

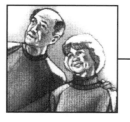

5. If oral agents do not improve blood glucose control after three to six months, it's unlikely that they will help and use of them should be stopped.

SIDE EFFECTS OF ORAL AGENTS

As with any medication, oral agents can have some side effects. Fortunately these problems don't happen very often, but you should be aware of what could happen. The most common side effect is probably low blood glucose (hypoglycemia). Since oral agents lower blood glucose, it could go too low if you skip or delay a meal or if you're on too large a dose. This isn't usually a serious problem and is more likely to occur if people are on insulin. If your blood glucose level is too low, you can eat small amounts of food to bring it back up.

Other possible side effects of oral agents include allergic reactions causing rash, hives, or upset stomach. You might also have bloating, cramping, and loss of appetite. If you have any of these symptoms, be sure to tell your health care team. In rare instances for some people, the combination of alcohol and oral agents can cause headache, facial flushing, and nausea. If this happens to you, you'll know you won't be able to drink alcohol while taking this drug.

You may have heard that oral agents can increase your risk for heart disease. This is not true. One study carried out in the 1970s reported a higher risk for a certain heart problem in people who already had serious heart disease, but studies since then have not found the same connection. The American Diabetes Association has investigated this question carefully and has determined that oral agents are safe.

INSULIN TREATMENT

If meal planning, exercise, and oral agents do not succeed in keeping your blood glucose near the normal range, you may need to stop using oral agents and begin injecting insulin.

A health care team may decide to use insulin therapy for a person with Type II diabetes for several reasons. One example would be obese persons who are not successful in losing weight. The excess weight may cause insulin resistance to be so high that blood glucose levels remain high even

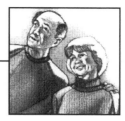

with a meal plan, more activity, and use of an oral agent. In such cases, insulin injections would be needed to keep blood glucose levels in the normal range. Another example would be someone who starts out with Type II diabetes but whose pancreas makes less and less insulin as the years go by. In such cases the person has moved closer to Type I diabetes and needs insulin to help keep blood glucose levels in the normal range.

Occasionally people with Type II diabetes need insulin therapy for short periods when situations require more insulin than the pancreas presently produces (for example, during times of stress or illness, such as a serious infection, heart attack, or surgery). Once the stressful period is over, the need for extra insulin usually disappears and shots are discontinued.

If your doctor has prescribed insulin injections to help control your blood glucose, it's important you read the section on controlling diabetes with insulin that starts on page 95. This information will help you avoid a problem such as an insulin reaction, which can occur when insulin injections are part of your health care plan.

MONITORING BLOOD GLUCOSE CONTROL

A key factor in evaluating the success of the health care plan in both Type II and Type I diabetes is blood glucose monitoring. Urine glucose testing will not give you the information needed to obtain and achieve blood glucose levels in the normal range. Listed below are some guidelines for blood glucose monitoring. Be sure to record the results of your blood glucose testing and discuss them with your health care team.

- If your health care plan requires you to inject insulin, it's best to test blood glucose three to four times a day—before meals and at bedtime.
- If you use meal planning, exercise, and/or oral agents, test blood glucose before breakfast, before your largest meal of the day, and 1 1/2 hours after that meal. Do this two to three days a week as long as your blood glucose levels stay in the normal range.

Another important method of evaluating long-term blood glucose control is the glycosylated hemoglobin test. This test measures the average glucose in the blood over the previous six to eight weeks. The results of this test, along with your regular blood glucose monitoring results, give you and your health care team an accurate measurement of overall blood glucose control.

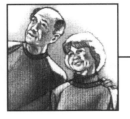

ROUTINE CARE OF TYPE II DIABETES

Persons with Type II diabetes should have certain expectations about their health care. Certainly one important expectation is the care needed to help maintain good blood glucose control. In the past, it was believed blood glucose control was the chief emphasis in treating Type II diabetes. However, interest in Type II diabetes and a group of health problems associated with it has increased lately.

People with Type II diabetes very often have a number of other problems as well. These include abnormal cholesterol levels, hypertension (high blood pressure), and obesity. In fact, these conditions are found together so often that it's been suggested they be grouped together because they are associated with a significantly increased risk for heart disease. The message for persons with Type II diabetes is that it's important to care for your diabetes, but it's also important to care for and treat these other associated problems, if present.

The key to successful management of your diabetes, and your general health, is to become part of your health care team. Be aware of your current health status and blood glucose control. The best way to do this is to schedule routine visits with your health care team. These visits should take place three to four times per year (more frequently if you have other immediate problems).

At each visit, certain key aspects of your health should be checked; for example your weight, blood pressure, heart sounds, eyes, and feet (paying particular attention to nerve responses and pulses). The health care team should review your blood glucose monitoring records with you and recommend changes if levels are often over your goals. A glycosylated hemoglobin test can also be done at each visit to evaluate your average blood glucose level over the past six to eight weeks. Your health care team can use your daily blood glucose results and glycosylated hemoglobin test results to decide if any changes need to be made in your health care plan.

Once a year you should have a complete physical examination. Special attention should be paid to blood cholesterol and triglyceride levels. Ideally, cholesterol levels should be below 200 mg and triglyceride levels below 150 mg. An EKG (electrical tracing of heart activity), chest X-ray, and other tests may be done to evaluate development of any potential long-term problems. Your kidneys should be checked through a urine and blood test, and the arteries in different parts of your body should be checked to determine if you're developing circulation problems. Your blood pressure should be evaluated (it may need to be taken several different times during

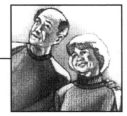

a visit to determine the true pressure). If blood pressure is over 140/90, your health care team should work with you in an aggressive program to bring it down below that level. Your eyes should be thoroughly examined once a year by a diabetes specialist or an ophthalmologist. In other words, it's important to receive an annual, in-depth evaluation of your total health.

SUMMARY

Type II diabetes is a serious disease. It affects millions of people in our society and has an enormous social, medical, and economic impact on lives. In the past, health professionals, and even persons with Type II diabetes, did not always give it the attention it deserved. We now know this was unfortunate, because the consequences of poor control and the chances for development of long-term complications are as great for Type II diabetes as they are for Type I diabetes. The outlook is rapidly changing, however, as the importance of good blood glucose control and good diabetes care for *all people with diabetes becomes more important.*

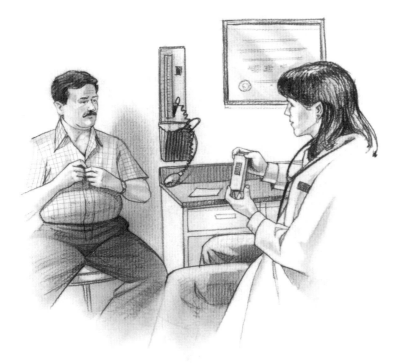

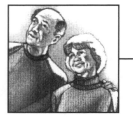

MONITORING YOUR KNOWLEDGE

1. List two factors that play a role in the development of Type II diabetes.

_____

_____

2. What are the first two approaches used to control Type II diabetes?

_____

_____

3. What are other treatment options for Type II diabetes?

_____

_____

4. Name three responsibilities of your health care team.

_____

_____

_____

Answers on page 233.

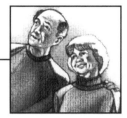

CHAPTER 13

Arlene Monk, RD, CDE
Marion J. Franz, MS, RD, CDE

Nutrition:
In Search of a
Reasonable Weight

Why are obesity and Type II diabetes related?

What are the steps involved in reaching and maintaining a
"reasonable weight"?

What's the difference between good and bad weight loss programs?

Many persons who develop Type II diabetes are overweight at the
time of diagnosis. Obesity can cause high blood pressure, increased
levels of blood fats (cholesterol and triglycerides), elevated blood
glucose levels, and other health problems. This is why one of the
nutrition goals of Type II diabetes is to help persons reach and
maintain a reasonable weight, which helps keep blood glucose and
blood fats in the normal range. This chapter provides information to
help you do this on your way to *living well* with Type II diabetes.

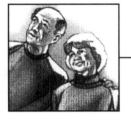

In Chapter 12 you learned about the connection between obesity and Type II diabetes. Insulin moves glucose into the cells with the help of receptor sites located on the outside wall of each cell. Obesity seems to decrease the number of these receptor sites, causing cells to become resistant to the action of insulin. Obesity also seems to cause changes within the cell, which add to the insulin resistance.

Your major goals in managing Type II diabetes will be lifestyle changes, including nutrition and eating behaviors, exercise, and mental well-being. If you can be successful in changing food intake and activity patterns, Type II diabetes can often be controlled without medication. However, if weight loss and meal planning alone are unsuccessful, an oral agent or insulin injections may be needed to keep blood glucose levels as near normal as possible. Regardless of the means of control, following a meal and exercise plan and monitoring blood glucose levels regularly are essential to good diabetes management.

Because heart disease and high blood pressure (hypertension) are associated with diabetes, it's important to reduce the total amount of fat and sodium in your meal plan. Diets high in fat (especially saturated fats and cholesterol) are associated with high levels of blood cholesterol, which is a risk factor for heart disease. Foods high in fat are also high in calories and contribute to obesity.

Scientific studies have shown that the amount of salt (sodium) in the average American diet contributes to high blood pressure, especially in persons who are genetically susceptible. Since people with diabetes appear to be especially susceptible to high blood pressure, and high blood pressure greatly increases the severity of diabetic complications, sodium reduction and weight loss are important. Together they can often bring blood pressure into the normal range.

REACHING A REASONABLE BODY WEIGHT

Reaching a reasonable body weight is best accomplished by combining several elements: a low-calorie meal plan, an exercise plan, and a plan for changing eating habits (especially the problem ones).

The best way to find out what weight is reasonable for your height and body frame size is to work with a professional who can help you determine a body weight that you feel is achievable.

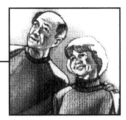

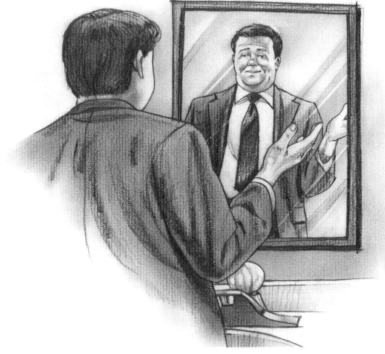

First you must set a weight goal. Often a 10- to 20-pound weight loss is all that's necessary to bring blood glucose levels back to normal. Next, you'll need a meal plan with a total caloric intake that will help you lose weight gradually. It's also important to examine eating behaviors that may be contributing to your weight problem. Changes in eating behaviors, such as improved food choices and distribution of food throughout the day, even without weight loss, may also help bring blood glucose levels back to normal.

Increasing your activity level is an important factor in blood glucose and weight control. A safe and moderate program of regular exercise can help:

- burn calories
- control appetite
- decrease body fat
- increase the amount of calories your body burns at rest
- replace stress eating

See Chapter 14 for more information on exercise and Type II diabetes.

ADJUSTING CALORIE LEVELS

Calories consumed above and beyond your body's needs are stored as energy reserves (fat). Fat is a very efficient means of storage, and the body

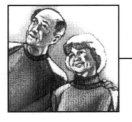

has an almost limitless capacity to accumulate fat. To lose fat, you must reverse the process—you must consume fewer calories than your body needs for energy. Since each pound of fat contains about 3,500 calories, to lose one pound of fat you must cut back your food intake by 3,500 calories or increase your energy level by 3,500 calories. Actually, the best way to lose weight is to combine calorie restriction with increased exercise.

Most people find that it's not too difficult to reduce their normal calorie intake by 500 calories per day, or 3,500 in one week. Adding 250 to 300 calories of exercise per day creates a negative energy balance of 750 calories per day. This will result in a reduction of 5,250 calories in a week, or one and a half pounds of fat. However, a realistic weight loss goal is usually 1/2 to 1 pound a week for persons over age 55 and 1 to 2 pounds for persons under age 55.

Keep in mind that it's more important to lose weight slowly and keep it off than to lose weight very rapidly and regain it again. For that reason, it's recommended that women eat a minimum of 1,200 calories a day and men a minimum of 1,500 calories a day. Meal plans at these caloric levels can be nutritionally adequate so that vitamin and mineral supplements will not be necessary.

Lest you become discouraged, research has shown that you can usually see dramatic improvements in your blood glucose levels by restricting your calorie intake and losing only five to 10 pounds. This again emphasizes the importance of slow but steady progress toward weight loss goals.

EVALUATING EATING HABITS

Remember, it's important to consider not only how much and what we eat, but also when and how we eat. Regular meal times are just as necessary for persons whose Type II diabetes is treated with insulin or diabetes pills as for persons with Type I diabetes.

Timing of meals and adjusting food for exercise are not as crucial if your Type II diabetes is treated with meal planning and exercise alone. However, you'll do better if you divide daily food into several meals and snacks. Well-planned breakfasts and lunches are especially important for controlling appetite throughout the day. The body appears to handle food better when it's divided into smaller meals and snacks. The insulin the pancreas is still making may be more effective if food is eaten in smaller amounts spread throughout the day.

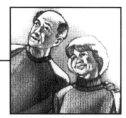

Our eating habits influence when and how we eat food. Some of these habits contribute to obesity. Let's look at eating habits and identify the good ones to keep and the not-so-good ones to change.

To begin to change something, we must first recognize and define the problem by becoming aware of what we do. Look at your eating habits as if through a magnifying glass and note every detail. To become aware of your eating habits, keep records for one to two weeks.

- Record everything you eat and drink except water.
- Record how long it takes to eat meals and snacks.
- Record where you eat and with whom.
- Record what else you do while eating.

What did you discover? What patterns do you see? Have you been fooling yourself into thinking you eat less than you actually do?

This self monitoring will help you develop awareness skills as well as an attitude that will be the base for making changes in your eating habits.

CHANGING EATING HABITS

Many behavior or habit changes evolve when you simply become more aware of a certain behavior. For example, eating more slowly allows you to feel full after your first serving. Sitting down in a specific place whenever you eat keeps you aware of the process of eating.

Once you've identified problems, the next steps are to learn ways to tune out the old and turn to something new. There are several ways to do this. Look at where the problem occurs and then look for ways to avoid the situation.

People in our society usually eat not because of physical hunger but because certain times, places, and even people become associated with food and eating. For example, if you are accustomed to reading the newspaper in the kitchen and nibbling because food is close at hand, you may have to find a different place to read the newspaper. Keeping food out of sight keeps it out of mind. It will be helpful to keep food out of rooms other than the kitchen, limit food intake to one specific place in your home, change your route if a particular store or vending machine is a problem, and clear the table immediately after you finish eating.

While it's best to avoid problem eating situations, it's not always possible to do so. We can't go through life avoiding all less-than-ideal situations. In this case, look for ways to change how you respond or react

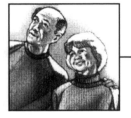

to the problem situation. For example, grocery shopping may be a necessity, but shopping on a full stomach and with a firm list can reduce the chances of impulse shopping. Planning daily menus helps reduce indecision at mealtimes. Proper planning can help you follow your meal plan and also reduce the tendency to overeat at parties or restaurants. Don't try to go without food all day to "eat as much as I want" later. You risk not only becoming hypoglycemic, but being so hungry when you arrive that you eat far more than you should or even want to.

If you regularly socialize, learn to respond to the waiter, hostess, and abundance of attractive foods in ways that allow you to enjoy yourself without overeating. Try leaving a bit of food on your plate without feeling guilty, and practice responding politely and firmly to people who try to encourage you to eat more than intended. Have an answer ready for the hostess who says have a little more. "Thank you, but I can't. One more bite would ruin a perfect meal."

As with diabetes control, behavior changes result from many small and repeated efforts. Changing habits is a process. This may be a slightly different mind-set, because many people follow a diet in an "all or nothing" fashion. Such thinking sets you up for failure. Look instead for gradual and permanent changes while allowing yourself some leeway. No one is ever totally in control or out of control. Set realistic goals for yourself and view your weight loss as the result of a series of accomplishments, each one an important step on the way to your goal.

TECHNIQUES FOR BEHAVIOR CHANGE

The following techniques show specific examples that have worked for others making changes in their eating habits. Pick those that can work for you and adapt them to fit your needs.

1. Slow down your eating speed. By eating slower you're less likely to finish off a second helping before your body has a chance to tell you it's satisfied with the first. To slow down the pace of eating:

   - Take 30 minutes for meals and 15 minutes for snacks.
   - Put down your utensil between bites. Savor each bite. Do not put your utensil back into food until you have swallowed what is in your mouth.
   - Count your chews per bite. Take at least 15 chews per bite.

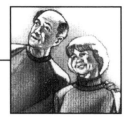

- When 3/4 of the meal is finished, stop eating for five minutes. Then if you feel like eating more, continue. If you don't feel like finishing, stop and congratulate yourself.
- If you want to take a second helping, wait 10 minutes before serving yourself seconds.

2. Eat in one location and set a full place setting for any food or beverage you take. This makes it difficult to "eat on the run" and reduces the number of places you associate with food. Make eating a special occurrence, and take time to enjoy it. As one person said, "No more eating in my car. I am important enough to give eating a special place in my day."

    - Do not participate in other activities (such as watching television, listening to radio, reading, or talking on the telephone) while eating. Without these distractions, you'll feel like you're getting more out of each mouthful.
    - Use a smaller plate or dessert plate for your meal rather than a full dinner plate. It will seem like you're getting more food than you really are.
    - Become aware of portion sizes. Use a scale and measuring cups as you begin and until you feel comfortable "eyeballing" your correct portion.
    - Do not serve food family style. Instead, serve your plate from the pots and pans in which the meal was cooked. You'll be better able to resist taking seconds with this technique.
    - Have someone else in the family clear the plates and put away leftovers. This reduces the temptation to nibble after you have finished your meal.
    - Keep your hands busy with a hobby such as wood carving or knitting if eating while watching TV is your problem.

3. Store food out of sight and out of reach. As you look around your house, what foods do you see? Are these problem foods? How can you "food proof" your house? Get rid of temptations.

    - Do not leave any food on the counter or table in plain view—this tests willpower too much. Use containers you can't see through.
    - Store food, especially problem foods, in an inconvenient place.
    - Spend less time in places or situations where you are surrounded by food.
    - Avoid buying food you tend to overeat, especially high-calorie foods. You'll be less likely to snack if it requires a walk to the grocery store rather than a walk to the kitchen.

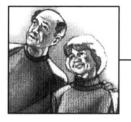

4. Change food buying and preparation habits. Do those extras you made for tomorrow's lunch have a way of becoming tonight's snack? Or do you say you buy the chips for the others when really they are for you?

- Write out a shopping list before you go to the supermarket. Stick to the list and don't buy extra items.

- Shop for groceries after meals, NOT while you are hungry. You're less likely to be attracted to foods not on your list when you shop with a full stomach. (This also does wonders for your grocery budget!)

- Avoid buying food you tend to overeat.

- Cut down the amount of food available to you at meals by preparing smaller portions. Prepare only one serving per person.

- If eating while preparing a meal is a problem, prepare the evening meal immediately after lunch or prepare the next evening's meal immediately after supper. Then, re-heat it before the meal. This will reduce the temptation to nibble.

5. Make specific plans to change eating habits.

- Take responsibility for your weight control. Give it priority. Set aside time each day to think ahead and plan your food intake for the next day.

- Develop the habit of eating three or more balanced meals daily. Never skip a meal. This could be dangerous if you take insulin or diabetes pills. Besides, most people find if they skip one meal, they just overeat at the next meal.

- Practice leaving a little bit of food on your plate without feeling guilty. Many people feel compelled to finish everything on their plate because of childhood "clean plate" training. This technique is especially important when eating in restaurants.

- Drink a glass of water, tomato or vegetable juice, or a cup of broth before meals to help curb your appetite.

- Keep intake of salt and beverages with caffeine to a minimum— both can indirectly affect weight and/or appetite.

- Keep a supply of low-calorie foods on hand—diet gelatin, raw vegetables, or diet pop.

- Don't feel compelled to eat because of social pressure. You can talk at the dinner table or at a party without eating.

- Give yourself rewards that aren't related to food for small units of weight loss.

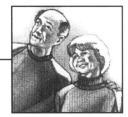

- Keep a written record of weekly weights. Don't weigh yourself too often. It's easy to become discouraged if you don't see results on the scale each day.

EVALUATING WEIGHT REDUCTION PROGRAMS

There are many ways to lose weight. Diets that tell you exactly what to eat and how much to eat will produce weight loss. So will a rigid limit of calories per day, or many of the gimmicky weight-loss programs available today. One problem with these methods is that they are often not nutritionally balanced, so you don't feel well while on the diet. The larger problem is that these diets come to an end and the person goes right back to the old eating habits that led to obesity in the first place. It's not uncommon for people to regain the lost weight plus more.

New and supposedly miraculous ways of losing weight are publicized everyday. They are popular because they promise ways that weight can be lost effortlessly and quickly. It's human nature to want to take the easiest route possible to a goal. When it comes to weight loss, we wish it would happen just by thinking about it!

Unfortunately, there is no magic, and the results go to those who work at it. When you are tempted by the new "diet of the week," be sure to run through this checklist before you commit yourself, your time, or your money:

- What will following this diet do to your diabetes?
- Does it sound too good to be true?
- Do you need to purchase "special" products or foods to follow this diet?
- Are any food groups eliminated from this diet?
- Could you follow this diet for the rest of your life, or even next year?
- What is the cost of this program?

Beware if you sense any doubts! You want to improve, not jeopardize, your health through weight loss.

Fad diets are:

Irrational. Most distort or ignore principles of good nutrition and defy the laws of nature. They may overemphasize one food or food group, assigning almost magical powers to it. They're often medically dangerous.

Deceitful. They often promise something for nothing. Beware of the "calories don't count" types of diets.

217

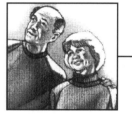

Limited. They often provide few food choices and are difficult to stick to for any length of time.

Off target. They often result in loss of muscle and body water instead of fat. The water is quickly replaced and the muscle tissue loss causes loss of body tone.

Expensive! There is usually some "special" product, food, or book necessary for the diet to be successful.

Very-low-calorie diets or very-low-calorie liquid diets are usually defined as less than 800 calories per day. Research is underway to determine the safety of such diets for people with diabetes and to find techniques that will help keep the weight off. It should be noted that very low-calorie diets are not recommended if a person has less than 50 pounds to lose, and they should never be used without very close medical supervision.

SUMMARY

To successfully manage Type II diabetes and control weight, follow these guidelines:

1. Improve your eating habits. Identify problem eating behaviors and set realistic goals to make gradual changes.

2. Moderately restrict calories. Consume 500 to 1,000 fewer calories per day in a nutritionally balanced meal plan.

3. Maintain a gradual weight loss, averaging 1/2 to two pounds per week, until you reach your weight goal.

4. Spread food intake throughout the day.

5. Participate in a regular exercise program to burn additional calories and increase mental and physical well-being.

6. Get support for your efforts—from family and friends, from a support group, and from your health care team.

7. When you reach your goal weight, keep the healthy eating and regular exercise habits as a permanent part of your lifestyle. Enjoy the new you!

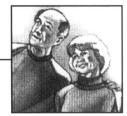

MONITORING YOUR KNOWLEDGE

1. Why is reaching and maintaining a reasonable body weight important if you have Type II diabetes?

_____

2. How is this best accomplished?

_____

3. List four things you can do to become aware of your eating habits.

_____

_____

_____

_____

4. List six techniques for behavior change that you think will work best for you.

_____

_____

_____

_____

_____

_____

Answers on pages 233 and 234.

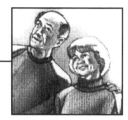

CHAPTER 14

Marion J. Franz, MS, RD, CDE
Jane Norstrom, MA

Routine Exercise:
The Answer to Improved Blood Glucose Control

What can routine exercise do for blood glucose levels in Type II diabetes?

How often and how hard must I exercise to see the benefits?

Where do I start?

Lifestyle changes that combine improved nutrition, safe and enjoyable exercise, weight loss, and blood glucose monitoring have been shown to be the best way to begin managing Type II diabetes. Although exercise has not been shown to improve overall blood glucose control for persons with Type I diabetes, it does appear to improve blood glucose control for persons with Type II diabetes. Routine exercise and weight control can eventually help reduce the need for or, in some cases, eliminate injected insulin or diabetes pills (oral hypoglycemic agents) from a management plan.

In this chapter we'll discuss the risks and benefits of exercise in the management of Type II diabetes. We'll provide information and tips to help you get started in a safe, effective exercise program and, most importantly, to help you stay motivated.

221

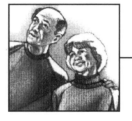

Routine exercise helps in the management of Type II diabetes because working muscles use and store glucose more effectively. Persons with Type II diabetes are frequently overweight. As a result, they become resistant to the insulin their body still produces. Exercise increases the body's sensitivity to insulin, so less insulin is needed to keep blood glucose levels normal. Exercise helps the muscles and liver store glucose better, which also helps lower blood glucose levels.

Research has shown that a combination of physical training and meal planning produces a greater increase in insulin sensitivity than meal planning alone. When an exercise program was added to a meal plan, muscle cells were able to store glucose better and blood glucose levels dropped. Even a single bout of high-intensity exercise (exercise done to the point of exhaustion) has been shown to improve blood glucose levels for up to 12 to 16 hours later in persons with Type II diabetes.

However, the benefits of exercise on blood glucose levels are short-lived. Exercise must be done regularly for it to help improve blood glucose control. For sustained improvement of blood glucose control, exercise must be performed three or more times a week. The benefits of exercise are lost when no exercise is performed for a three-day period. The more you exercise, the more improvement you'll see in your diabetes control. Studies have shown that frequently repeated activity is more important than high-intensity activity.

OTHER BENEFITS OF EXERCISE

Exercise helps reduce your risk for heart disease, which is a major threat to people with Type II diabetes. Routine exercise decreases the amount of triglycerides and cholesterol in the blood and increases the amount of HDL cholesterol (the good cholesterol) in the blood, which helps protect against heart disease.

Exercise can also be a way to burn excess calories and help with weight loss. Approximately 3,500 calories are stored in one pound of fat. Therefore, to lose one pound of fat, you must (1) reduce your calorie intake by 3,500 calories, (2) increase your activity level by 3,500 calories, or (3) combination of both. Decreasing your calorie intake by 500 calories a day and adding 250 calories of activity gives you a deficit of 5,250 calories in one week, or a loss of 1-1/2 pounds of fat.

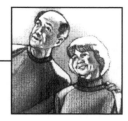

The chart "Using Up Calories" (below) will give you an idea of how much exercise you need to do to burn 250 calories. These calorie estimates are general averages; how many calories you actually burn depends on how hard and how skillfully you perform the activity. As you can see, it takes a significant amount of exercise to lose weight by exercise alone, so you also have to watch what you eat!

USING 250 CALORIES THROUGH EXERCISE

Activity	Minutes Needed to Burn 250 Calories		
	129 lbs (54.5 kg)	150 lbs (68 kg)	220 lbs (90 kg)
Aerobic dancing (doesn't include warm-up and cool-down)	27	22	16
Bicycling			
(6 mph)	71	57	43
(12 mph)	27	22	16
Bowling	100	83	71
Calisthenics	69	56	42
Dancing			
(slow)	89	71	54
(fast)	27	22	16
Golf (walking with bag)	54	43	32
Running or jogging			
(5 mph)	34	27	20
(7.5 mph)	24	19	14
(10 mph)	18	15	11
Skiing (cross-country)	38	31	23
Racquetball	42	34	25
Swimming (fast, freestyle)	36	29	22
Tennis			
(singles)	42	34	25
(doubles)	71	57	43
Walking			
(3 mph)	74	58	44
(4 mph)	49	39	29
(upstairs)	32	26	19

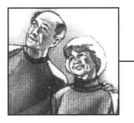

A bonus to this calorie reduction is that a routine exercise program also increases your *metabolism rate,* which is the number of calories your body burns when at complete rest. Furthermore, in people who exercise regularly more calories are changed into heat instead of fat. These beneficial effects extend well beyond the actual exercise period.

This bonus does not automatically cause weight loss, however. With exercise there will be an increase in lean body mass (muscle), which may result initially in a small increase in body weight. In fact, you may not notice any weight loss, but your clothes may fit better. This means you've lost some of your fat and gained lean body mass. When you stop a routine exercise program, the percentage of body fat again increases rapidly.

You may lose several pounds during an exercise session, especially in hot and humid weather. This is not fat loss. It is body water lost from sweating and must be replaced by drinking plenty of fluids. If you do not replace the water lost during exercise you can become dehydrated. This can lead to serious problems.

When exercising, remember to monitor food intake carefully. Although exercise helps control appetite in some persons, in others it can increase appetite and caloric intake. Be careful not to increase food intake. Some people compensate for the extra calories used during and immediately after exercise by being less active than usual at other times of the day. This can be a problem especially if calories are severely restricted.

GUIDELINES FOR EXERCISING SAFELY

If you take insulin or an oral agent to help control blood glucose levels, be aware of the precautions discussed in Chapter 9. However, since your body is still producing some insulin, your blood glucose levels will not be as unstable with exercise as those in the person whose pancreas is no longer producing any insulin. You will not generally need to eat extra food before or after exercise.

Because people with Type II diabetes often have a higher incidence of coronary heart disease that they are not aware of, it's a good idea to check with your doctor if you have any questions or concerns before beginning an exercise program.

If you've been sedentary for a number of years and have a weight problem, it's important to start with a mild exercise program and gradually increase your level of fitness. At first you may find you're unable to exercise

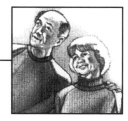

continuously. But once you try, you'll find even small changes can make a difference. An exercise program that gradually increases in intensity is the most successful and safest for persons with Type II diabetes.

The most efficient way to burn fat is to exercise continuously for at least 20 to 30 minutes (long duration) at a perceived exertion level of "somewhat strong" (see chart on page 57), which results in no shortness of breath (low intensity). This type of exercise uses stored fat as the major energy source. Exercise under 2 to 3 minutes (short duration) that causes shortness of breath (high intensity) uses stored carbohydrate as the major energy source and is not as helpful for weight control.

For weight management, do aerobic exercise for at least 25 to 30 minutes, five to six times a week. Begin gradually, with five- to 10-minute exercise sessions. The goal is to burn 250 to 300 calories per session. Exercise should be done in the 60 to 75% target heart rate zone. At less than 60%, exercise has little effect on glucose levels. If you have Type II diabetes, it's important that you begin your exercise program in the 60% target heart rate zone and gradually increase your target pulse. The following chart lists target heart rates in the 60 to 75% target range for persons with Type II diabetes.

Age	Beats/10 Sec.	Beats/Minute
30	19–23	114–143
35	18–23	111–139
40	18–22	108–135
45	17–22	105–131
50	17–21	102–128
55	16–20	99–124
60	16–20	96–120
65	15–19	93–116
70	15–19	90–113
75	15–18	87–109
80	14–18	84–105
85	14–17	81–101

My target heart rate is _____ beats per 10 seconds.

TARGET HEART RATE IN THE 60–75% RANGE OF MAXIMUM HEART RATE

Adapted, with permission, from *Managing Type II Diabetes: Your Invitation to a Healthier Lifestyle,* by Monk A, et al. Minneapolis: Diabetes Center, Inc., 1988:70.

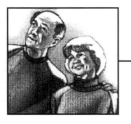

Exercise should be low-impact to prevent injury to bones and joints. Low-impact exercises are done with at least one foot touching the floor at all times. There is no jumping or jarring to put stress on joints. Exercise recommended for weight loss includes brisk walking, swimming, bicycling, and low-impact aerobic dance.

Muscle strengthening exercises, such as weight lifting, have been shown to result in significant improvements in blood glucose levels. They increase muscle mass, and muscles use more glucose than fat does. However, avoid strenuous weight lifting and isometric exercises. They increase blood pressure and can cause or aggravate kidney and eye problems.

If you manage your diabetes by meal planning alone, you won't need to eat extra food before, during, or after exercise, except when exercise is exceptionally vigorous and long. In that case, extra food may be just as beneficial to you as it is to persons who do not have diabetes.

Support from family or friends is important in any exercise program. It's easy to get discouraged when improvement comes much slower than you would like. That's why a group exercise class can be especially helpful. Joining a class commits you to a certain time, and other group members can offer encouragement. It's important to find an exercise class at an appropriate level for you. For instance, if everyone in the group has been exercising for a while and knows all the right moves, it may be easier for you to become discouraged, fatigued, and quit.

RISKS AND PRECAUTIONS

Blood glucose regulation during exercise for persons with Type II diabetes is not significantly different than for persons who do not have diabetes.

Hypoglycemia

During mild to moderate exercise, elevated blood glucose levels fall toward normal but not lower, so hypoglycemia caused by exercise rarely occurs. However, if you inject insulin or use oral agents you may be at risk for low blood glucose after exercise. Your blood insulin levels may be higher than normal during exercise and, as a result, your liver may not release enough glucose to prevent hypoglycemia. Therefore, you may need to decrease or even omit the oral agent or insulin before exercise. Check with your health care team if you're uncertain about how to do this. The other option is to increase food intake after or before exercise. However, care must be taken to not overeat at these times.

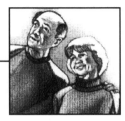

Medications or Medical Problems

Special precautions should be taken if you use drugs or alcohol that can produce hypoglycemia. Beta-blocking agents (used to treat high blood pressure) can prevent responses that normally correct hypoglycemia. Check with your doctor to see if any medications or drugs might interfere with exercise.

Exercise testing may be particularly important for persons who experience *silent ischemia,* which is a reduced ability to feel pain in the chest and heart area because of nerve damage (neuropathy) caused by diabetes. Persons who are not aware of angina pectoris (pain or a sense of heaviness or squeezing in the chest) are at greater risk of having a heart attack.

If you have neuropathy in your feet or decreased circulation in your legs and feet, you should avoid forms of exercise that could involve trauma to the feet. Injuries can occur and go undetected, especially if nerve damage is present. Have the nerve sensitivity and circulation in your feet checked before starting an exercise program.

Wearing the proper shoes can help prevent foot injuries. Always look at your feet after exercise, paying attention to any areas that are red, hot, blistering, swollen, or tender. Seek medical help immediately if such problems exist.

Exercise may worsen diabetes complications that are already present. This is particularly true of eye, kidney, and nerve damage. Nerve damage can block the body's ability to feel pain from overdoing exercise or from injury. Additionally, blood pressure during exercise may rise higher in persons with diabetes than in persons without diabetes, which can worsen problems with eyes and kidneys.

GETTING STARTED

It's important to be serious about beginning an exercise program but not to the point where you overdo it. Although exercise requires a life-long commitment of time and effort, you still want it to be fun. Don't try to do too much too soon. If you haven't exercised regularly for a number of years, it's going to take a while to regain what it took years to lose. Keep the following guidelines in mind as you start your exercise program.

1. It's very important to start slowly and gradually increase the amount of time you exercise each day until you reach your desired time goal.

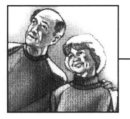

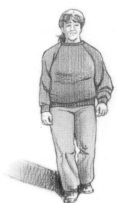

2. Put your emphasis on aerobic exercise (exercise that is lower in intensity and longer in time). This type of exercise burns calories more effectively.

3. For weight control, it's important to exercise more often than if exercising just for cardiovascular fitness. Work up to doing some type of aerobic exercise five to six days each week.

4. Choose an activity you enjoy. Vary your activities.

5. Exercise at a time of day that's best for you. You'll be more likely to stick with it.

EXERCISE EXTENDERS

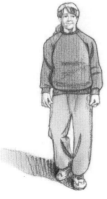

Besides participating in a routine exercise program, it's important to increase your overall activity level as often as you can. Here are some suggestions.

- Take a walk during your lunch hour, but don't skip lunch. Bring a bag lunch, eat, and then get out for a walk. Or walk to a nearby park and eat your lunch there.

- Park at the farthest end of the parking lot and walk to your destination. You can do this at shopping centers, supermarkets, or work.

- Walk up a couple of flights of stairs rather than taking the elevator.

- Walk whenever possible in your neighborhood—when going to visit neighbors, to the corner drug store, or to buy a newspaper, and so on.

- If you take a bus, get off a few blocks early and walk the rest of the way.

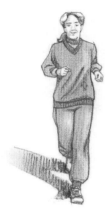

- Take a quick walk around your house or apartment during TV commercials. Reports show that during an average hour of TV programming 10 minutes are devoted to commercials. If you watch TV for three hours you can work in about 30 minutes of walking. Or better yet, turn off an uninteresting program and take a 30-minute walk.

- Take exercise breaks instead of coffee breaks during work or school.

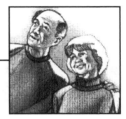

TIPS TO HELP YOU EXERCISE

It's easy enough for us to remind you that routine exercise is an important part of a healthy lifestyle. However, the only exercise helpful to you is what you actually do. These eight tips can help you start and continue an exercise program. They can help you take control of your situation and do something about it.

1. *Visualize.* See yourself as a person who feels good, looks good, and has energy. Think about your positive aspects, not your negative ones.

2. *Reject excuses.* If your excuse is that you are just too tired to exercise after work, then go for a 20-minute walk at lunchtime.

3. *Be prepared to make sacrifices.* It takes time to fit exercise in, and you'll need to make decisions and set priorities. You might have to miss your favorite TV shows if your exercise class meets at those times.

4. *Establish goals and rewards.* Come up with some short-term, intermediate, and long-term goals and reward yourself when you reach them. You may find it helps to chart your progress daily. For example, you could chart how many miles you walk in a year or the distance you swim in three months.

5. *Find an exercise partner*—a neighbor, spouse, friend, or class, or even an exercise video. Exercise is often more fun if you have someone to do it with. Exercising with someone helps you stick to your program.

6. *Build in variety.* It's important to find several fitness activities, indoor and outdoor, to participate in. Boredom sets in quickly if your program lacks variety. You might swim on Monday, walk on Tuesday, do an exercise video on Wednesday, and so on.

7. *Plan your exercise time.* Set aside time during the day for exercise. Many people find it helpful to actually schedule exercise as an "appointment" on their daily calendar. Make it a high priority so the time you've scheduled doesn't get used for something else.

8. *Make it fun.* This is really the key to success. Are you enjoying your exercise? Is it play? If it isn't, what can you do to make it fun? Be creative. Explore your options. Learn a new skill—it can be very rewarding.

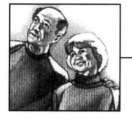

IT'S YOUR TURN

Consider each of these tips separately and think of how you can make them work for you. Make a list of activities that you enjoy doing or that you feel you do well. Then list the activities you would like to learn. Next, list all the excuses you use to avoid exercise. See if you can come up with ways to counter each excuse. If your excuses tend to be other activities, like watching TV or going out, you'll have to decide which is more important. List possible exercise partners, then contact them and arrange a schedule. Think of things you can do alone if your partner can't join you.

SUMMARY

Exercise is important for persons with Type II diabetes. It increases your body's sensitivity to insulin, helps your muscles and liver store glucose, helps burn excess calories, promotes weight loss, and improves blood glucose control.

We know that beginning an exercise program can be difficult, especially if you've never exercised before. But it's a very important part of treating your diabetes—as important as meal planning, weight loss, and medication. We want you to take it seriously and proceed with caution. Exercise with the approval of your health care team. Monitor your progress. Seek out an exercise class if you need structure, support from others, and accountability. It all can help ensure progress and success.

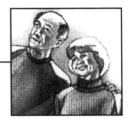

MONITORING YOUR KNOWLEDGE

1. How does exercise help in the management of
Type II diabetes?

_____

2. To be of benefit, exercise must be done how often?

_____

3. What is the most efficient way to burn fat with exercise?

_____

4. List the activities you enjoy doing, or feel you do well.

_____

_____

_____

5. List the activities you would like to learn.

_____

_____

_____

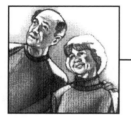

6. List the excuses you use to avoid exercise.

_____

_____

_____

7. List ways to counter excuses.

_____

_____

_____

Answers on page 234.

ANSWERS

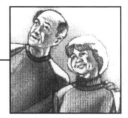

CHAPTER 12

1. *Heredity and obesity* are two factors that play a role in the development of Type II diabetes.

2. The first two approaches used to control Type II diabetes are *meal planning and exercise.*

3. *Oral hypoglycemic agents (diabetes pills) and injected insulin* are two other treatment options. If blood glucose levels do not respond to meal planning and exercise alone, an oral agent may be added to your treatment plan. In order for them to work, your own pancreas must still be producing insulin. If meal planning, exercise, and oral agents do not succeed in keeping your blood glucose levels near the normal range, you may need to stop using oral agents and begin injecting insulin.

4. Expect your health care team to:

- *Provide the medical care needed to help you maintain good blood glucose control.*

- *Provide medical care and treatment for other associated problems, including abnormal cholesterol levels, high blood pressure, and obesity.*

- *Check your weight, blood pressure, pulses, heart sounds, eyes, and feet at yearly visits.*

- *Review your blood glucose monitoring records.*

- *Order a glycosylated hemoglobin test at each visit.*

- *Perform a compete physical examination once a year.*

- *Schedule an examination of your eyes by an ophthalmologist.*

CHAPTER 13

1. If you have Type II diabetes, it's important to reach and maintain a reasonable body weight *because obesity causes the body to become resistant to the action of insulin. Insulin moves glucose into the cells with the help of receptor sites on the outside wall of each cell. Obesity seems to decrease the number of these receptor sites, causing cells to become resistant to the action of insulin. Obesity also seems to cause changes within the cell, which add to the insulin resistance.*

2. Reaching and maintaining a reasonable body weight are best accomplished *by combining several elements: a low-calorie meal plan, an exercise plan, and a plan for changing eating habits (especially the problem ones).*

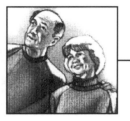
3. To become aware of your eating habits, *keep records for one to two weeks.*

- *Record everything you eat and drink except water.*
- *Record how long it takes to eat meals and snacks.*
- *Record where you eat and with whom.*
- *Record what else you do while eating.*

4. I choose the following behavior change techniques because I think they will help me change some of my problem eating habits.

_____

_____

_____

_____

CHAPTER 14

1. Exercise helps in the management of Type II diabetes *because working muscles use and store glucose more effectively. Exercise increases the body's sensitivity to insulin so less insulin is needed to keep blood glucose levels normal. Exercise helps the muscles and liver store blood glucose better, which also helps lower blood glucose levels.*

2. To be of benefit, exercise must be done *regularly (three or more times a week). The benefits of exercise are lost if no exercise is performed for a three-day period.*

For weight management, aerobic exercise should be done for at least 25 to 30 minutes, five to six times a week. Exercise should be done in the 60 to 75% target heart rate zone.

3. The most efficient way to burn fat with exercise is *to exercise continuously for at least 20 to 30 minutes (long duration) in a way that results in no shortness of breath (low intensity).*

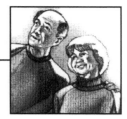

4. I enjoy doing and feel I do well at the following activities (fill in blanks).

_____

_____

_____

5. I would like to learn the following activities (fill in blanks).

_____

_____

_____

6. I use the following excuses to avoid exercise (fill in blanks).

_____

_____

_____

7. I can counter my excuses in the following ways (fill in blanks).

_____

_____

_____

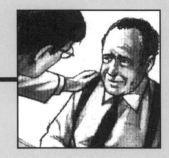

Long-Term Problems

Education and Prevention

CHAPTER 15

Richard M. Bergenstal, MD

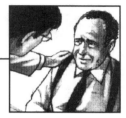

Long-Term Problems:

Three Links in the Chain of Prevention

What do I need to know about the problems associated with diabetes?

How do I know if the long-term problems of diabetes are beginning?

What can I do to decrease my risk for developing problems?

Diabetes, like many other diseases, can affect several systems in the body and cause problems. This chapter is an introduction to the long-term problems, or complications, of diabetes. It focuses on three links in the chain of prevention, delay, and effective management of these problems: education, early detection, and regular follow-up. The chapters that follow provide more details on diagnosis and treatment of each long-term problem.

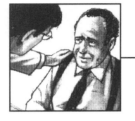

Since the discovery of insulin in 1921, people with diabetes are living longer and longer. We know that many people have had diabetes for more than 50 years yet still live long, healthful lives. What we don't know is why the long-term problems of diabetes don't develop in some people no matter what they seem to do, whereas some of these problems do develop in others who take excellent care of their diabetes.

Today, doctors and researchers are learning more about how to help people with diabetes live longer, healthful, productive lives. Much of this challenge has involved recognizing, treating, and looking for ways to prevent or delay the complications (problems) of diabetes. It's important that you learn as much as you can about these problems. Only then will you realize that significant medical advances have been made to help you reduce your risk for developing them.

The chain of action for managing diabetes has three links that can be used to effectively delay or prevent the complications.

- *Education* involves learning about the complications of diabetes, what causes them, and how you can prevent them. That's what this chapter is all about.

- *Early detection* involves learning to recognize the earliest symptoms and signs, as well as knowing and keeping track of changes in the results of your laboratory tests. Being aware of what you feel can help you recognize early symptoms. Changes noted in your physical examination and laboratory tests can be early signs of problems that may be developing. The charts at the end of this chapter will help you know what changes you need to be aware of.

- *Regular follow-up* involves setting up a schedule of office visits to work with your health care team to minimize your risk for a particular complication. Your chain of prevention becomes stronger as you work alongside professionals who can help you.

EDUCATION: GATHERING INFORMATION ABOUT COMPLICATIONS

To strengthen the link of education, you must first know the complications associated with diabetes. They can be divided into three groups: immediate, intermediate, and long-term. This section of the manual focuses on long-term problems.

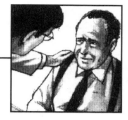

Two of the *immediate problems* of diabetes—hyperglycemia (high blood glucose) that can lead to ketoacidosis (extremely high blood glucose), hypoglycemia (low blood glucose) that can lead to severe hypoglycemia (unconsciousness from low blood glucose levels)—were discussed in Chapter 11. These immediate problems can develop within minutes to days and usually go away if recognized early and treated promptly.

Blurry vision can also result if blood glucose levels are temporarily too high. As blood glucose levels return to more normal levels, the blurry vision improves.

Infections can also cause blood glucose levels to become elevated. For prevention of infections, ask your health care team about your need for flu shots. Flu shots are recommended yearly (in the fall) for certain people with diabetes. This shot helps prevent or minimize types of flu or influenza. Influenza is a type of flu that often results in a long illness, during which it is difficult to control one's diabetes. It also raises the risk for developing pneumonia. A flu shot does not prevent common colds. Also ask about pneumonia shots (pneumovax). This shot is given once in a person's lifetime. It prevents the most common type of bacterial pneumonia (pneumococcal pneumonia), often called walking pneumonia. It's recommended for some people at high risk for infections, including some people with diabetes.

Intermediate problems can become a concern over months to years but can usually be prevented with proper treatment. These problems include delayed growth and physical development in children and adolescents and are discussed in Chapters 8 and 31. Pregnancy is also a concern for women who have diabetes. The good news is that with good diabetes control before and during pregnancy, complications associated with pregnancy can also be prevented. Pregnancy is discussed in Chapter 26.

Diabetes can sometimes gradually damage various organs in the body, including the eyes, kidneys, and heart. It also damages body systems, such as the nervous system and blood vessel system. Such complications usually take years, even decades, to develop, which is why they're called *long-term problems*. The goal is to reduce risk factors associated with these problems and learn the earliest ways to detect them and the best ways to treat them.

Small blood vessel (microvascular) damage is primarily responsible for problems in the eyes and kidneys. Large blood vessel (macrovascular) damage can cause heart attacks, strokes, or poor blood circulation to the legs. Damage to the nervous system can result in reduced sensitivity to touch, temperature, and pain in any part of the body, especially the feet and hands. The feet in particular need special care because their condition depends on a combination of healthy large blood vessels, small blood vessels, and nerves.

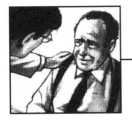

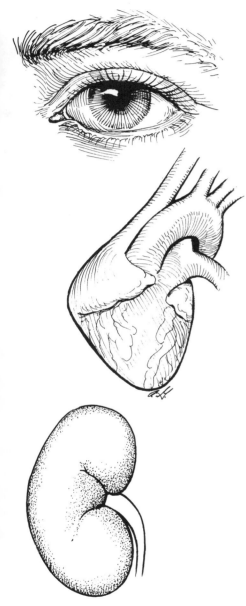

Long-term problems can affect the eyes, heart and blood vessels, kidneys, nerves, and feet

HOW BLOOD GLUCOSE LEVELS RELATE TO LONG-TERM PROBLEMS

Education can also help you understand how high blood glucose levels can have a major influence on the development of long-term problems. It is hoped that "tight control" of blood glucose levels will prevent or slow the development of long-term problems. Most diabetes experts agree that good blood glucose control appears to slow the development of complications. They also admit that the perfect study to prove this has not yet been done. High blood glucose levels can damage various systems in the body in several ways.

High blood glucose levels and other related factors can thicken the lining (basement membrane) of small blood vessels (capillaries). This appears to damage the small blood vessels by making them leak and unable to supply needed nutrients to tissues. It is most evident in the eyes and kidneys.

When blood glucose levels are high, excess glucose can attach to proteins in the body and may cause some other complications. For example, glucose attaching to proteins in the tissue of the hands or the joints may lead to stiff hands or a type of arthritis.

Certain tissues are able to change the glucose that passes through them into an alcohol form of sugar called sorbitol. As blood glucose levels go higher, more sorbitol accumulates, which disrupts the normal functioning of these tissues. Sorbitol accumulation in nerves appears to be partly responsible for nerve damage sometimes experienced by people with diabetes. It may also build up in the kidneys, eyes, and large blood vessels. Drugs (aldose reductase inhibitors) that prevent glucose from being changed into sorbitol are now being tested. (This sorbitol does not come from food sorbitol.)

OTHER RISKS RELATED TO LONG-TERM PROBLEMS

Education can make you aware of other risk factors for developing long-term problems. It's important that you do what you can to reduce or eliminate any of these risk factors.

High blood pressure can greatly increase the damage caused by high blood glucose levels. The kidneys, eyes, and heart are very sensitive to high

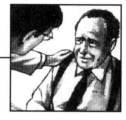

blood pressure, particularly if high blood glucose levels have already caused some weakening of the tissues. Acceptable blood pressures vary somewhat with age but in general should not be above 140/90. The top figure (systolic) is the pressure on blood vessels when blood is being pumped through them by the heart, and the bottom figure (diastolic) is the pressure when the heart is resting.

Many *medications* and methods are used to control high blood pressure. Medications should be selected carefully for the person with diabetes, because some of them may increase blood glucose levels or have other undesirable effects. Some can increase levels of fats in the blood or make it difficult to recognize an insulin reaction (hypoglycemia).

The two major fats (lipids) carried by the blood—*cholesterol and triglycerides*—have been shown to increase the risk for development of heart and blood vessel (cardiovascular) disease. These fats may be high because of a genetic trait, excessive amounts of fat in the diet, and/or high blood glucose levels. Whatever the cause, it's important to lower the levels into the normal range. The average American range for blood fat levels is too high, so ask your health care team to test your blood for these fats and, if necessary, help you learn how to reduce them to healthy levels.

Smoking can greatly increase the risk of developing heart and blood vessel disease. It's especially harmful in anyone with another risk factor for heart and blood vessel disease, which includes everyone with diabetes, high blood pressure, and high blood fat levels. The risk for heart disease is reduced promptly and greatly when a person stops smoking.

Being *overweight* increases the risk for developing high blood pressure, Type II diabetes, and high blood fat levels. Since all of these factors are also known to increase the risk for cardiovascular disease, it makes sense to avoid obesity as a preventive measure, especially when one has diabetes.

Certain effects must be understood and planned for if persons with diabetes are to drink alcoholic beverages. *Drinking large amounts of alcohol* can damage nerves and/or increase nerve problems already present because of diabetes. Impotence and numbness in the feet are especially common when a person with diabetes regularly drinks large amounts of alcohol.

Even though we know a lot about factors that could contribute to the complications of diabetes, these problems are also likely to be determined by *genetic factors*. So if a family member has had a heart attack, pay particular attention to your risk factors and take positive steps to lower them.

Since long-term problems take many years to develop, it stands to reason that *the longer you have diabetes* the more at risk you are for developing one of these complications. Yet there are people who've had diabetes for 50 years with only minor complications.

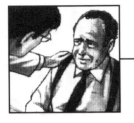

EARLY DETECTION: RECOGNIZING EARLY SIGNS AND SYMPTOMS

Once you're aware of what problems can be found with diabetes and you know some of the causes, the next step is to learn the earliest way to detect these problems. You can watch for signs and symptoms and your health care team can perform tests for you. Often, your health care team can use early detection methods to tell you a complication is starting, even before you feel anything related to it. If a complication is detected early, there is often an effective treatment available that can slow it down or hopefully even prevent any progression.

Early detection methods used by your health care team may include asking the right questions about how you feel (symptoms), looking for changes in the physical examination (signs), or performing the appropriate laboratory blood test or diagnostic test. The tables at the end of this chapter show some of the earliest symptoms, signs, and laboratory tests used to detect problems in the areas most commonly affected by diabetes—the eyes, kidneys, nerves, heart, and blood vessels.

REGULAR FOLLOW-UP: AN IMPORTANT LINK

With education, early detection, aggressive intervention, and regular follow-up, many of these problems can be minimized. The tables include suggested time intervals for follow-up visits with your health care team.

One of the blood tests your doctor does at your follow-up visits is called a glycated or glycosylated (which means to attach glucose onto) hemoglobin. As glucose circulates in the bloodstream it becomes attached to a protein in the red blood cell called hemoglobin. Measuring the percentage of hemoglobin that has glucose attached to it can provide a fairly good estimate of a person's average blood glucose levels during the past six to eight weeks.

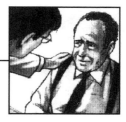

SUMMARY

The next six chapters continue the discussion of the long-term problems of diabetes. Each chapter ends with a list of things you can do to prevent the specific problem from developing. They also include a list of what your health care team can do to prevent or manage the problem.

Remember, education, early detection, and regular follow-up are your strongest links in the chain of prevention.

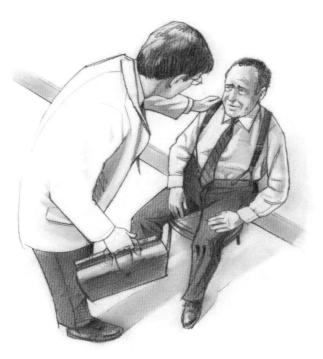

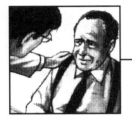

EARLY DETECTION AND FOLLOW-UP OF LONG-TERM PROBLEMS IN DIABETES

	You	**Your Health Care Team**
Symptoms (what you feel)	*Report:* • fatigue, nausea, itching • chest pain • less tolerance for exercise • shortness of breath • leg cramps when walking • black-outs or temporary weakness • blurry vision • changes in visual acuity (sharpness) • double vision • floating spots in your eyes (floaters) • pain, burning, tingling, or numbness in feet or hands • impotence (loss of erections in men) • stomach bloating • diarrhea, constipation • slow bladder emptying • dizziness when standing	*Ask about:* All of these early symptoms
Signs (what you find on physical examination)	*Look for:* • edema (fluid accumulation, most commonly found around the ankles) • inability to tell hot from cold • numbness in feet • blisters or calluses • loss of hair growth on feet and hands • feet that are red when hanging down and white when elevated	*Check your:* • heartbeat • pulse in neck (carotid) • pulses in feet, arms, and legs • blood pressure (check for drop when moving from lying to standing position) • blood pressure for new elevation (especially if over 140/90) • feet for ulcers or thick calluses • feet for vibration sensation (reduced tuning fork test) • reflexes • legs for signs of edema • visual acuity (sharpness) • small blood vessels in the back of the eyes with an ophthalmoscope

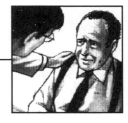

	You	Your Health Care Team
Laboratory or Diagnostic Tests	*Test:* • blood glucose (self monitoring) • blood pressure (self monitoring, if recommended)	*Test:* • blood cholesterol and triglycerides • circulation in legs and neck (using Doppler sound waves) • urine for very small amounts of protein (microalbumin) • urine for protein (dipstick method), or for protein or creatinine clearance (24-hour urine sample) • electrical conduction of nerves (if necessary to verify damage) • for impotence in men and evaluate for stomach, bladder, or intestinal problems (as needed) • heart function (ECG, if necessary) • exercise capabilities (exercise stress test, if necessary) *An eye specialist should:* • dilate eyes to evaluate blood vessels • check pressure in eye • check lens of eye (cataracts) • photograph eyes to evaluate changes • do fluorescein angiogram (inject dye into an arm vein, then look to see if dye leaks from blood vessels in the back of the eyes)

EARLY DETECTION AND FOLLOW-UP OF LONG-TERM PROBLEMS IN DIABETES (CONTINUED)

247

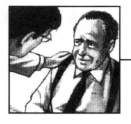

EARLY DETECTION AND FOLLOW-UP OF LONG-TERM PROBLEMS IN DIABETES (CONTINUED)

	You	**You**
Follow-Up (emphasize if early changes are detected)	*Be sure to:* • have regular check-ups with health care team • see eye specialist yearly • exercise routinely • follow your meal plan (low salt, low fat) • report foot infections or damage • stop smoking • purchase shoes that fit properly • avoid excess alcohol, which also causes nerve damage • report symptoms of urinary tract infections right away (burning urge to empty bladder frequently, but only able to urinate small amount) • have urine protein checked yearly • ask which medications can be taken safely • discuss if insulin dose is appropriate	*Follow up with:* • regular check-ups (every three months) • referrals to specialists for eye, kidney, foot, nerve, blood vessel, or control problems • blood pressure checks at each visit • annual blood cholesterol and triglyceride tests • foot checks at each visit (monitor infections and injuries closely) • ECG and exercise stress tests, if necessary • evaluation for wrist (carpal tunnel) and trigger finger problems • treatment for urinary tract infections • low-protein diets if kidney problems arise • careful monitoring of medications that may cause harmful side effects • eye checks in pregnant patients • referral to ophthalmologist for patients planning pregnancy

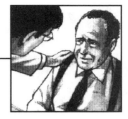

CHAPTER 16

Priscilla M. Hollander, MD
Leonard Nordstrom, MD

Heart Problems:
Steps to Reduce Risk Factors

"The essence of life is a healthy heart."
Proverbs 14:30

How does heart disease develop?

What is atherosclerosis?

Can heart disease be prevented?

Over the years researchers have discovered certain conditions, called *risk factors*, that increase a person's chance for developing heart and blood vessel (circulatory) problems. This chapter explains why heart disease is such a common problem in our society, especially for people with diabetes. It suggests specific steps to help you and your family identify and improve risk factors when possible. By supporting each other in these efforts, your family can take giant steps toward a life of vitality and fitness.

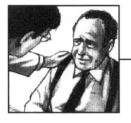

THE CIRCULATORY SYSTEM

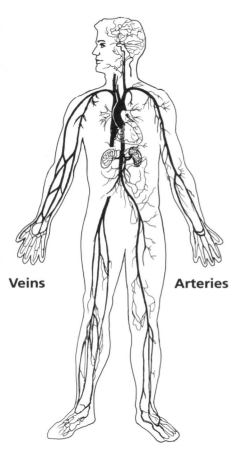

Veins   **Arteries**

Veins are shown on left side of the drawing and arteries are shown on the right

Many parts of the body are crucial for it to function properly. This is especially true of the heart and blood vessels (the *circulatory* or *cardiovascular system*). Circulation of blood throughout the body supplies oxygen and nutrients to the organs and allows them to do their jobs. If the heart is unable to pump enough blood throughout the body, or if a blood vessel is blocked, the affected areas quickly lose their ability to function and serious problems may result.

People can do several things to keep their heart and blood vessels healthy and working efficiently. The best way is to pay special attention to how risk factors apply to you. That way your heart can continue providing vital nutrients and oxygen to your body for a long and active life.

HEART DISEASE AND DIABETES

Heart disease is the most common cause of death in the United States. It's also the number one cause of death among people with diabetes and can be found in people with both Type I and Type II diabetes. Heart attacks may also occur at an earlier age in people with diabetes than in the general population. Women in the general population tend to be protected from heart attacks until menopause. The reasons for this protection are unclear, but it appears to be lost for women with diabetes. The rate of heart attack is the same for both men and women with diabetes at all ages. In fact, studies show that persons with diabetes may have two to four times the risk for a heart attack as persons without diabetes.

HOW HEART DISEASE DEVELOPS

Damage to large blood vessels appears to be the main cause of heart disease and other circulatory problems, such as heart attack, high blood pressure (hypertension), poor blood circulation to the brain (cerebral vascular disease, or stroke) and poor blood circulation to the arms and legs (peripheral vascular disease). The type of blood vessel damage that results in these problems can occur in anyone, but in people with diabetes it seems to occur at a faster rate.

Damage to small blood vessels can also cause problems, such as poor circulation to the eyes and kidneys. However, these blood vessel changes do not occur in people who do not have diabetes.

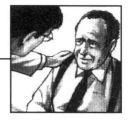

Most blood vessel damage is probably caused by *atherosclerosis*, or "hardening of the arteries," but the exact causes are not completely understood. Atherosclerosis occurs when the walls of the blood vessels gradually thicken and harden. It may happen in the large blood vessels as well as the small blood vessels. In some blood vessels atherosclerosis may lead to actual blocking of the artery. If this happens, the tissue supplied by these blood vessels may die.

It appears that certain blood vessels in the body are more likely to be affected by atherosclerosis. One such group, the *coronary arteries*, supplies blood to the heart. If these blood vessels become narrowed or blocked, damage to the heart muscle or a heart attack may result.

Coronary artery disease is characterized by chest pain called *angina*. As the vessels that supply the heart start to close off, the supply of oxygen and nutrients to the heart muscle is decreased and may cause damage that results in chest pain. At first this pain usually occurs during exercise or activity—when the heart is working harder. However, as more of the heart muscle becomes affected, the chest pain can occur at any time. This doesn't always signal a heart attack; it's a warning that there is a problem in the arteries that supply the heart. If the arteries go on to become completely blocked, the heart muscles supplied by these blood vessels may die and the person is likely to have a heart attack.

Blockage of arteries that supply the heart can be reversed in a number of ways. If you experience angina, see your health care team immediately for an evaluation and cardiac testing. Cardiac testing may consist of a stress test and/or a heart scan. During a stress test, you are linked to a heart monitoring machine while exercising on a treadmill. If the heart monitor shows certain changes during the test, it can confirm that the heart is damaged.

If the stress test is abnormal or if chest pain is severe, the doctor may suggest a *cardiac catheterization*. In this test, you are hospitalized and you undergo a special procedure that involves flushing dye through the arteries around the heart. Pictures are taken, and if enough heart blockage is seen, one of several procedures may be suggested to open up the blood vessels.

The oldest, and perhaps most common, procedure used to open up blood vessels is called a *cardiac bypass*. In this operation new blood vessels are surgically implanted to bypass the blocked blood vessels. A newer technique is called *angioplasty*. In this procedure a probe is passed into the blood vessel to chip away at the accumulated cholesterol plaque. The newest technique, which is still experimental, uses a laser beam to remove the plaque. For persons who don't have extreme blood vessel blockage or are not suitable candidates for surgery, medications such as *calcium channel blockers* or *beta blockers* may be used to help dilate or expand the arteries and keep them open.

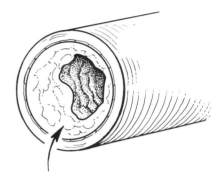

Fatty deposit in an artery

251

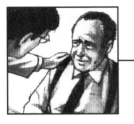

Another form of heart disease that can affect anyone but often accompanies diabetes is called *cardiomyopathy*. In cardiomyopathy, the small blood vessels that supply the heart become blocked by atherosclerosis. If they're blocked long enough, the heart muscle becomes scarred and weak and cannot expand and contract well enough to pump blood to all parts of the body. This problem generally does not cause chest pain or a heart attack.

If enough of the heart muscle loses its ability to pump blood, the heart will begin to fail. Fluid will accumulate in different areas of the body, especially in the lungs, causing shortness of breath and swollen ankles. The problem, called *congestive heart failure*, is difficult to treat. However, medications can help. *Lanoxin* (digoxin) may make the heart muscle beat stronger and improve circulation, and *diuretics* can help remove fluid from the body. These medications may also be helpful to persons with cardiomyopathy.

HIGH BLOOD PRESSURE (HYPERTENSION)

Anyone can have high blood pressure, but it's more common in people with diabetes. In fact, about two thirds of adults with diabetes have hypertension. It has been shown to increase the incidence of heart disease, and it speeds the rate of atherosclerosis in large blood vessels and probably small blood vessels as well. Therefore, everything possible should be done to prevent high blood pressure. If it does develop, it should be treated early and aggressively.

Control of blood pressure is important for persons with diabetes. High blood pressure increases the risk for stroke, heart disease, and kidney disease and can worsen eye problems. In the past, 140/90 was considered the top of the normal blood pressure range. Some research indicates that it might be important for people with diabetes to have even lower blood pressure, with a top goal of 135/85. More studies are needed to confirm the best blood pressure range for people with diabetes. Your health care team will help you to determine the best treatment and goals for you.

Many medications are available to treat high blood pressure. However, it's important to note that some of them may interfere with blood glucose

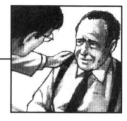

control in people taking insulin. Diuretics are pills that decrease fluid volume and rid the body of excess salt. However, in some people they cause blood glucose levels to increase. The medications most likely to cause problems are called beta blockers. Beta blockers lower blood pressure by blocking the effects of adrenalin on blood vessels. Adrenalin is a key agent in setting off the symptoms of an insulin reaction. When its effects are blocked, a person may not have the warning signs of low blood glucose and may have a severe insulin reaction or even lose consciousness.

This side effect doesn't happen to everyone who takes insulin and uses beta blockers. Because these medications can be very useful in treating heart disease and hypertension, they may be prescribed for persons using insulin. It's important to watch closely at first to see if a medication is going to cause problems. If problems occur, the medication should be replaced with another (see Chapter 24).

STROKE (CEREBRAL VASCULAR DISEASE)

Another area of concern is poor circulation to the blood vessels that supply the brain. Blockage of a blood vessel in the brain can cause a cerebral vascular accident or, as it's more commonly known, a stroke. As with many of the circulatory system problems, strokes are possible in people with or without diabetes. However, the incidence is higher in people with diabetes.

The effect of blockage of a particular blood vessel depends on its location in the brain. Various parts of the brain control different parts of the body. Sometimes strokes may affect only speech, other times they may affect the ability to use part of the body, such as a hand or a foot. The most common form of stroke may leave persons paralyzed on one side of the body. Atherosclerosis can play a role in the development of strokes. Plaque may build up in a blood vessel and close it off. If this happens in one of the two *carotid arteries* (the main vessels that supply blood to the brain), part of the plaque may rip off and may be carried to the brain, where it can block a smaller vessel and cause a stroke.

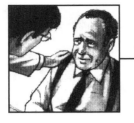

POOR CIRCULATION TO THE EXTREMITIES (PERIPHERAL VASCULAR DISEASE)

Poor circulation to the extremities, or peripheral vascular disease, involves both the small and large blood vessels of the legs and feet and is very common in people with diabetes. Blockage of the large blood vessels in the legs may cause discomfort or pain in the thigh or calf muscles when a person is standing, walking, or even exercising. The extent of pain depends on how much blockage there is. With slight blockage, a person may be able to walk a long distance before noticing pain. The pain and discomfort usually go away when the person stops and rests for a minute and the blood supply to that area is re-established. However, the pain usually returns after the person starts the activity again.

Treatment of peripheral vascular disease can be difficult. Some medications may help expand the blood vessels. Another approach is to bypass a damaged blood vessel and put in a new one to help restore circulation.

PREVENTING OR SLOWING ATHEROSCLEROSIS

A number of things can speed the process of atherosclerosis. Avoiding or treating these risk factors can help reduce a person's chance for developing serious problems with the large and small blood vessels. Preventable risk factors include smoking, high levels of cholesterol and triglycerides in the blood, obesity, and hypertension.

Smoking. Smoking is a very serious risk factor for both heart disease and peripheral vascular disease. People who smoke have two to four times the rate of heart attack and ten times the rate of peripheral vascular disease experienced by nonsmokers. Therefore, if you smoke it's crucial that you quit. Of course, the best thing is to not start smoking, but unfortunately some people find themselves trapped by this addiction. We cannot stress enough how important it is to stop smoking. If you have tried to quit without success, ask your health care team for a referral to a reputable program that will help you succeed.

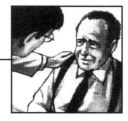

Cholesterol and Triglycerides. High levels of cholesterol and triglycerides have been definitely associated with increased incidence of atherosclerosis and heart attacks. A number of recent studies support these findings. In fact, it has been shown that as blood cholesterol levels increase above the 200 mg/dl level, the incidence of heart attacks increases. It's interesting to compare the low rate of heart disease in countries such as Japan, where dietary fat intake is low, with the high rate of heart disease in countries such as the United States and Finland, where fat intake is high. A high level of fat intake, especially foods containing large amounts of saturated fats and cholesterol, is known to be one important factor.

Some people have a genetic tendency to develop high levels of triglycerides and cholesterol and are at great risk for heart disease at a relatively early age. They need to not only follow a healthy meal plan in terms of fat intake, but also take special medication to help lower their cholesterol and triglyceride levels. All people, especially those with diabetes, who cannot lower their cholesterol into the 200 mg/dl range by meal planning alone need to be evaluated and considered as candidates for taking medications to lower cholesterol. This is an important subject to discuss with your health care team, because both age and history of heart disease play a role in determining your need for medication.

Obesity. Long-term studies have shown that obesity is a risk factor for heart disease. It also promotes hypertension and can worsen diabetes, both of which increase a person's risk for developing heart disease. Therefore, people who are overweight should set a goal to lose weight and get as close to their desirable weight as possible.

Hypertension. Prevention of high blood pressure is an important part of reducing risk for heart disease. This includes keeping salt intake at recommended healthy levels, exercising regularly, avoiding obesity, and having blood pressure checked regularly to make sure hypertension can be treated promptly if it develops.

Diabetes is also considered a risk factor for heart disease. As already stated, people with diabetes have an increased rate of heart disease. The question is: Does good control of blood glucose play a role in preventing heart disease, as is the case with other complications associated with diabetes? This is not a well-studied area. Some preliminary findings indicate that improved blood glucose control may indeed lower blood pressure and slow the progress of atherosclerosis, thus reducing the risk for heart disease.

It's safe to say that good blood glucose control and good overall diabetes control are important to reducing the risk for heart disease. The other risk factors must also be reduced if possible, and this is important not just for the person with diabetes but for everyone.

255

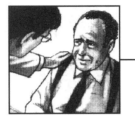

SUMMARY

A healthy heart and blood vessels are obviously very important for continued good health. A healthy lifestyle with good control of diabetes, a nutritious meal plan, prevention or control of hypertension, no smoking, and regular exercise can lead to a healthy heart and to a healthful and long life.

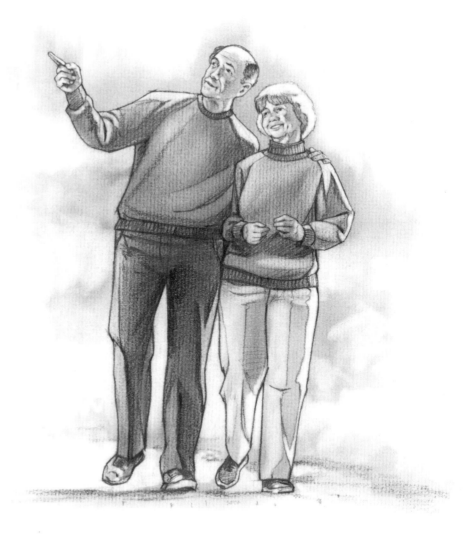

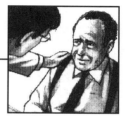

WHAT YOU CAN DO

1. Don't smoke.
2. Reduce intake of foods high in fats, especially saturated fats and cholesterol.
3. Reduce intake of foods high in sodium (salt).
4. Make moderate exercise a regular part of your lifestyle.
5. Maintain a reasonable weight within the recommended healthy range.
6. Maintain good control of blood glucose levels.
7. See your health care team regularly to monitor your success at caring for your diabetes and maintaining a healthy heart.

WHAT YOUR HEALTH CARE TEAM CAN DO

1. Refer you to a program to help you stop smoking if you smoke.
2. Test your blood annually for levels of cholesterol and triglycerides and help you learn how to lower them if the cholesterol level is higher than 200 mg/dl or the triglyceride level is higher than 150 mg/dl.
3. Check your blood pressure at each visit and begin a treatment plan to lower it if it's higher than 140/90 on repeated tests.
4. Help you plan a safe and effective individual exercise program.
5. Help you lose body fat if necessary.
6. Review your blood glucose testing records and glycosylated hemoglobin and make changes in your management plan if your blood glucose levels have not remained in the desirable range.
7. Test your heart function and blood circulation to all parts of your body at least annually if you are over age 30 or have had diabetes for more than ten years.

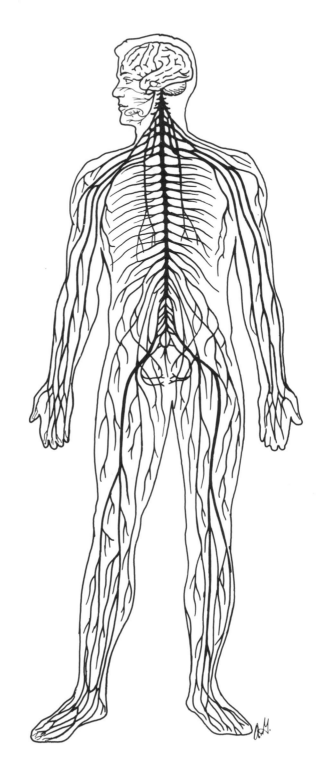

THE NERVOUS SYSTEM

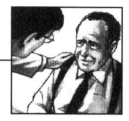

CHAPTER 17

Priscilla M. Hollander, MD

Nerve Problems:
Protecting the Body's Communication System

How does diabetes cause damage to nerves?

How are painful neuropathies treated?

Why is early detection of nerve problems important?

Damage to nerves (*neuropathy*) is very common in people with both Type I and Type II diabetes. Studies indicate that neuropathy may develop at some time in many people with diabetes. This damage can distort messages traveling along certain nerves or not allow the messages to pass at all. In this chapter you'll learn about the different nervous subsystems that can be damaged by diabetes, how to detect the symptoms of neuropathy, and appropriate treatment.

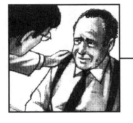

Of all the systems in the human body, the nervous system is one of the most marvelous. This network of nerves is the body's communication system, much like how a network of telephone lines can be a country's communication system. The nervous system is so extensive that its branches reach every part of the body. It funnels messages to and from the brain, allowing coordination of the body's many functions. Some nerves carry messages of sensations such as pain, touch, or temperature; others carry instructions from the brain to the legs, feet, hands, and internal organs.

Neuropathy does not always cause obvious symptoms, but when it does they may include pain, loss of sensitivity, or loss of function. Symptoms of neuropathy tend to develop gradually and then increase in intensity, although occasionally symptoms may appear quite suddenly. Symptoms may be severe for a while and then disappear or they may last for a few weeks to months. In some cases, neuropathy can persist for months to years.

HOW DIABETES CAUSES DAMAGE TO NERVES

We're beginning to understand how diabetes causes damage to nerves, but much is still not known. Some evidence suggests that diabetes affects small blood vessels that supply the nerves with oxygen and nutrients. If these supply lines are damaged, some nerves do not receive the oxygen and nutrients they need to maintain themselves and do their work of carrying messages.

Diabetes can also cause damage to the wall around the nerves. Nerves are insulated with a coating of fat. Like the insulation around a telephone wire, the fat protects the nerve from outside damage. Diabetes has been shown to cause a breakdown, or even disappearance, of the layer of fat around nerves. When this happens the nerve is "short-circuited." In other words, messages passing along the nerve wall will be either distorted or blocked. In some cases the nerve may even transmit false messages.

The nervous system is divided into three main subsystems.

- The *cranial nervous system* supplies nerves that go to various areas of the head, such as the eyes, ears, face, and jaw.
- The *autonomic nervous system* includes nerves that go to the internal organs, such as the heart, stomach, intestines, and blood vessels.

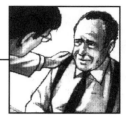

- The *peripheral nervous system* includes nerves that go to the extremities, such as the arms, hands, legs, and feet, as well as to the muscles in the abdomen and back.

Although in theory any nerve in the body can be affected by diabetes and cause symptoms of neuropathy, certain nerves in each of the above three subsystems seem to be involved more often.

CRANIAL NERVOUS SYSTEM

Two sets of cranial nerves seem to be most often affected by diabetic neuropathy. One is the group of nerves that goes to the eye muscles. Each eye has six muscles. Their job is to move both eyes at the same time so you see only one image. If the eyes fail to move in unison, you have double vision. This problem usually occurs suddenly. For instance, if a nerve to one of the muscles is damaged by diabetes, that muscle's action may be slowed or even stopped. Luckily this seems to be a temporary problem that usually disappears, although it may take up to several months to clear. Until it clears, wearing a patch over one eye helps.

The other cranial nerves that may be affected are the right and left facial nerves. These nerves control the lower eyelids as well as facial expressions (grimaces, smiles, and so on). If there is a problem with a nerve on one side of the face, that side of the face may actually sag. The lower eyelid will droop and the outside of the person's smile will also droop. This problem is called Bell's palsy. It may occur in people who do not have diabetes but is much more common in people with diabetes. Fortunately, like the problem with the eye muscles, Bell's palsy is often temporary. It's rare for these problems to leave any permanent changes.

AUTONOMIC NERVOUS SYSTEM

In some ways, the autonomic nervous system can be described as the silent system. We don't have conscious control over these nerves as we do for parts of the cranial and peripheral nerves. We cannot command our hearts to beat faster the same way we can command our legs to move more quickly. However, the autonomic system is very important, which becomes evident when damage occurs and causes problems.

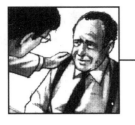

One of the most common areas affected by diabetes is the digestive system (stomach and intestines). Nerve damage to the stomach usually causes it to empty more slowly than it should. This can lead to a feeling of fullness, which may cause nausea and occasional vomiting. The problem can be present all the time or may occur once in awhile. Often it seems to be worse in the early morning before or following breakfast.

The medical name for this neuropathy is *gastroparesis*, which means "slow emptying" or "paralysis of the stomach." The condition can sometimes be difficult to diagnose, because a number of diseases cause the same symptoms. One of the best ways to diagnose gastroparesis is to have someone swallow a barium dye, which outlines the stomach. A series of x-rays is then taken and used to evaluate whether there is a problem with the way food is passing through the stomach.

Gastroparesis can be difficult to treat, but several approaches may be helpful. One is to eat smaller meals. Another is to evaluate diabetes control and, if necessary, improve poor control. A third approach is medication. Unfortunately, only one medication that may help is presently available. It's called Reglan (metoclopramide), and it actually speeds the rate at which stomach muscles contract to help digestion occur normally. It's usually taken about half an hour before meals and sometimes at bedtime. Reglan doesn't work for everyone, but it can be helpful for some persons. Presently, other medications are also being tested.

The intestine is another problem area in the digestive system. Diabetes can affect the large and small intestines in two different ways—diarrhea or constipation. Diarrhea caused by diabetes often occurs at night, but it certainly can occur during the day as well. Bowel movements can be sporadic and often occur with little warning. The medical approach to this problem is a balanced meal plan plus conservative use of antidiarrhea agents, such as Lomotil or Pepto Bismol. Treatment for constipation involves a balanced meal plan with an appropriate amount of fiber, physical activity, and careful use of various laxatives.

In the genitourinary system, autonomic nerve problems may cause the bladder to have problems emptying when it's full of urine. This happens because of damage to the nerves that usually give a signal of pressure when it's time to urinate. Therefore, a person may not urinate often enough, which can cause enlargement of the bladder and worsen the problem. Often an evaluation by a urologist is helpful to assess the severity of the bladder problem. Certain medications, such as Urecholine, can help increase complete emptying. A constant assessment for urinary tract infections and prompt treatment are important in slowing damage to the bladder and kidneys. Another genitourinary problem common in men with diabetes involves with the function of the penis, causing impotence, an inability to have erections (see Chapter 21).

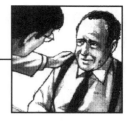

Autonomic neuropathy can also affect the nerves that lead to the heart. Damage to the principle nerve that influences the pace of the heart can cause problems with heart rate. Persons with diabetes may have elevated fasting pulse rates or slight irregularities in their heart rate from damage to this particular nerve. It's still unclear what effect this has on the heart. An EKG (heart tracing) can sometimes pick up the slight irregularities in heartbeat. These irregularities can be used as an early warning of damage to the autonomic nervous system before other symptoms appear.

The final major problem area in the autonomic nervous system relates to nerves that go to the blood vessels. Neuropathy can cause low blood pressure in certain areas of the body, especially upon rising from a sitting or lying position. The amount of blood in the blood vessels must constantly be regulated to maintain a healthy blood pressure throughout the body. As you move from lying or sitting to a standing position, blood must be shifted so the right amount is in the right place at the right time. You may have experienced a momentary twinge of dizziness after going very quickly to a standing position. This is because it takes a little time for your body to move some blood from your feet to your head.

Your body is able to shift blood by sending messages along various little nerves to the blood vessels, telling them when to contract and expand. If these nerves are damaged, they don't work as quickly and it takes longer to shift blood volume. When you get up suddenly, it may take so long to shift blood from the feet to the head that you get quite dizzy and may even fall. This problem is called *postural hypotension*, which means that blood pressure is momentarily low because of a change in body posture. People with this problem can usually avoid dizziness by not standing quickly after sitting or lying for some time. There are also medications that can help the blood vessels shift blood.

PERIPHERAL NERVOUS SYSTEM

Two main types of neuropathy can occur in the peripheral nervous system. One involves a number of nerves at the same time (*peripheral polyneuropathy*), and the other involves only one nerve (*peripheral mononeuropathy*).

Peripheral polyneuropathies are the most common of all neuropathies. They generally affect the feet and/or legs and occasionally the hands and/or arms. There are two main symptoms of this type of neuropathy. One is a "pins and needles" feeling of tingling, numbness, and/or burning. The

263

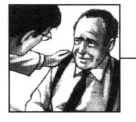

symptoms may be most noticeable at night and are usually found in both feet. When the problem occurs in both feet/legs or both hands/arms it's called *symmetrical* (both sides of the body) neuropathy. The numbness from this problem can interfere with the ability to feel pain. This can be serious because you may injure your foot or hand and not even notice it. If an infection occurs and is untreated, problems such as gangrene could result.

Symmetrical neuropathies can be quite painful. The pain is usually worse at night and has been compared to an electric shock, a burning sensation, or even a toothache. The painful neuropathy may come on very quickly or very slowly. Once it occurs, it usually lasts from six to 18 months and then may disappear. This contrasts with the numbness and tingling, which may go on for months or even years.

Occasionally an *asymmetrical* (one side of the body) painful neuropathy may develop. This usually occurs in one of the thighs and may also cause loss of muscle and muscle weakness in the area. Again, this problem is usually temporary and passes in three to six months. It's important to use specific exercises and other methods to help prevent loss of muscle strength in the affected area.

Peripheral mononeuropathies (affecting only one nerve) most often affect a nerve in the chest or abdomen. Pain from the nerve may be confused with other medical problems such as appendicitis, kidney stones, or heart disease. This makes the problem difficult to diagnose. Like the other painful neuropathies, it usually lasts from three to six months and then may disappear.

Peripheral neuropathies can be diagnosed and confirmed using a test called an *electromyelogram (EMG)*. This test records the speed of nerve impulses as they move along a specific nerve. In diabetes, the nerve impulse is usually slow and has other abnormal characteristics. An EMG is done by a neurologist (a nerve disease specialist).

TREATMENT OF PAINFUL NEUROPATHIES

Some methods of treating specific problems related to neuropathies have already been discussed. The focus in this section is on methods of reducing the pain that sometimes accompanies the peripheral neuropathies. Pain can vary from quite mild to very severe, and it may be continuous or sporadic.

Several medications that were first developed to treat other conditions have been useful in reducing or eliminating the pain of neuropathy. One group of medications (eg, Dilantin and Tegretol) was first developed to treat seizures. Amitriptyline (Elavil) and phenothiazines were developed

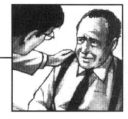

primarily to treat problems with depression. Elavil has been used individually and in combination with Prolixin, which is an example of the phenothiazine group, to successfully treat neuropathies. However, the Elavil and Prolixin combination does have side effects and in some persons may cause dizziness and sleepiness. It's not really clear how either groups of medications reduce neuropathic pain.

One new approach to treatment of painful neuropathies is the use of an ointment called capsaicin. This can be applied to the feet and legs several times a day.

Strict diabetes control is another important way to reduce neuropathic pain. As mentioned in the section on peripheral neuropathy, the speed of nerve impulses is slowed in people with neuropathy. But, improvement in blood glucose control has been shown to help the nerve impulses regain their normal speed.

If both good blood glucose control and medications do not provide relief from pain, it may be necessary to use temporary pain killing medications, such as acetominophen (eg, Tylenol) or aspirin, or antiinflammatories (eg, Motrin). For the most severe episodes of pain it may be necessary to use one of the weaker narcotics, such as codeine, or even stronger narcotics. These narcotics must be used under close supervision of a health care team. Painful neuropathy may persist for months, but in most cases it eventually disappears.

New advances in the treatment of neuropathy may be near. Several experimental drugs may help block the nerve damage caused by diabetes. These drugs fall into a category called *aldose reductase inhibitors*. They may actually block or reduce the effects of chemical reactions in diabetes that may be damaging to nerves. It's hoped that these drugs may prevent the development of neuropathy caused by diabetes and possibly help repair damage that has already occurred.

SUMMARY

It's important that your health care team check the function of your nerves as part of routine diabetes care. This can be done by testing the reflexes in your upper and lower body and by checking your feet and hands for decreased sensation to pin prick and vibration. Your health care team should ask if you have had any vision problems, trouble emptying your bladder, problems with impotence, or any numbness, tingling, or unusual pain in any area of your body. Some of these may be symptoms of neuropathies, but neuropathies can mimic almost any other pain.

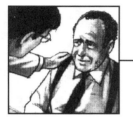

WHAT YOU CAN DO

1. Maintain good blood glucose control.
2. Tell your doctor about any tingling, numbness, loss of feeling, muscle weakness, pain or other unusual sensations.
3. Ask your doctor to investigate any persistent digestive, urinary, or sexual problems.
4. If medications are prescribed, take them exactly as directed.
5. If you have loss of feeling in any part of your body, be especially careful to avoid injury to that area, and check it daily for infections or other problems.

WHAT YOUR HEALTH CARE TEAM CAN DO

1. Use glycosylated hemoglobin tests and your blood glucose testing records to help you maintain good blood glucose control.
2. Ask you regularly about symptoms of neuropathy.
3. Check the function of your nerves as part of routine care.
4. Refer you for diagnostic tests if symptoms occur.
5. Prescribe medication and pursue other methods of coping with painful neuropathy.
6. Teach you how to avoid problems that can occur with loss of sensitivity, muscle weakness, and other possible effects of neuropathy.

CHAPTER 18

Janet Swenson Lima, RN, MPH
Stephen H. Powless, DPM
Ellie Strock, RN,C, CDE

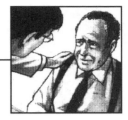

Foot Problems:
Keeping Feet For a Lifetime

Why is foot care so important if you have diabetes?

How can you prevent foot problems?

What does proper daily foot care involve?

Most of us don't think about our feet all that much, yet we use them every day for walking, working, and carrying out our daily lives. We tend to take our healthy feet for granted. Yet for people with diabetes, proper foot care is a serious matter, and a lifetime with healthy feet cannot be taken for granted. This chapter explains how diabetes can cause foot problems and provides information on keeping your feet healthy with a few minutes of care each day.

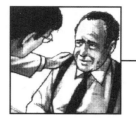
P roper foot care is an important part of the health care plan for people with diabetes. Diabetes can cause foot problems that may result in serious damage, or even amputation, if not caught early and treated promptly. Most of these problems and amputations could be prevented through good foot care, early identification of problems, and proper treatment.

HOW DIABETES AFFECTS YOUR FEET

High blood glucose levels from diabetes can contribute to neuropathy (nerve damage), blood vessel disease, and infection. When it comes to your feet, any of these problems can cause major damage if the right steps aren't taken to prevent or detect them.

Neuropathy (Nerve Damage)

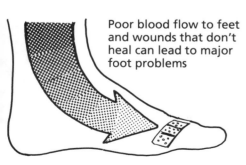

Damage to these nerves may result in numbness or pain and lead to more severe foot problems

The nerves in your feet are very important. They send messages to the brain, alerting you to injuries, telling you that blisters are forming, giving you early warnings of problems in shoe fit, and keeping your skin soft and moist to ward off dryness, cracking, and infection. If these messages can't get through, you may not realize problems are developing until it's too late.

Symptoms of neuropathy include numbness, tingling, burning or pain in the hands or feet, difficulty with balance, and loss of feeling. Neuropathy can also weaken the foot's muscles and shorten its tendons, which can change the shape of your foot.

Blood Vessel Disease

Poor blood flow to feet and wounds that don't heal can lead to major foot problems

Healthy blood vessels help keep your feet warm and healthy, heal wounds, and fight off infection. Blood vessels expand and contract in response to the body's needs. For instance, if your feet are cold, your blood vessels contract. If your feet are warm or need extra blood to heal a wound, your blood vessels expand.

Damaged blood vessels become hardened and lose their ability to expand and contract, resulting in poor blood flow to the feet. Symptoms of poor blood flow include leg pain while at rest or at night, pain in the calf while walking that goes away at rest, wounds that don't heal, and feet that are cold to the touch.

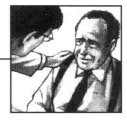

Sometimes the blood vessels that carry blood to the foot are alright, but the smaller vessels within the foot are damaged. This reduces the amount of oxygen and nutrients that reach the cells in the feet, and may cause poor healing of a wound or contribute to infection.

Infection

The white blood cells of the body attack germs to help fight infections. High blood glucose levels prevent those white blood cells from doing their job. As a result, wounds take longer to heal and small infections can become big problems.

If a wound isn't healing because of poor blood supply, it may spread through the foot and even into the bone. The infected tissue kills healthy tissue around it, causing gangrene, which is a Greek word for "gnawing death of tissue." Gangrene is hard to treat and sometimes results in amputation of the foot, lower leg, or other affected areas.

Good foot care can help prevent the problems that may lead to amputation. Good diabetes care, especially good control of blood glucose, is essential to keeping your feet healthy. So is awareness of common foot problems that may turn into major complications if not detected and treated properly.

COMMON FOOT PROBLEMS

Many common foot problems that are no big deal to people without diabetes can be a great threat to people with diabetes. Because of poor blood flow or loss of feeling in the feet, a minor injury or problem (such as ingrown nails, blisters, calluses, corns, or athlete's foot) can escalate into a severe one. Keep in mind that any foot injury can be the beginning of a serious problem and needs to be brought to the attention of a *podiatrist* (foot specialist) or your health care team immediately.

Corns, Calluses, and Blisters

Corns and calluses are thickenings of the outer layer of skin caused by repeated rubbing and pressure on the same area of the foot. If not properly treated, corns or calluses may act like a stone in the shoe, putting constant pressure on the sensitive tissue and causing it to become injured or bruised.

Such an injury may cause an ulcer or sore, which can become infected. Often the infection may not be seen because the callus or corn is covering it

269

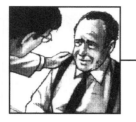

and may not be felt because of nerve damage. Fluid draining from the corn or callus may be the first sign of a problem. This must be treated immediately by a podiatrist or your health care team.

Blisters are formed when shoes rub and irritate the skin. Do not try to pop or drain a blister; this would allow germs to enter and an infection could develop. Wash the area gently and protect it from further irritation. If the blister seems to heal slowly or becomes inflamed, contact your health care team promptly.

Ingrown Nails

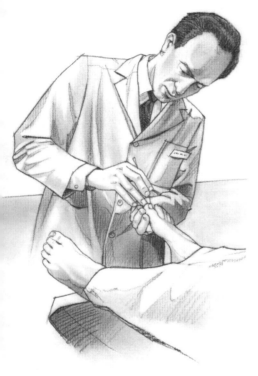

An ingrown nail is an edge or border of the nail that cuts into the skin next to it. It can be caused by injury, improper nail trimming, "bathroom surgery," curved nails, and poorly fitting shoes.

An ingrown nail may be painful, red, or swollen or drain fluid. It can become infected easily and needs to be treated immediately. Your podiatrist or health care team can take care of this by removing part of the nail and prescribing antibiotics to prevent or treat related infection.

Cracked Skin and Athlete's Foot

Nerve damage can cause your skin to become dry and cracked. Cracks give bacteria a place to enter, and a serious infection may develop. Dry, cracked skin can be treated with lotions.

Athlete's foot is a fungal infection that is usually found between the toes and may spread to the toenails. Symptoms include cracking and peeling of skin between the toes and/or bottoms of the feet, pain, itching and/or bleeding between the toes, and thickening and crumbling of the toenails. Careful washing of the feet and drying between the toes can help prevent athlete's foot. Your health care team may prescribe a lotion or powder to heal the infection.

Plantar Warts

Plantar warts are caused by viruses and may be very hard to get rid of. They occur on the bottom of the foot and may look like a circular callus. Do not use commercial wart removers to treat the wart unless your health care team tells you to—they may prescribe other medications.

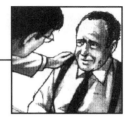

Bunions and Hammertoes

Bunions are enlargements of the joint at the base of the big toe and are usually inherited. Wearing shoes with a wide toe area can help prevent irritation of the skin surrounding the bunion. Sometimes surgery is necessary to remove the extra bone.

Hammertoes are formed when muscles in the foot become weakened and the tendons shortened, causing the toes to buckle under. This may be inherited, but it can be caused by neuropathy or wearing shoes that are too short. Shoes with a large toe area help prevent corns from forming on tops of hammertoes. Sometimes surgery is necessary to realign the bones.

CARING FOR YOUR FEET

As you can see, it's a good idea to take care of your feet. Be sure to exercise. For instance, walking is a good, safe way to stay in shape and improve blood flow. But be careful of calluses or foot injuries and wear proper-fitting shoes and socks. It is most important to develop an effective program of foot care based on:

- prevention
- early identification of problems
- prompt treatment
- proper daily foot care

Prevention

Prevention of foot trouble begins with good health habits. For people with diabetes this means, first and foremost, maintaining normal levels of blood glucose and blood fats (cholesterol and triglycerides). It also means not smoking, because nicotine causes blood vessels to become smaller, which decreases blood flow to your feet.

Prevention also means being aware of the risk factors for developing foot problems. Foot problems have a greater risk for developing in people with diabetes than in people without diabetes. For instance, the risk increases if you:

- are over age 40
- are overweight
- have had diabetes for more than ten years
- have poor circulation or loss of feeling in your feet or hands

271

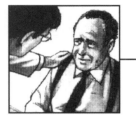

- have had changes in the shape of your feet, such as bunions, or hammertoes, or because of arthritis
- have already had foot infections or an amputation

You can't do anything about your age or the length of time you've had diabetes. But you can control your blood glucose levels and quit smoking. The more you're at risk, the more important it is to take steps to prevent problems with your feet. Remember the following important "don'ts":

1. Don't soak your feet routinely. Soaking dries and cracks your skin, inviting infection.
2. Don't smoke. Smoking decreases circulation and can worsen foot problems.
3. Don't expose your feet to extremes of hot or cold. Be sure to test the temperature of bath or shower water with your wrist or elbow before stepping in.
4. Don't use hot water bottles, heating pads, or electric blankets. They could easily burn your feet.
5. Don't use commercial wart or corn removers. They can damage your skin.
6. Don't wear tight shoes or stockings. They can restrict blood flow and create pressure on the lower legs and feet.
7. Don't go barefoot, even in the house.

Early Identification

The best thing you can do for your feet is give them a lot of attention. Daily inspection is the key to early identification of foot problems. Examine the skin between and on the bottom of your toes. Look for signs of cracking, peeling, redness, or irritation. If you can't see the bottoms of your feet, use a mirror. Look for sores, blisters, drainage, or redness, all of which might indicate infection.

Watch for changes in the shape of your foot, which can be caused by weak muscles or shortened tendons due to diabetes-related nerve damage. Check carefully every day for corns, calluses, ingrown toenails, ulcers, cracks, or injuries. These can become infection points.

Don't try to "doctor" your foot problems with sharp instruments, pumice stones, or commercial corn or wart removers. They can make matters worse. Leave the doctoring to your health care team. When you see a problem developing, get prompt professional help. That's the third major step in preventive foot care.

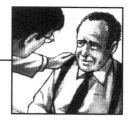

Prompt Treatment

Treat minor injuries promptly. Clean the area with mild soap and water, and dry thoroughly. Apply an antibiotic cream, such as Bacitracin, and cover with clean gauze. Check the area at least once a day.

Even if your feet feel fine, make it a point to have them examined every few months by a specialist who understands the relationship between diabetes and foot problems. Remember, the cost of an examination is much smaller than the cost of losing a foot. Your podiatrist or health care team will work with you to plan your personal foot care program. With daily care, you can prevent foot problems.

Daily Foot Care

At home, foot care should be part of your daily routine.

Cleansing. Wash your feet every day in your bathtub or shower using warm water and mild soap. Dry them gently with a soft towel. Then let them air dry before putting on socks and shoes. Don't soak your feet regularly. Soaking removes natural oils from your skin, drying it out and causing it to crack.

Lotions. If your feet are dry or cracking, moisten the skin with an emollient lotion, such as Aquacare, Carmol-10, Eucerin, Atrac-tain, or a product recommended by your podiatrist or health care team. Be sure to leave the area between your toes dry to prevent fungal infection.

Nail Care. Keep your toenails cut straight across, using a long-handled toenail clipper. Do not cut the nails shorter than the ends of your toes or cut into the corners. If nails are cut too short you may accidentally injure the skin around the nails. If necessary, smooth the rough edges gently with a cardboard emery board. A metal file has sharp edges that could injure the skin. Have excessively thick or brittle nails treated by a podiatrist. If you need help with ingrown or other problem toenails, see your podiatrist or health care team.

Footwear. Finally, shoes that fit well can help prevent many foot problems, such as corns, calluses, ingrown nails, blisters, and ulcers. A roomy, well-made walking or athletic shoe is best. When buying shoes, look for:

- *soft leather uppers* that will mold to your foot and allow it to breath
- *soft insole and inner lining*, without rough areas or thick seams that can irritate your skin
- *a firm sole* to encourage a "rocking" walk that helps lessen pressure on the balls of your feet

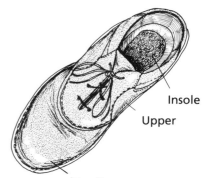

Insole

Upper

Toe Box

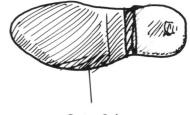

Outer Sole

273

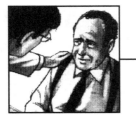

- *a wide toe box* that allows your toes to wiggle around. Avoid narrow or pointed styles that can cause corns and calluses
- *enough length* to allow a half inch beyond your longest toe when standing

Don't wear the same shoes every day. Try to alternate shoes every other day. Remember to wear the correct shoe for each activity.

Choose your socks carefully, too. Wear thin, soft cotton or wool-blend socks that cushion your feet and protect them from pressure. Avoid socks with seams, creases, or elastic bands that may reduce circulation. You may find that cotton-soled nylons help control excess perspiration. Wearing cotton footlets inside the stockings also works well.

SUMMARY

With a few minutes of care each day, you can help prevent foot problems from occurring or turning into serious complications. By knowing how diabetes affects the feet and by taking the proper precautions, you'll be well on your way to keeping your feet for life.

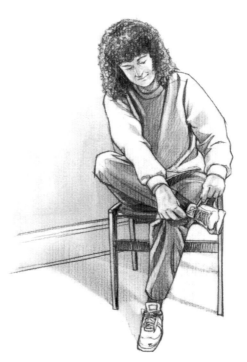

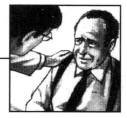

WHAT YOU CAN DO

1. Check your blood glucose regularly and maintain normal levels of blood glucose and blood fats.
2. Check your feet daily.
3. Wear well-made, well-fitting shoes.
4. See your health care team every three to four months. Have your feet examined at every visit. Taking off your shoes and socks will remind them to check your feet.
5. Call your health care team or podiatrist immediately if you see any sign of infection (redness, swelling, drainage, warmth) or if you have any problems or questions.

WHAT YOUR HEALTH CARE TEAM CAN DO

1. Help you maintain normal levels of blood glucose and blood fats and reduce other risk factors for foot problems.
2. Advise you in selecting proper, safe shoes.
3. Teach you how to care for your feet and prevent minor problems from becoming serious.
4. Examine your feet at every visit and ask you about any foot problems you've had as well as any leg pain when you stand, sit, or walk.
5. Check the blood flow to your feet and test your ability to feel light touch or other sensations in your feet and legs. If you have poor blood flow or sensitive areas, advise you how to avoid injury and what to look for during daily checks of the affected areas.

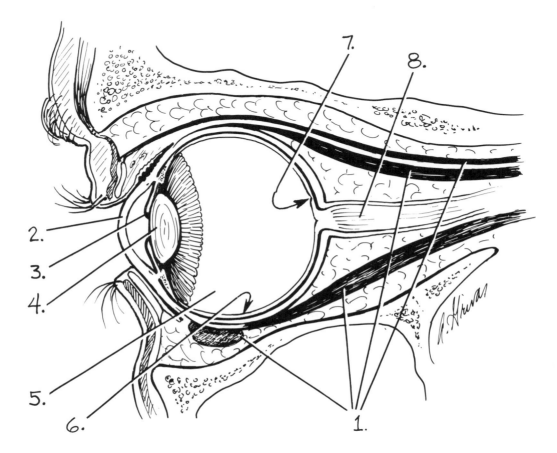

PARTS OF THE EYE
1. Eye muscles
2. Cornea
3. Iris
4. Lens
5. Vitreous
6. Retina
7. Macula
8. Optic nerve

CHAPTER 19

William J. Mestrezat, MD

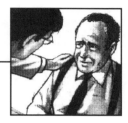

Eye Problems:
Improving the Outlook by Early Detection

How often should I have my eyes examined?

Why is it important to see an ophthalmologist?

What is laser treatment?

Eye disease is one of the most serious complications of diabetes. It is a major cause of blindness in people between the ages of 20 and 74, and it is the reason 50,000 Americans are legally blind. However, there is now evidence that new eye treatment methods and good diabetes control can greatly improve these statistics and the outlook for people with diabetes. This chapter discusses eye problems caused by diabetes and provides the latest information on prevention, early detection, and timely and effective treatment.

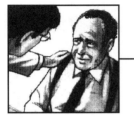

If you have Type I or Type II diabetes, it's very important to have your eyes examined regularly. Eye problems can develop after about five years in Type I diabetes and at any time in Type II diabetes.

The statistics may be frightening, but remember that they include people who've had diabetes for the last 20 to 30 years. Until recently, these people did not have the latest treatment methods available to them.

Today the outlook is better. New treatment methods can help eye disease in its early stages. Doctors that are trained to detect changes in the eyes of people with diabetes can provide annual check-ups. Your health care team may refer you to an ophthalmologist, who is a specialist in diseases of the eye. This doctor will set up a regular schedule of appointments and advise you on how to prevent eye problems from developing.

HOW DIABETES AFFECTS THE EYES

Diabetes can affect all parts of the eye. But to understand these problems, you first need to understand the parts of the eye (lens, eye muscles, cornea, vitreous, and retina) and their functions. The chart below provides terms and definitions to help you.

Cornea: clear window in front of the eye that lets light enter

Eye Muscles: turn eyes in various directions to look at objects

Iris: colored part of the eye that acts like the opening on a camera and adjusts the amount of light entering the eye through the pupil

Lens: focuses light onto the retina

Macula: a small area at the center of the retina onto which light rays are focused

Optic Nerve: carries picture from the retina to the brain by means of electrical impulses

Retina: inner lining at the back of the eye that develops a picture through a chemical reaction and sends it along the optic nerve to the brain for interpretation

Vitreous: clear jelly-like substance that fills the inside of the eye and is loosely attached to the entire surface of the retina

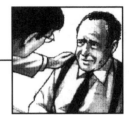

Refer to the eye diagram as you read about each part of the eye and how diabetes can affect it.

THE LENS

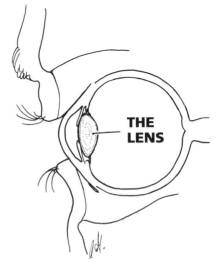

The lens of the eye focuses light onto the retina so images can be seen clearly. Blurred vision is one of the most common eye problems caused by diabetes. It sometimes occurs with changes in blood glucose level, especially during times of poor control. When blood glucose levels rise, the lens takes in glucose and water, causing it to swell. Because of the swelling, light rays can no longer be focused on the retina and vision is blurry. After several weeks of high blood glucose levels, the lens returns to its normal shape and vision improves. When blood glucose falls, the lens shrinks, again blurring vision.

Blurred vision from lens changes will correct itself in two to six weeks. Treatment consists of controlling and stabilizing the blood glucose level. Glasses should not be prescribed during these episodes because they may not be needed when the lens stabilizes.

Cataracts are a more serious problem involving the lens. Normally the lens is clear, allowing light rays to pass through it. Cataracts are areas in the lens that block or change the direction of light rays. This blurs vision and sometimes causes glare.

Cataracts are more common and occur at an earlier age in people with diabetes. If a cataract is caught early enough it is sometimes reversible with good blood glucose control. But if a cataract progresses to the point that vision is significantly impaired, surgery is the only effective therapy.

THE EYE MUSCLES

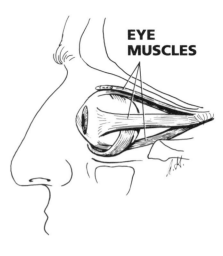

Each eye has six muscles that work together to turn the eye in all directions. The muscles are controlled by nerves coming directly from the brain. These nerves can be affected by diabetes just like any other nerve in the body. When this happens, the affected nerve stops turning the eye normally and, depending on which nerves are affected, different directions of gaze are lost.

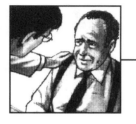

The major symptom of eye muscle problems is double vision, especially when looking in certain directions. There may also be severe pain. People with this problem should have a complete neurological examination to make sure the double vision is caused by diabetes and not some other problem. If this examination is normal, no treatment is needed. The double vision almost always goes away in four to eight weeks and usually does not recur. A patch can be worn over one eye until the problem clears.

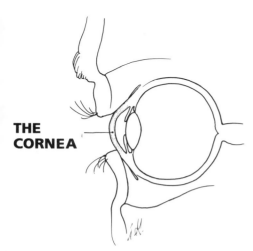

THE CORNEA

THE CORNEA: WINDOW OF THE EYE

The cornea is a clear window in front of the eye that lets light enter. In people who've had diabetes for many years, the cells on the front surface of the cornea are not as well attached to the underlying cells as they are normally. As a result, these surface cells can come off with minor force, such as rubbing the eyes hard. Loss of these cells is called *corneal erosion*. People who have problems with corneal erosion could have great difficulty wearing contact lenses. This is seldom a problem for people who have had diabetes for only a few years.

Symptoms of corneal erosion include pain (usually severe), sensitivity to light, and excessive production of tears. The treatment consists of wearing a tight patch over the eye, use of antibiotic drops or ointments, and frequent follow-up visits to the eye doctor. Corneal erosion can heal slowly and can become infected.

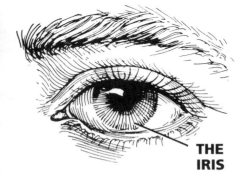

THE IRIS

THE IRIS

The iris is the colored part of the eye that acts like the opening on a camera to adjust the amount of light entering the eye through the pupil. Diabetes can cause abnormal blood vessels to form on the iris, which can cause a severe form of glaucoma. There are no symptoms of this condition until it produces very high pressure in the eye, causing pain and blurry vision.

Abnormal blood vessels on the iris are often discovered before they can grow to the point of causing high pressure in the eye. In that case they can be treated using a laser method, which will be described in the section about retinal problems. If glaucoma develops, special eye drops and medications can be used to lower the eye pressure. Sometimes surgery is needed if the medications and laser treatments do not control the problem.

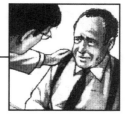

THE RETINA

The retina is the inner lining of the back of eye that develops a picture through a chemical reaction and sends it along the optic nerve to the brain for interpretation. Problems with the retina are called *retinopathy*. They are potentially the most serious eye problems caused by diabetes.

The first problem that usually occurs in the retina starts when the smallest blood vessels, or capillaries, become plugged. As a result, other blood vessels widen and leak. This is called *background diabetic retinopathy*. As the vessels continue to leak blood, fluids, and fat, the retina becomes wet and its ability to receive images is hurt. At least mild forms of these changes can be seen in the eyes of 80% of people who have had either Type I or Type II diabetes for 25 years. These changes may not cause any symptoms and they may not get any worse.

Background retinopathy usually does not cause significant loss of vision unless there is leakage into the macula, the area of the retina used for detailed vision. Such leakage can cause swelling of the macula, or *macular edema*. This is the most common cause of blurred vision from diabetes. It may go away when high blood glucose and/or blood pressure levels return to normal, or it may need to be treated with laser therapy.

Background retinopathy is diagnosed by looking into the eyes with an ophthalmoscope. Occasionally, it's necessary to take a special series of photographs called a *fluorescein angiogram*. This is the best way to study the blood vessels of the retina and show plugged-up capillaries and the exact location of leakage (if there is any). The fluorescein angiogram is done by injecting a special dye into the arm, which circulates to the eye. The photographs are taken over a 15-minute period.

Treatment of retinopathy involves several considerations. First, it's commonly believed that good diabetes control helps prevent retinal problems and, if they do occur, slows the progression. High blood pressure and kidney disease are known to make retinopathy worse, so it's important that they are treated.

If specific areas of retinal blood vessel leakage are detected and if they are threatening significant loss of vision, laser treatments are used. The laser is a highly concentrated beam of light produced by electrically charging either argon or krypton gas. The beam of light is bounced back and forth between mirrors until it is extremely intense. An ophthalmologist aims the beam by looking through a special microscope-like viewer and releases brief pulses of laser light to burn tiny areas of the blood vessel. This seals the blood vessel so the retina can dry itself and function normally. Laser

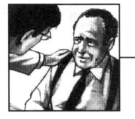

treatments are usually done in an ophthalmologist's office once the eyes are dilated. The treatments take only a few minutes and can usually be done with minimal, if any, eye discomfort.

A large national study conducted by the National Institutes of Health, called "The Early Treatment of Diabetic Retinopathy Study," showed that laser treatment for macular edema reduces the chance for vision loss by half. The study also showed that laser treatments are better at keeping vision from worsening than they are at restoring vision, so it's important to catch conditions early, before they cause significant vision loss. Sometimes laser therapy done while the vision is still excellent will keep it that way.

If background retinopathy worsens and is not controlled, it can result in what is called *proliferative retinopathy*. This is when abnormal blood vessels form in the retina in response to the loss of capillaries. The abnormal blood vessels bleed easily and can cause large eye hemorrhages and severe loss of vision. This is usually seen in people who've had diabetes for more than 20 years. The abnormal blood vessels show no symptoms until they bleed.

Controlling medical problems such as high blood pressure and kidney disease is important for people who have proliferative retinopathy. Laser treatments need to be done in most of these patients because of the great risk for eye hemorrhage. The laser treatments destroy the areas of capillary loss, which reduces the formation of abnormal blood vessels. After laser treatment, the abnormal blood vessels usually shrink or go away.

THE VITREOUS

The vitreous is a clear, jelly-like substance that fills the inside of the eye and is loosely attached to the entire surface of the retina. When abnormal retinal blood vessels bleed, they bleed into the vitreous. Symptoms vary from dark floating spots in the vision field to almost total darkness, depending on the amount of bleeding.

Most vitreous hemorrhages clear on their own, although it can take months. Limited activity and sleeping with the head elevated on two to three pillows are important so that the blood will settle to the bottom of the eye, where it will not affect vision. It is then absorbed gradually by the body. When the blood has cleared enough so the retina is visible, laser treatment is usually begun.

If the blood still affects vision after it has been given a reasonable chance to clear on its own, surgery is usually performed. This procedure is

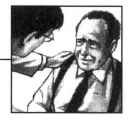

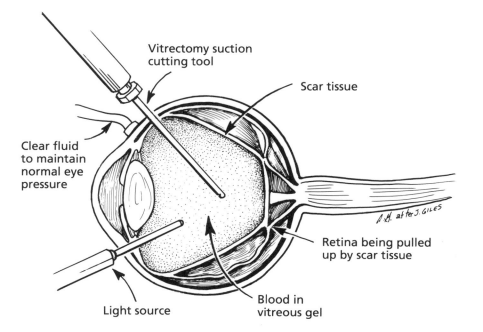

Vitrectomy suction cutting tool

Scar tissue

Clear fluid to maintain normal eye pressure

A.A. after J. GILES

Retina being pulled up by scar tissue

Light source

Blood in vitreous gel

With a vitrectomy, blood and vitreous are removed with specially designed instruments

called a *vitrectomy*. The blood and vitreous are removed with specially designed instruments using an operating room microscope. The vitreous is replaced with a saltwater solution that is made to be as close to normal eye fluid as possible.

Normally, the vitreous is loosely attached to the retina. In people with diabetes, this adhesion can become strong. The vitreous can form scar-like bands that pull on the retina and cause it to detach. This is called *traction retinal detachment*. The detached part of the retina does not function because it loses part of its blood supply. Blurry vision occurs when the macula is detached, but if the macula is not detached there are usually no symptoms.

Many people who have traction retinal detachments also have vitreous hemorrhages. The blood in the vitreous makes it impossible to tell with an ophthalmoscope whether there is a traction retinal detachment. An ultrasound test is a painless office procedure that sends sound waves through the blood in the eye to give a picture of the back of the eye. It can show whether a traction retinal detachment is present behind the vitreous blood.

Traction retinal detachments are repaired by first doing a vitrectomy. Special small scissors are then inserted into the eye and the traction bands are cut. When the traction is relieved, the retina reattaches itself and usually starts to function again.

283

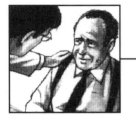

SUMMARY

Diabetes can cause serious problems in all parts of the eye, but only a small percentage of people with diabetes experience serious complications. Temporary vision problems can be caused by changes in blood glucose levels; however, these changes do not always progress to loss of vision.

It's hoped that good blood glucose control and control of other medical problems, such as high blood pressure, can prevent serious eye problems from developing. Since problems can be present in eyes with good vision, it's important to have regular eye examinations even if vision is normal. The key to prevention, early detection, and timely and effective treatment is to have your eyes examined regularly by a doctor who is trained to detect eye changes related to diabetes. Remember, YOU are the most important person caring for your diabetes. Your actions and those of your doctor may save your vision.

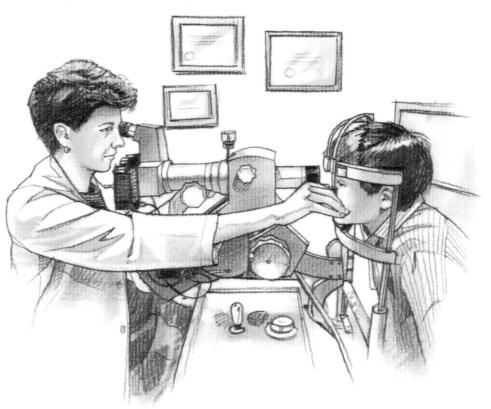

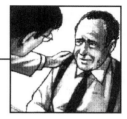

WHAT YOU CAN DO

1. Maintain good control of your blood glucose levels, testing your blood several times a day to make sure it is as close to normal as possible. Contact your health care team if blood glucose levels are high or low and you cannot control them.

2. See your health care team regularly—at least four times a year or more often if problems occur.

3. Have your vision checked and your eyes dilated and examined at least once a year by a doctor trained to detect diabetic eye changes.

4. See an ophthalmologist promptly if eye changes are detected.

5. Don't smoke.

WHAT YOUR HEALTH CARE TEAM CAN DO

1. Ask if you have any vision problems at each visit.

2. Put drops in your eyes and examine them at least once a year.

3. Have you read an eye chart at least once a year.

4. Check your blood pressure at each visit and if it is high, start treatment right away.

5. Have you see an ophthalmologist at least once a year if you have had Type I diabetes for more than five years or if you have Type II diabetes.

6. If changes are found in your eyes, have you see an ophthalmologist who is experienced in detecting and treating diabetic retinopathy.

Glomeruli are closely packed small blood vessels in the kidney that can be damaged by diabetes

Glomerulus

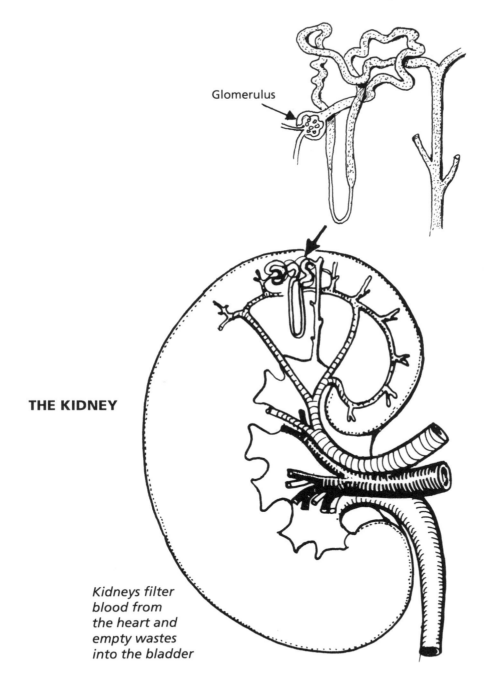

THE KIDNEY

Kidneys filter blood from the heart and empty wastes into the bladder

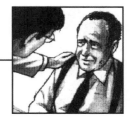

CHAPTER 20

Donald A. Duncan, MD

Kidney Problems:
Using the Prevention and Treatment Threesome

How can diabetes cause kidney damage?

What can be done to prevent it?

How is kidney disease treated?

Kidney disease is another of the more serious problems caused by diabetes. If not detected early and treated promptly, it can lead to kidney failure or even death. Fortunately, a great deal of research is underway to find the causes and improve the treatment of kidney disease. This chapter discusses how kidney disease develops and progresses as a result of diabetes, and how it can be prevented and treated using a three-pronged approach—control of blood glucose, prevention of high blood pressure, and reduction of protein in the diet.

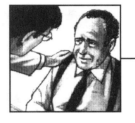

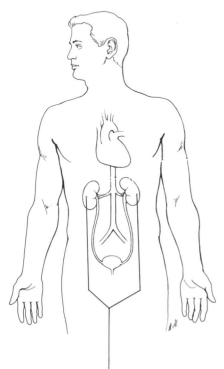

Kidneys filter blood from the heart and empty wastes into the bladder

In the United States today, between 25 and 30% of persons starting chronic dialysis or receiving a kidney transplant need these forms of treatment because of kidney disease caused by diabetes. Over the years, considerable progress has been made in helping prevent or delay the development of kidney disease and in treating it if it does develop. Hopefully, this will result in a much lower incidence of kidney failure in people who have diabetes.

HOW KIDNEY DAMAGE OCCURS

The kidneys are two organs located in the lower back, near the spine and in front of the lowest ribs. Each is filled with about one million tiny clumps of very closely packed small blood vessels called *glomeruli*. Their job is to filter waste products from the blood and make urine.

Diabetes can harden and narrow the arteries (arteriosclerosis) that supply the kidneys. It also can damage the glomeruli. The glomeruli become scarred and blocked and can no longer effectively filter waste products from the blood. This causes *uremia*, which means "urine in the blood."

There is considerable evidence that high blood glucose plays a significant role in damaging the glomeruli. However, it's not known why some people with diabetes are more susceptible than others to kidney damage as a result of high blood glucose levels.

SYMPTOMS AND SIGNS OF KIDNEY DISEASE

Kidney damage develops very gradually. If it's going to occur, kidney failure usually begins 15 to 20 years after the diagnosis of diabetes. If symptoms are detected early enough, progression can be slowed in most cases. Then several more years may pass before total kidney failure occurs. These large amounts of time can be used to do everything possible to reduce the extent of kidney damage. It's often necessary to work with a kidney disease specialist to get the best results.

Usually the first indication of kidney disease is *proteinuria*, or the appearance of protein (mostly albumin) in the urine. The protein, which we all carry in our blood, leaks through the damaged glomeruli and appears in the urine. It's detected during a routine urine test. The presence

288

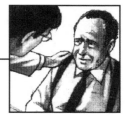

of albumin in the urine causes no discomfort, and a person is not aware of its presence unless the urine is tested.

As the amount of albumin lost into the urine increases, the level of albumin in the blood falls below the normal range of 3.5 to 5.0 gm/100 ml. Then some of the water in the blood vessels seeps out into the skin to produce a swelling called *edema* (your grandparents called it dropsy). After a person has been lying down all night, the eyes, face, and hands become swollen. After being in an upright position all day, the fluid moves downward to cause swelling of the legs and feet. Other diseases, such as heart failure, can also produce edema.

A combination of high protein levels in the urine, low blood albumin levels, edema, and an associated increase in blood fat levels is characteristic of a kidney disorder known as *nephrosis*. Diabetes causes but one of the several types of kidney disease that can result in nephrosis.

As damage to the glomeruli continues, uremia develops. The first symptoms of uremia are weakness, loss of appetite, nausea, and then vomiting. Uremia is diagnosed when a blood sample shows the presence of larger amounts of the waste products that the kidney normally gets rid of. The two waste products usually measured are urea (often expressed as BUN, or blood urea nitrogen) and creatinine. Normal values are 5 to 25 mg/100 ml of serum for BUN and 0.5 to 1.5 mg/100 ml of serum for creatinine.

As the uremia progresses, other symptoms occur. These include itching, easy bleeding, and mental confusion. When more than 95% of both kidneys are destroyed, death will occur unless the person is treated with an artificial kidney machine or peritoneal dialysis or given a kidney transplant.

Kidney disease in diabetes is complicated by high blood pressure (hypertension). At first it produces no symptoms to make the person aware of its presence, but it may be detected during a physical examination. Usually it occurs about the time protein appears in the urine. Only when blood pressure is very high does it cause symptoms such as headache, shortness of breath, visual disturbances, dizziness, or even stroke.

The combination of narrowed arteries and blocked glomeruli causes high blood pressure in the great majority of people with diabetes who have kidney disease. In turn, high blood pressure causes more damage to the smallest arteries (arterioles) in the kidneys. This speeds the loss of kidney function.

Infection is another contributing factor to kidney disease in diabetes. The bladder and kidneys of people with diabetes seem to be more prone to invasion by bacteria than those of people who do not have diabetes. A bladder infection usually produces an urge to urinate frequently. Often this is every 15 to 30 minutes. Urination may be painful, and sometimes the urine is bloody. An infection of one or both kidneys produces back pain near the lowest ribs, chills, high fever, and often cloudy urine.

289

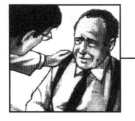

PREVENTION AND TREATMENT

Considerable research in recent years suggests that good blood glucose control prevents, or at least slows, the development of kidney disease. This is understandable, since much of the damage to the glomeruli appears to result from excessive glucose in the blood attaching to the protein-containing structures in the glomeruli. Several studies have suggested that good blood glucose control may reverse the very earliest stages of proteinuria (albumin in the urine). Once kidney disease becomes more evident with development of greater proteinuria and uremia, it unfortunately is too late for good blood glucose control to reverse the process. The best we can hope for then is that better control will at least slow down the progression of kidney disease. There is no specific drug available to heal kidney disease in diabetes.

Prevention or control of high blood pressure definitely decreases damage to the small arteries in the kidneys. Today many excellent drugs are available for the treatment of high blood pressure. One group, called ACE (angiotensin converting enzyme) inhibitors, appears to be of special value to people with diabetes. Also, control of kidney infections through the use of antibiotics or sulfa preparations preserves kidney function.

As kidney disease progresses, certain dietary changes become necessary. Restricting salt (sodium chloride) in the diet reduces both blood pressure and the amount of fluid retained by the body. Drugs that increase urination (diuretics) also can be used to help eliminate excess fluid from the body.

When the kidneys begin to fail and waste products (such as urea and creatinine) accumulate in the blood, it's helpful to decrease the amount of protein in the diet. This decreases the formation of those waste products, which helps decrease the person's nausea, vomiting, and weakness. Also, studies suggest that in addition to making the person feel better, a low-protein diet actually slows the progression of kidney disease itself. Most people eat 80 to 100 grams of protein daily. In the presence of kidney failure plus nephrosis and the loss of large amounts of protein in the urine, protein intake is reduced to about 60 grams per day. In the presence of kidney failure without nephrosis, protein intake is reduced to as low as 40 grams per day.

Generally, the daily insulin dose decreases as kidney failure develops. This is caused both by weight loss as a result of poor appetite and by a prolonging of insulin action time, which occurs with uremia.

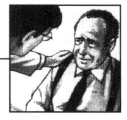

DIALYSIS

Dialysis, the artificial filtration of waste products from the blood, becomes necessary when approximately 90% of total kidney function is lost. Dialysis does not cure kidney disease, but it does prevent death from uremia. Two methods of dialysis are available: *hemodialysis* (use of an artificial kidney machine) and *peritoneal dialysis* (filtering through a tube inserted into the abdomen).

In hemodialysis, blood flows from a person's arm through a plastic tube to a filtering device called the dialyzer. The dialyzer removes the waste products from the blood and returns the "cleaned" blood to the person. Most people undergo hemodialysis treatments for three to four hours three times each week.

In peritoneal dialysis, a plastic tube (catheter) is surgically inserted through the abdominal wall into the peritoneal cavity. The peritoneal cavity is the space enclosed by the peritoneum, a thin membrane that lines the abdominal wall and intestinal tract. The peritoneum then acts as a filtering surface through which waste products in the blood can pass. A procedure often used today is CAPD, or continuous ambulatory peritoneal dialysis. In this procedure a person runs two liters of a specially prepared salt solution (dialysate) into his or her abdominal cavity, leaves the solution in for four to six hours, then drains it out. This is done four times a day, seven days a week.

Whether hemodialysis or peritoneal dialysis is used is a matter of personal preference. Both methods accomplish the same purpose, which is to remove the waste products of uremia from the blood.

It is usually recommended that dialysis be started when the remaining kidney function is about 10% of normal. Waiting until less than 10% of kidney function remains increases the risk of advanced eye disease, which often is associated with advanced kidney failure in persons with diabetes.

TRANSPLANTATION

Today, the most satisfactory approach to treating end-stage kidney failure in persons with diabetes is to replace (transplant) the diseased kidneys with a healthy human kidney. This is especially true for the person who loses kidney function before the age of 65. Older people often do better staying on dialysis. Most people are first treated with dialysis. Then, after their

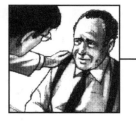

condition has been stabilized, they are considered for a transplant.

The diseased kidneys are usually left in place unless they are infected or are causing severe hypertension that cannot be controlled with drugs. The transplanted kidney is added as a third kidney. It is placed in the lower abdomen on one side of the urinary bladder.

Transplant patients must take anti-rejection drugs for the remainder of their lives. A person is less likely to reject the kidney if it comes from a living family member (related donor transplant) than if it comes from a deceased unrelated donor (cadaver transplant). However, recent figures from the University of Minnesota show that even when the kidney is received from an unrelated donor, 80% of transplant patients still have their new kidneys functioning well two years later. The likelihood of rejection of the transplanted kidney decreases considerably after the first two years. Some people with diabetes have kept their transplanted kidneys for more than 15 years and continue to do well.

If a transplanted kidney is rejected, a person fortunately can return to dialysis and then receive a second or even a third transplant. Unfortunately, after many years a transplanted kidney may develop the same disease that destroyed the original kidneys. Pancreas transplants appear to be one answer to this problem. Although still considered experimental by some, the success rate of pancreas transplants is improving rapidly. Already evidence suggests that a successful pancreas transplant prevents recurrence of damage in the newly transplanted kidney if blood glucose levels are kept as near normal as possible 24 hours a day.

SUMMARY

To reduce the risk for kidney disease, people with diabetes should do everything possible to control blood glucose levels and prevent high blood pressure. Once kidney disease develops, reducing protein in the diet can also be helpful. Considerable progress has been made in helping people with diabetes prevent or delay the development of kidney disease and in treating it if it does develop. Present research should result in even more progress in the very near future.

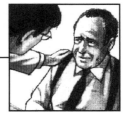

WHAT YOU CAN DO

1. Ask you health care team about the health of your kidneys.
2. Work with your health care team to control your diabetes and keep blood glucose levels as close to normal as possible.
3. Guard against high blood pressure by lowering salt intake, maintaining a healthy weight, and exercising regularly. Have high blood pressure treated right away if repeated measurements show pressures of 140/90 or higher.
4. If kidney problems develop, decrease protein in your diet.
5. Be on the lookout for kidney infections (manifested by an urge to urinate frequently, painful urination, or mid-back pain associated with fever). Infections should be treated promptly.

WHAT YOUR HEALTH CARE TEAM CAN DO

1. Talk to you about how diabetes and kidney damage are related.
2. Help you learn to test your blood glucose and keep levels as close to normal as possible.
3. Check your blood pressure at each visit and suggest ways you can prevent or treat high blood pressure.
4. Check a urine sample at least once a year for early signs of kidney damage. A blood sample can be checked if signs of possible kidney damage are found.
5. Ask you about symptoms of kidney and urinary infections.
6. Refer you to a specialist if kidney damage develops.
7. Refer you to a dietitian for advise on salt and protein restriction.

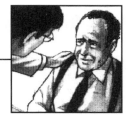

CHAPTER 21

Clyde E. Blackard, MD
Joe Nelson, MA, LP
Janet Swenson Lima, RN, MPH
Ellie Strock, RN, C, CDE

Sexual Problems:
Communicating and Seeking Help

Should someone over age 50 still be interested in sex or should I just let it go?

If I have trouble with erections, does it mean I have a deep-seeded psychological problem?

What is impotence, and what treatments are available?

When people begin to experience problems with their sexuality they sometimes have trouble asking for help, especially if they've been unable to express themselves well before. This chapter is designed to provide you with some answers to questions you might have regarding your sexuality and difficulties you might be experiencing. It's also designed to encourage you to seek the help you might need to resolve a problem. If nothing else, let this chapter reassure you that your interest in your sexuality is a normal and healthy part of your functioning, as it is for all human beings.

295

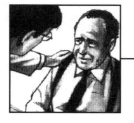

Our sexuality is an extremely important part of who we are, from the time we are born until the day we die. It's really a part of us to be cherished and enjoyed rather than to be ashamed of and avoided. If you're worried that someone might catch you reading this chapter, rest assured that many, many people join you in the concern you have about your sexuality.

NORMAL SEXUAL FUNCTIONING

When a man is sexually excited, signals pass from the brain, along the spinal cord, to the nerves and blood vessels in the penis. The arteries and spongy tissue inside the penis dilate with blood and the penis expands, causing an erection. Normally, this expanded and enlarged penis can be inserted into the vagina. But problems at any stage in the process can result in impotence.

As you can see from the description of normal sexual functioning, it's amazing that we're able to function as well as we do. The need for cooperation among nerves, blood vessels, and psychological functioning helps us understand why diabetes can have an impact on sexual functioning. Several major sexual dysfunctions are associated with diabetes. For women, those dysfunctions seem to be associated with nerve damage that causes difficulty with lubrication and/or difficulty reaching orgasm because of decreased nerve sensitivity. For men, the two primary dysfunctions are retrograde ejaculation (the inability to ejaculate despite having an orgasm) and impotence.

These disorders can be quite distressing. They can create strains in relationships and for the person experiencing the problem. However, of the sexual disorders associated with diabetes, impotence is by far the most common and certainly the most studied. So, for practical purposes, this chapter will focus on impotence.

It's important to note that having diabetes and a problem with impotence doesn't necessarily mean the two are related. It's also important to note that the three problems outlined above are not the only sexual dysfunctions a person with diabetes can experience. If you're having some difficulty with anything about your sexual functioning, be sure to get an evaluation to determine exactly what the problem is, what's causing it, and what you can do about it.

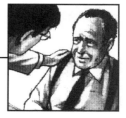

IMPOTENCE

Impotence is defined as the inability to achieve and maintain an erection adequate for vaginal penetration to the mutual satisfaction of both partners. More than 10 million men in the United States are impotent. This figure may be low because a vast number of men have not reported the problem to their doctors. We know that about half of the men with diabetes in this country are or will become impotent.

Impotence related to diabetes usually results from nerve damage (neuropathy). With some men, diabetes damages the nerves that carry signals to the blood vessels of the penis. Poorly controlled diabetes may damage some of the blood vessels needed for an erection. If the nerve signals are blocked or the blood vessels damaged, the penis does not expand and there is no erection. In some cases, problems with the nerves and blood vessels may work together to cause impotence.

In the past it was thought that about 90% of impotence had a psychological cause. Now, with the help of more information and better medical testing, more than half of the cases of impotence are believed to have physical causes and the rest have psychological or emotional causes. Besides diabetes, other physical causes include hormone imbalances, blood vessel and heart diseases, kidney problems, nervous system disorders, stroke, certain medications, and surgery for injury to the pelvis, back, or spinal cord. Heavy use of cigarettes and/or alcohol can also cause impotence.

Many men believe that aging alone is a cause of impotence. This is a myth, because impotence isn't normal in men of any age. It is normal for older men to need more stimulation to get an erection, but the ability to get an erection has no age limit.

DIAGNOSIS

Over the last ten years, many advances have been made in the diagnosis and treatment of impotence. If you're having problems with impotence, it's important that you have a thorough medical evaluation, including:

- a medical and sexual history by your health care team
- a complete medical examination by a doctor, preferably a urologist
- a thorough examination of your sex organs, to make sure the blood vessels, nerves, and tissues of the penis are working normally for erections to occur

297

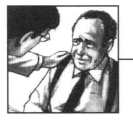

- a thorough evaluation of the circulation, blood pressure, and nerve function in the penis (circulation should be checked with a Doppler machine, which amplifies the sound of the blood going through the blood vessels in the penis)
- a rectal examination, to check for prostate problems
- blood tests to check your hormone levels and diabetes control
- a review of all medications you are taking to see if they are causing or contributing to impotence

The doctor may also inject a small amount of medication, namely Papaverine, into the penis to cause an erection. This test can help determine the cause of impotence.

Four to five erections normally occur during a night's sleep. Your doctor may do tests to measure nighttime erections. The absence of rigid nighttime erections indicates a physical cause of impotence. Depending on the cause of impotence, other blood flow studies or an overnight sleep test at a hospital may be done.

Although physical problems contribute to or cause 50% or more of the problems with erections, it's helpful if psychological evaluations are done along with physical evaluations. Many people find this to be quite threatening and feel defensive when they are questioned. They feel their problem is physical, and they really don't want people to ask questions about their relationships or emotional status. In the past, couples have gone through months of counseling only to discover the problem is physical and not psychological. On the other hand, some have received physical treatment when the problem could have been resolved through brief counseling and psychotherapy. Therefore, a complete diagnostic evaluation, including the psychological components, is important.

When considering issues that may be contributing to a problem with erections, it's important to first look at a couple's relationship. Is there open and honest communication? Or is the relationship very closed and guarded and lacking expression of feelings? Sometimes men who cannot express anger directly have problems with erections because of this anger. It's also not unusual to find that strained, emotionally unstable relationships outside of the bedroom are the same in the bedroom as well.

The next step is to evaluate a man's psychological and emotional functioning related to sex. The kinds of questions that are important to ask are:

1. Are you experiencing a great deal of anxiety and tension as you approach your partner?
2. Are you still turned on sexually by your partner?

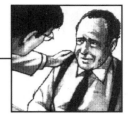

3. Are there other stressors or issues that are coming into your mind at the time you should be focusing on your sexual feelings with one another?

4. Are you experiencing any serious depression or problems with a generalized anxiety that may be disrupting your ability to focus on sensual things?

It might seem unusual to ask questions about what exactly a couple does sexually. However, one area that seems to be a common problem is the difference in a couple's expectations of sexual functioning and what they actually do. It's odd that one of the most important areas in our lives, our sexuality, is one we receive no training in whatsoever, yet we are expected to perform as experts from the moment we first learn about it. You may find that even if communication is not causing the problem, it's still helpful to learn about normal sexual functioning for you and your partner and communicate what you want and need from each other.

A less frequent, but still possible, cause that needs evaluation concerns early childhood experiences and your feelings about sexuality during your formative years. As you can see, with a sexual dysfunction many possible areas need evaluation. Often, evaluation reveals that a man has a mild physical problem that, combined with a psychological component, contributes to creating a problem with erections. When this happens, either physical or psychological treatment (or a combination of both) is necessary to truly help a couple deal with the issue.

TREATMENT

Treatment of impotence should be based on the cause. If the impotence is caused by something psychological, sex therapy or counseling may be recommended. If it's caused by something physical, many treatments are available. Adjusting or changing medications may help some people. If low male hormone (testosterone) levels are a problem, hormone injections may help. And in recent years, many men with impotence have begun using a drug (Papaverine) that causes an erection when injected into the spongy tissue of the penis.

For some men, penile implants may be recommended. These devices are surgically placed inside the body and allow men to have an erection by pumping a fluid into the implant. Penile implants work best for men who have normal sexual desire, cooperative partners, and the ability to ejaculate and have orgasms even though they're unable to have erections. A new

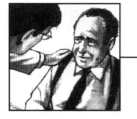

method of treatment that does not require surgery, medication, or injections involves any of the new vacuum devices. These devices work by way of a pump that creates an erection.

Even if impotence is caused by a physical problem, counseling may still be needed along with medical treatment to help with issues in the relationship and to improve self-confidence. The other choice is not to have any treatment at all. That is up to you.

From a psychological perspective, three primary methods are used to treat erection problems. After the exact nature of the problem is evaluated, the treatment is tailored to the problem. For intrapersonal problems (problems within yourself), individual psychotherapy would be recommended as the method of treatment. For problems related to communication between the couple, counseling or marital therapy for the couple might be indicated. If the problem is related to anxiety focused on sexual contact or behavioral problems within sexual contact, then sex therapy, called *Sensate Focus*, would be the primary method of treatment. Sensate Focus requires that both partners in the couple be involved in the treatment. It often involves not only structural behavioral assignments but also some counseling regarding communicating each other's needs. Sensate Focus is documented in many different books and articles and has proven to be a very effective method of treating sexual dysfunctions, particularly those related to impotence.

If you've never been involved in counseling before, you might think it's something that will tear you apart and cause you to look at deep-seated problems you've never wanted to look at in the past. On the contrary, sexual counseling is designed to help you regain the enjoyment you have lost. It focuses on the sensual aspects of your relationship and creates an atmosphere in which you can get pleasure out of your sexual contact rather than disappointment and anger. Keep in mind that once you have had a diagnostic evaluation and received recommendations for treatment, you still have the right to choose to do nothing or continue as you have in the past. Many couples report that although they chose not to receive the recommended treatment, their communication improved, they felt better about their relationship, and they began to have some restoration of their sexual contact.

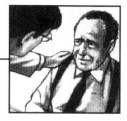

SUMMARY

It's absolutely normal and essential for human beings to find a way to express themselves sexually throughout their lives. That's why problems with sexuality can be difficult. Communication is the first step in getting help for a problem. Discuss it with your partner. Although the topic may be difficult to discuss, the payoffs for starting the discussion can be tremendous. If you have difficulty talking with your partner, at least begin to discuss the problem with your doctor, health care team, or someone you trust to give you an honest response about whether or not help is available for you. If your doctor has difficulty talking about sexuality, ask for a referral to someone who is able and willing to talk to you about your sexual functioning. Don't accept "There is no hope for you" as an answer until you have explored all of the avenues possible and have made that decision for yourself.

We hope this chapter has provided you with the encouragement and permission to seek help for a problem that you might be experiencing in order to renew a part of you that all of us find very important, our sexuality.

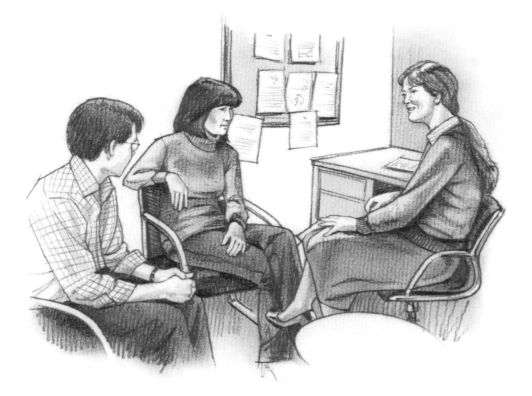

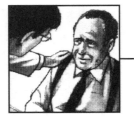

WHAT YOU CAN DO

1. Keep your blood glucose levels as near normal as possible.
2. Talk with your partner about the problem. Make a joint decision about what you want to do.
3. Discuss the problem with your health care team to find out what is available for treatment.
4. Educate yourself by reading about the topic and attending information meetings.

WHAT YOUR HEALTH CARE TEAM CAN DO

1. Ask you if you're having any problems with your sexuality.
2. Listen to your concerns about your sexuality problems.
3. Provide information and help you decide what options you may have.
4. Perform baseline tests to determine the cause of the problem.
5. Refer you to a specialist or a clinic that assesses and treats the problem.

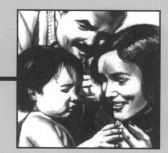

Advanced Management and Special Concerns

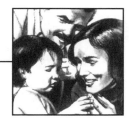

CHAPTER 22

Marion J. Franz, MS, RD, CDE
Nancy Cooper, RD, CDE

Meal Planning:
Adding Flexibility

Do you enjoy eating out in restaurants?

What are aspartame, acesulfame-K, and sucralose?
Is it safe to use them?

Are fructose, sorbitol, or hydrogenated starch hydrolysates better
to use than sucrose?

How do you use the information from food labels?

Does alcohol raise or lower blood glucose levels?

For people with diabetes, meal planning provides nutritious, healthful
food choices to help control blood glucose and blood fat levels. If
you're armed with the right information, meal planning can be
enjoyable and the eating can be downright good! This chapter
shows you how to add flexibility to your meal plans without
compromising the nutritional standards or blood glucose control
necessary for good diabetes management.

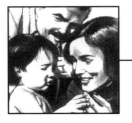

One of the keys to success in living well with diabetes will be your ability to add flexibility to your meals. The more you learn about nutrition, the exchange lists, and diabetes management, the more you can experiment with different foods and meals without upsetting your blood glucose control. Before long, you'll be able to add flexibility and interest to your meals as well as stay within your meal plan, whether you're eating at home or away.

EATING AWAY FROM HOME

When eating at a restaurant, cafeteria, or someone else's home, bring your common sense with you. You can follow your meal plan and enjoy yourself at the same time. The following guidelines can help.

- Know your meal plan. Know how many exchanges you have for each meal and make selections appropriately.

- Watch portion sizes. If portion sizes are too large for your meal plan, share your entree, ask for a "doggie bag," or leave the food. It's more important to keep your diabetes under control than to clean your plate!

- Ask how foods are prepared. How foods are cooked affects their exchange value. For example, foods fried in deep fat, such as chicken and shrimp, contain an additional starch/bread exchange and one or two additional fat exchanges per serving. Meat weight listed on a menu refers to the portion size before cooking. Meat loses about a fourth of its size in cooking, so an eight-ounce steak is approximately six, not eight, meat exchanges after it is cooked.

- Request that condiments, such as salad dressings, gravy, sauces, and so on, be served on the side so you can control the amounts.

- Know which food groups can be exchanged for other food groups. For example:
    — 1 fruit = 1 starch and/or 1 starch = 1 fruit
    — 1 nonfat milk = 1 starch plus 1 lean meat (It really should be one nonfat milk and 1 fat exchange; however, when you eat out you'll probably find that you're short of fat exchanges. Save up as many fat exchanges as you can from other times of the day to use for the meal eaten out. You might even try to be careful of fat exchanges the next day as well!)

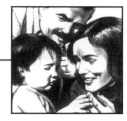

- Know how to adjust your meal and insulin injection times. People who take insulin injections must remember to eat on schedule. To make adjustments in meal times and/or insulin injections, see Chapter 10.

- For people whose Type II diabetes is controlled by meal planning alone, timing of meals is not as essential. But when eating away from home, it's important to continue to watch your portion sizes. Eat half of the portion and take the rest home for lunch the next day in a doggie bag, or split the portion with a friend.

- Use diet and low- or reduced-calorie products when available. Some restaurants now have diet syrup, jams, and jellies and low- or reduced-calorie salad dressings. These items may not appear on the menu but may be available if you ask for them.

- Oops! If you feel you have indeed "blown it," remember that you can exercise! Granted, it takes a lot of exercise to burn many calories, but dancing, bicycling, or a brisk walk can help.

- When dining away from home, it's helpful to do some planning. Plan where you will eat, what you will eat, and how much you will eat.

Where: It helps if you're familiar with the menu of the restaurant. The more choices on the menu, the more apt you are to find choices appropriate for you.

What: Decide ahead of time what you're going to order. By doing this you won't be as tempted by inappropriate food choices. Be the trendsetter—order first, so you won't be tempted as you listen to what others are ordering!

How Much: Judging portion sizes by "eyeballing" them will help you decide how much to take home and save for another meal.

By planning, understanding your meal plan, and correctly judging portion sizes, you can enjoy dining away from home while keeping your diabetes in control.

SWEETENING FOODS WITHOUT USING SUGAR

There are two alternatives to sugar: low- or non-caloric sweeteners and caloric sweeteners.

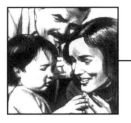

Low- or Non-Caloric Sweeteners

Low- or non-caloric sweeteners are usually intensely sweet, so only very small amounts of them are needed. Examples are saccharin, aspartame (brand name NutraSweet®), acesulfame-K (brand name Sunette®), and sucralose. They are the primary alternatives to sugar (sucrose). Some of these products may contribute a very minimal amount of calories, but given the way they are used in a meal plan the amount of calories contributed is negligible.

Saccharin. Although saccharin has been used for about 80 years in the United States, in 1977 it was designated by the Food and Drug Administration (FDA) as a possible cancer-causing agent. More recent studies have shown that saccharin is not a health threat to humans. The policy of the American Diabetes Association is that, in light of current evidence, the use of saccharin is safe for people with diabetes.

Aspartame. Aspartame is marketed as a tabletop sweetener called Equal™. Under the brand name NutraSweet, aspartame is used in a variety of food products. Aspartame is limited in use due to its instability in heat—it loses its sweetness if cooked or baked.

As with saccharin, questions have also arisen about the safety of aspartame (Equal or NutraSweet). Before it was approved by the FDA for use in foods, aspartame underwent more than 100 scientific studies during the past 20 years. According to the FDA, "few compounds have withstood such detailed testing and repeated close scrutiny."

The only documented harm from aspartame affects people with a very rare inherited disease called phenylketonuria, or PKU. This is why a warning to people with PKU appears on all foods containing Equal or NutraSweet.

Acesulfame-K. Acesulfame-K (Sunette) is a manmade sweetener with a high degree of stability when exposed to heat. It's marketed as a tabletop sweetener called Sweet One™. Acesulfame-K has been reviewed and determined to be safe by regulatory authorities in more than 20 countries. Its safety is supported by more than 50 studies conducted over 15 years.

Sucralose. Sucralose is the first sugar substitute made from sugar. It's the only substitute to combine the taste of sugar with excellent stability in processed foods and beverages. It has no calories and can be used virtually anywhere sugar can be used, including in cooking and baking. Sucralose retains its sweetness over long storage periods and at elevated temperatures. Extensive studies have been conducted and evaluated to show and support that sucralose is safe for humans to use.

Other low- or non-caloric sweeteners may be available in the United States in the near future, including cyclamate and alitame. If cyclamate is reapproved, it will probably be used for most purposes in combination with

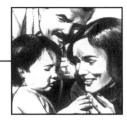

other sweeteners because of its relatively low sweetness intensity. Alitame is a highly intense sweetener with a sugar-like taste and good heat stability.

A variety of sweeteners allows for more low-calorie food products. With several low- or non-caloric sweeteners available, each can be used in the applications for which it is best suited. Sweetener limitations can often also be overcome by combining them.

Another term to be familiar with is *accepted daily intake (ADI)*. According to the FDA, ADI is the amount of sweetener that can be used by humans over a lifetime and still be considered safe by a factor of at least one hundred-fold. This is about 1/100 of an amount shown to have no toxic effects in animals. The ADI is usually reported as an amount per kilogram of body weight (2.2 pounds equals 1 kg), which ends up being a very large amount of a sweetener. For example, 50 mg/kg is the ADI for aspartame. For a 110-pound (50 kg) person, this represents twelve 12-oz cans of 100% aspartame-sweetened soda pop or seventy-one packets of Equal per day for a lifetime. As you can see, the ADI is based on a very generous safety factor.

Alternative Caloric Sweeteners

Various caloric alternatives to sucrose are also available. The majority of them have the same number of calories as sucrose. Pure crystalline fructose, high fructose corn syrups, sorbitol, and other sugar alcohols fall into this category. Different sugars have names that end in "ose," while sugar alcohols are made from sugars and have names that end in "ol." Fructose and sorbitol have been used in Europe as alternatives to sweeteners, such as sucrose, that contain glucose.

Pure Crystalline Fructose. Fructose is a commercial sugar that is sweeter than sucrose, although its sweetness actually depends on how it's used in cooking. If used in products that are cold and acidic in nature, it tastes sweeter. If used in products that require heat, such as baking, it's usually not sweeter than sucrose. It is suitable for baking, canning, and freezing.

In people with well-controlled diabetes, foods containing fructose cause a more modest increase in blood glucose levels than do foods containing sucrose. However, use of fructose is not recommended for people in poor control of their diabetes, because with an insulin deficiency, it is readily changed to glucose. Fructose is also equal to sucrose in caloric value, so it must be counted as part of the total caloric intake.

High Fructose Corn Syrup (HFCS). HFCS is a combination of fructose and dextrose (glucose). The two most used commercial products are 55% and 90% HFCS respectively. The remaining percentage is from glucose. Studies show HFCS has an effect on blood glucose similar to that of sucrose.

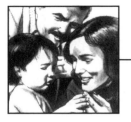

Hydrogenated Starch Hydrolysates (HSH). HSH is produced by a series of chemical reactions that begin with cornstarch. This produces a series of products containing mixtures of polyols (sugar alcohols). The sweetness varies from 25 to 50% of sucrose and is suitable for use in a wide variety of candies. Compared with glucose, it increases blood glucose less in persons with Type I and Type II diabetes. This is because of decreased absorption, but the caloric savings appear to be low.

Sorbitol. Sorbitol is the most commonly used sugar alcohol. It is readily converted to fructose and is similarly used by the body. One of the major problems with sorbitol is that it may cause diarrhea in some people. Also, many products sweetened with sorbitol end up with as many or more calories than the product they are replacing because of the added fat used to dissolve the sorbitol and give the food a creamy texture.

Mannitol. Mannitol is commonly used as a bulking agent in powdered foods and as a dusting agent for chewing gum. Excessive consumption may also cause diarrhea.

It should be remembered that all of these sweeteners contribute calories to the meal plan and are not "free foods."

USING FOOD LABELS IN MEAL PLANNING

Labels on foods can help you decide which foods are appropriate for your meal plan and how to use them correctly. To best use the information on labels, first look at the list of ingredients. Ingredients contained in the largest amount by weight will be listed first.

A phrase that often appears on labels is "nutritive sweetener." This identifies a sweetener that contains calories. Examples include invert sugar, corn syrup, dextrin, molasses, sorghum, honey, maple or brown sugar, sorbitol, mannitol, xylitol, hydrogenated starch hydrolysates, and concentrated fruit juices. If the label contains the phrase "non-nutritive sweetener," it indicates that the sweetener contains few or no calories. Examples include saccharin, aspartame (Equal or NutraSweet), acesulfame-K (Sunette or Sweet One), and sucralose.

Dietetic products are those in which some ingredient has been restricted or changed and a substitution has been made. Dietetic, diet, and dietary mean the same thing when used on labels. They do not necessarily mean the product is low in calories or useful for people with diabetes. If used,

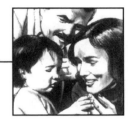

they must be counted in the meal plan as other products are, since they are generally not free foods. Dietetic products must comply with the nutrition information format because of their nutritional claims.

Dietetic products that might be useful include artificial sweeteners, diet soda, and canned fruits without added sugar. Dietetic products that may be useful as free foods include diet syrups, diet or low-sugar jams or jellies, sugar-free hard candies and sugar-free gum. Always check the caloric content to be sure these products do not contain more calories than you expect.

Dietetic products to be wary of include dietetic ice cream, cookies, candy bars, and cakes. Many of these products are actually higher in calories than the products they are replacing. Although they are frequently made with sorbitol, the fat content of these products is usually greater than in regular food products. Other considerations in the use of dietetic foods may be cost and quality of the product.

After you have checked the ingredients list, look for nutritional information. This information can help you fit the product into your meal plan. Nutritional information on a food product label must follow a standard format and include:

- serving size and number of servings per container
- number of calories per serving
- grams of carbohydrate, protein, fat, and saturated fat per serving
- number of calories from fat per serving
- milligrams of cholesterol per serving
- milligrams of sodium per serving
- grams of dietary fiber per serving
- percentage of vitamins A and C, iron, and calcium per serving

Knowing the number of calories per serving can be helpful in deciding how to fit a product into your meal plan. If a food contains less than 20 calories per serving, it's considered a "free food" and may be used either at mealtime or at snacktime but is not counted in the meal plan. However, free foods that contain calories should be limited to one per meal or not more than three or four per day.

By looking at the other nutritional information on the label, you can estimate how many exchanges are in a serving of a food, which will help you include it in your meal plan. Pay particular attention to the grams of carbohydrate, protein, and fat, although the grams do not need to be exactly equal to the exchanges in your meal plan. In most meal plans, variations of a few calories or grams of protein, carbohydrate, or fat are not significant.

Use the following table and example to convert information from a label to the exchange system.

311

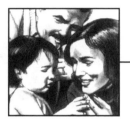

AMOUNTS OF NUTRIENTS IN FOOD EXCHANGES

Exchange	Calories	Carbohydrate	Protein	Fat
1 starch/bread	80	15 gm	3 gm	trace
1 lean meat	55	—	7 gm	3 gm
1 medium fat meat	75	—	7 gm	5 gm
1 high fat meat	100	—	7 gm	8 gm
1 vegetable	25	5 gm	2 gm	—
1 fruit	60	15 gm	—	—
1 milk (skim)	90	12 gm	8 gm	trace
1 fat	45	—	—	5 gm

STEPS FOR CONVERTING NUTRITIONAL LABELING TO EXCHANGES

The following label is from a 10-oz box of frozen pizza.

```
Nutritional Information Per Serving
Serving size ..............1/2 pizza (5 oz)
Servings per container....................2
Calories.......................................350
Protein....................................17 gm
Carbohydrate..........................33 gm
Fat............................................16 gm
```

To make it easier to convert label information to the exchange system, follow these steps:

1. Check the label for the information you need to convert to the exchange system. You need:

Serving size ....1/2 pizza (5 oz)
Calories.......................................350
Protein ....17 gm
Carbohydrate ....33 gm
Fat ....16 gm

2. Check the serving size. Is this a reasonble size for your use?

3. Compare the label information with the carbohydrate, protein, fat, and calories on the exchange table. First, look at the amount and source of carbohydrate in the food product. In this case, you'll be converting the carbohydrate to starch/bread exchanges. Note in the exchange table that 15 gm of carbohydrate and 3 gm of protein equal 1 starch/bread exchange. This means that the 30 gm of carbohydrate plus 6 gm of the protein in your pizza serving equal 2 starch/bread exchanges.

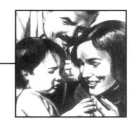

	Carbohydrate	Protein	Fat
1/2 pizza	33 gm	17 gm	16 gm
2 starch/bread exchanges	30 gm	6 gm	—

4. Next, subtract the grams of protein you used in figuring the starch/bread exchanges from the total amount of protein in the serving size. Then convert the remaining grams of protein to meat exchanges. Use the medium-fat meat exchange values from the exchange table.

	Carbohydrate	Protein	Fat
1/2 pizza	33 gm	17 gm	16 gm
2 starch/bread exchanges	30 gm	-6 gm	—
		11 gm	16 gm
2 medium-fat meat exchanges		14 gm	10 gm

5. Next, subtract the grams of fat in the meat exchanges from the fat contained in the serving size. Then convert the remaining grams of fat to fat exchanges.

	Carbohydrate	Protein	Fat
1/2 pizza	33 gm	17 gm	16 gm
2 starch/bread exchanges	30 gm	-6 gm	—
		11 gm	16 gm
2 medium-fat meat exchanges		14 gm	-10 gm
			6 gm
1 fat exchange			5 gm

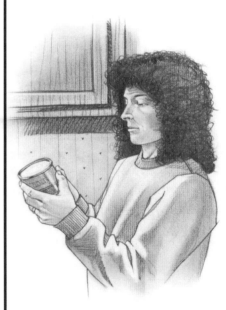

6. If you eat 1/2 of this 10-oz pizza, you use the following exchanges from your meal plan:

2 starch/bread, 2 medium fat meat, 1 fat

7. Final check:

	Carbohydrate	Protein	Fat	Calories
1/2 pizza	*33 gm*	*17 gm*	*16 gm*	*350*
Exchanges:				
(2 starch/bread,	*30 gm*	6 gm		
2 medium-fat meat, 1 fat)		+14 gm	10 gm	
		20 gm	+5 gm	
			15 gm	*355*

8. If the difference between the grams per serving and the grams accounted for by the exchange system is less than half of an exchange, you do not need to count those extra grams.

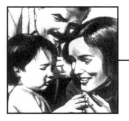

HOW ALCOHOL AFFECTS DIABETES

The decision to use or not use alcoholic beverages is an individual one. To make this decision, you need to know how alcohol affects blood glucose levels and the rest of your body.

Alcohol is broken down by the liver, but the liver can process less than one ounce of alcohol per hour. Alcohol cannot be converted to glucose by the liver, but it can be used as a source of energy. If the calories from alcohol are not used as an immediate energy source, they are converted to fat and triglycerides.

The metabolism of alcohol does not require insulin. In fact, alcohol increases the effect of insulin. The presence of alcohol in the blood has also been shown to prolong the effects of a single injection of insulin.

Overall, alcohol lowers blood glucose levels, especially if it has been some time since food was eaten. In that case, blood glucose is initially supplied by the breakdown of carbohydrate stored in the liver (glycogen) and later by the liver's conversion of protein to glucose. Alcohol inhibits this conversion of protein to glucose, which can cause hypoglycemia. Furthermore, release of "stress hormones" that raise blood glucose levels becomes blunted, increasing the risk for hypoglycemic reactions becoming more severe.

Hypoglycemia can occur even before a person is aware of being mildly intoxicated. If food has not been eaten with the alcoholic beverage or for several hours before, two ounces of alcohol is enough to produce hypoglycemia. Also, persons in poor control of their diabetes or who have exercised strenuously usually have depleted carbohydrate stores and so are at special risk for hypoglycemia.

Even when alcohol is consumed with food, the hypoglycemic action of alcohol may persist from 8 to 12 hours after the last drink and may occur after only a drink or two. At this point, the body needs to convert protein to blood glucose but alcohol blocks the process.

On occasion, alcohol can cause blood glucose levels to become elevated. This may be because alcohol affects judgment, making it difficult for a person to follow a meal plan. However, this hyperglycemia is usually temporary and is followed several hours later by a drop in blood glucose to below-normal levels.

Alcohol is a concentrated source of calories, yielding seven calories per gram. For comparison, carbohydrate and protein contribute four calories per gram and fat contributes nine calories per gram. Alcohol provides energy but no other essential nutrients. An ounce and a half of 80 proof

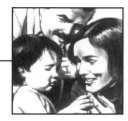

liquor contributes about 100 calories. Sweet wines and beers also contain carbohydrates, so they have additional calories.

When diabetes is well controlled, the blood glucose level is not affected by the moderate use of alcohol if it is consumed shortly before, during, or immediately after eating. However, certain conditions indicate that alcohol should not be used, for example:

- alcohol abuse
- elevated triglyceride levels
- gastritis
- pancreatitis
- certain types of kidney and heart diseases
- frequent hypoglycemic reactions
- gestational diabetes
- Type I diabetes with pregnancy

Check with your health care team to determine whether any of these contraindications applies to you. Alcohol also interacts with barbiturates and tranquilizers, sleeping pills, antihistamines, cold remedies, and a number of other drugs. Avoid these combinations.

GUIDELINES FOR THE USE OF ALCOHOL

Many persons with diabetes can include alcohol with their meal plan by following some simple guidelines. These guidelines refer to occasional use of alcoholic beverages, which is defined as approximately two "equivalents" (drinks) not more than once or twice a week. If alcohol is used daily, the amount must be limited and the calories counted in the meal plan.

The guidelines listed below can help persons with diabetes make informed decisions about the use of alcohol.

- Drink alcohol only if your diabetes is in good control. Drinking alcohol when you are in poor control can make control even worse. Your health care team can advise you on how to balance your food intake, exercise, and medication to achieve better blood glucose control, and they will tell you if there is some reason you should avoid alcoholic beverages. To keep control of your diabetes, know the effect of alcohol on blood glucose levels.
- Drink alcohol in moderation. It's best to limit the amount to no more than two of the following equivalents, or drinks, each day. Each contains approximately the same amount of alcohol.

315

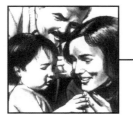

— 1.5 oz of distilled spirits (hard liquor such as whiskey, scotch, rye, vodka, gin, cognac, rum, dry brandy)

— 4 oz of dry wine

— 2 oz of dry sherry

— 12 oz of beer, preferably light

- For persons of normal weight who require insulin, two of the above equivalents can occasionally be used as an "extra." No food should be omitted because of the possibility of alcohol-induced hypoglycemia and because alcohol does not require insulin to be metabolized. However, even this amount of alcohol can cause hypoglycemia if not accompanied by food.

- Persons with Type II diabetes for whom weight is a concern must count the calories from alcohol in their meal plan. Calories are best substituted for fat exchanges because alcohol is metabolized in a manner similar to fat (each of the above equivalents is equal to two fat exchanges). Avoid or limit alcohol consumption if you need to shed excess pounds. Since alcohol provides calories (without the benefit of other nutrients), most of which your body stores as fat, losing weight may become more difficult when you drink, even occasionally.

- Never drink on an empty stomach or after vigorous exercise. Alcohol makes you especially vulnerable to hypoglycemia, so be sure to drink only with a meal, directly before, or shortly afterward. Remember that alcohol may also promote hypoglycemia the "morning after."

- Sip slowly and make a drink last a long time. Even one drink is enough to give your breath the smell of alcohol. Since symptoms of alcohol intoxication and hypoglycemia are similar, it's easy to mistake low blood glucose for intoxication, which may delay necessary treatment.

- Avoid drinks that contain large amounts of carbohydrate. Liqueurs and cordials are sweet and may have a sugar content as high as 50%. Beer and ale contain malt sugar, which should be substituted in the meal plan. Light beer is recommended because it has approximately 3 to 6 grams of carbohydrate per 12-oz can in contrast to regular beer, which has 13 grams of carbohydrate per can.

- Don't let a drink make you careless. Alcohol can have a relaxing effect and may dull judgment. Be sure meals and snacks are taken on time and selected with usual care. Too much alcohol may lead to further dietary indiscretion. Avoid hypoglycemia the morning after drinking alcohol by setting your alarm before you retire to help you get up, test, and eat your usual breakfast.

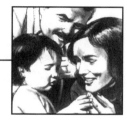

- Carry identification. Visible identification should be carried or worn when drinking away from home. An insulin reaction can appear too much like intoxication to take any chances.

The "Alcoholic Beverages" table provides information on the average alcohol, carbohydrate, and calorie content of alcoholic beverages and exchanges for Type II diabetes.

ALCOHOLIC BEVERAGES

Beverage	Serving	Alcohol (gms)	Carbohydrate (gms)	Calories	Exchanges for Type II
Beer					
regular	12 oz	13	13	150	1 starch, 2 fat
light	12 oz	11	5	100	2 fat
near	12 oz	1.5	12	60	1 starch
Distilled Spirits					
80 proof (gin, rum, vodka, whiskey, scotch)	1 1/2 oz	14	trace	100	2 fat
dry brandy, cognac	1 oz	11	trace	75	1 1/2 fat
Table Wines					
dry white	4 oz	11	trace	80	2 fat
red or rose	4 oz	12	trace	85	2 fat
sweet	4 oz	12	5	105	1/3 starch, 2 fat
light	4 oz	6	1	50	1 fat
wine cooler	4 oz	13	30	215	2 fruit, 2 fat
Sparkling Wines					
champagne	4 oz	12	4	100	2 fat
sweet Kosher	4 oz	12	12	132	1 starch, 2 fat
Appetizer/Dessert Wines					
sherry	2 oz	9	2	74	1 1/2 fat
sweet sherry, port, muscatel	2 oz	9	7	90	1/2 starch, 1 1/2 fat
cordials, liqueurs	1 1/2 oz	13	18	160	1 starch, 2 fat
Cocktails					
Bloody Mary	5 oz	14	5	116	1 vegetable, 2 fat
Daiquiri	2 oz	14	2	111	2 fat
Manhattan	2 oz	17	2	178	2 1/2 fat
Martini	2 1/2 oz	22	trace	156	3 1/2 fat
Old Fashioned	4 oz	26	trace	180	4 fat
Tom Collins	7 1/2 oz	16	3	120	2 1/2 fat

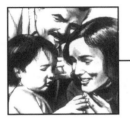

ALCOHOLIC BEVERAGES (CONTINUED)

Beverage	Serving	Alcohol (gms)	Carbohydrate (gms)	Calories	Exchanges for Type II
Mixes					
mineral water	any	—	0	0	Free
sugar-free tonic	any	—	0	0	Free
club soda	any	—	0	0	Free
diet soda	any	—	0	0	Free
tomato juice	1/2 cup	—	5	25	1 vegetable
Bloody Mary mix	1/2 cup	—	5	25	1 vegetable
orange juice	1/2 cup	—	15	60	1 fruit
grapefruit juice	1/2 cup	—	15	60	1 fruit
pineapple juice	1/2 cup	—	15	60	1 fruit

SUMMARY

The more information you have about food and nutrition, the more flexibility you'll be able to introduce into meal planning. It can help you control blood glucose and blood fat levels and provide healthy, nutritious, and tasty meals.

The International Diabetes Center has written several other sources of nutrition information that can make meal planning and dining more convenient and healthy for everyone. See the back of the manual for ordering information on these books.

- *Exchanges for All Occasions* provides information about eating out in restaurants, useful tips for meal planning while traveling, ideas for holiday menus, information on food labeling and alternative sweeteners, and information on how to modify your own recipes to lower fat and calories and increase fiber.

- *Convenience Food Facts* contains nutrient values for more than 1,500 name-brand processed food products. The nutrient tables list the product name; serving size; number of calories; grams of carbohydrate, protein and fat; milligrams of sodium; and exchange value.

- *Fast Food Facts* includes the same nutrient information for menu items from popular fast-food restaurants.

- *The Joy of Snacks* is a cookbook designed to help you prepare easy, nutritious snacks that make eating fun.

- *Diabetes Actively Staying Healthy* can help you make decisions about exercise and food adjustments.

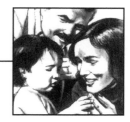

Armed with the information from this manual and other nutrition publications, meal planning can be enjoyable. After all, the proof of the pudding is in the eating!

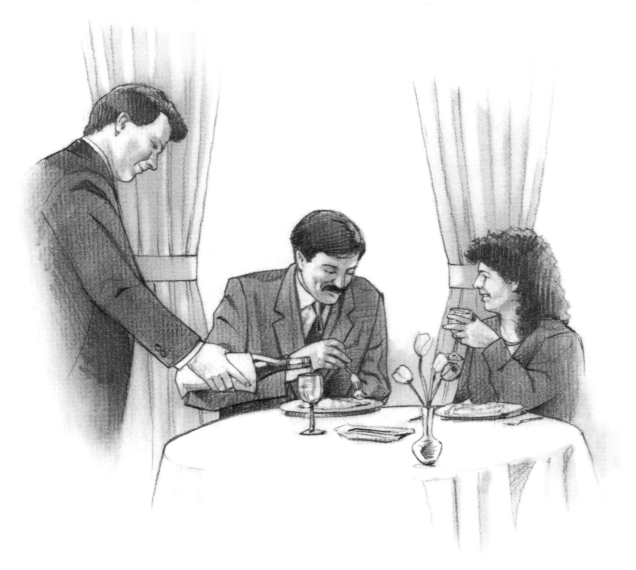

CHAPTER 23

Randi S. Birk, MA, LP

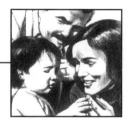

Stress Management:
Learning to Cope With External and Internal Stressors

What causes stress in your life?

Can stress be managed?

What is the relationship between stress and diabetes?

How does stress affect blood glucose levels?

Each of us is like the strings on a violin—if there is no tension on those strings, there will be no music. Similarly, if we have no stress—no challenge—in our lives, we may become bored and even ill. Yet, if we keep tightening the pegs on that violin, the strings will surely snap. And if we keep adding more and more stress to our life, at some point we will "snap" in the sense that we may experience a physical or emotional problem. As you read this chapter, try to identify the right level of stress for you—the level at which you can "play well" and yet not be overwhelmed.

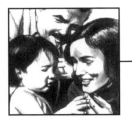

S tress is *"the non-specific response of the body to **any** demand made upon it."* This definition was first introduced by Canadian endocrinologist Hans Selye. "Non-specific" means our body responds in the same way, regardless of the type of stress we experience. However, the key word in this definition is "any."

Typically, people think stress is caused by negative experiences, such as being stuck in traffic, a confrontation with your boss, or an approaching deadline. Selye suggests that stress can result from any out-of-the-ordinary demand. This means that experiences we usually consider positive, such as marriage, family, and even vacation, may also produce stress. He calls these positive stresses *eustress*; negative stresses are *distress*. It's distress that most of us refer to when we talk about stress. But it's important to remember that even positive experiences, when they are out of the ordinary, can create stress.

People vary widely in how much stress they can tolerate. Some thrive on a great deal of stress. They say, "My job is so stressful, but I love it!" Stress seems to stimulate and challenge them. Others have difficulty coping with this much stress and prefer quieter lifestyles. We cannot totally eliminate stress from our lives. As Selye states, "The person without any stress—is dead." We can, however, manage stress and help keep it in a healthy and even positive range.

HOW DOES STRESS MANAGEMENT RELATE TO DIABETES CARE?

The relationship between diabetes and stress is twofold. First, diabetes may cause stress. This certainly won't surprise you. Living with a chronic illness that demands a complex schedule of medical care, involves the potential of immediate and long-term problems, and affects the entire family creates a whole range of stresses. Second, stress can affect diabetes. Most people report higher blood glucose levels during periods of stress. However, this is not universal. Others note that their blood glucose actually drops when they experience stress. The best approach is a personal scientist approach: test your blood glucose when you feel stressed and see what happens. There probably will be some effect. Therefore, because diabetes can add stress and because stress can affect diabetes, stress management is an important tool to help you manage your diabetes.

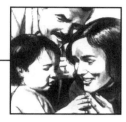

HOW STRESS AFFECTS YOUR BODY

The stress response occurs automatically whenever we view something as a threat. The threat doesn't have to be physical, it may be a threat to our ego, our values, and so on. The stress response begins deep inside our brain, in the master gland of emotion called the *hypothalamus*. The hypothalamus controls the stress response as well as the relaxation response, which we'll discuss later. Within six seconds, the hypothalamus sends a message to the pituitary gland, which in turn sends a message to the adrenal glands located above the kidneys. The adrenal glands then release adrenalin (and cortisol), stress hormones that have a tremendous effect on the body.

Think about the last time you had an outpouring of adrenalin. You probably felt your heart pounding faster and your breathing becoming shallow and rapid. Your blood pressure and blood glucose levels may have been elevated (although for some people blood glucose levels actually drop). You also may have noticed that your senses were sharper and your pupils were dilated, which is why lights seem too bright and noises seem too loud. Meanwhile, the stress hormones are directing your blood flow to nourish the areas most critical in meeting "the threat"—the brain and major muscles. This is accomplished by opening some blood vessels (vasodilation) and closing others slightly (vasoconstriction). But since you have only so much blood volume, some areas receive less blood than normal, in particular your digestive tract and extremities (hands and feet). This is why your hands feel cold and clammy when you're under stress. You've heard the expression "cold feet"? Well, they literally are.

Considering what's happening to your body, what are you ready for? Fight or flight! Your body is preparing to fight off the threat or flee the situation. This response clearly had evolutionary value. Back when our ancestors were cave people, if a big old saber-toothed tiger sauntered in looking for dinner, they had to be ready fast to either fight it off or flee. Today we don't encounter many saber-toothed tigers. Instead we experience situations in which it's inappropriate to either fight or run. We must learn new, more effective ways of managing our stress. If we don't, those stress hormones will continue to keep us in a "red alert" state and we'll become exhausted. We'll also be vulnerable to a number of the ill effects of stress.

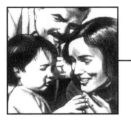

CAUSES OF STRESS

A *stressor* is anything that triggers the fight or flight response, or any demand that may cause stress. There are two broad forms of stressors, external and internal.

External Stressors

External stressors come from our environment—from outside ourselves. Think about those things in your environment that cause stress for you, such as taxes, bills, phone messages, too much to do in too little time, traffic, and so on. External stressors include both major stressful events (such as a job change) and minor, everyday irritants (hassles). Psychologists now believe that people can handle the major stressful events in their lives, rallying energy and coping adequately. Instead, they suggest it's the daily "hassles" that take the most significant toll by creating ongoing stress. Think about your hassles. Then compare these to your "uplifts" (positive, nice events that make you feel good). Do you have more hassles, more uplifts, or are they fairly even. Identifying your external stressors is an important first step in discovering what you can do to manage stress.

Internal Stressors

Internal stressors come from within us. Generally we're less aware of these stressors, but they're likely to play an even greater role in the creation of stress in our daily lives. There are many broad areas of internal stressors, and this chapter focuses on four: values and beliefs, errors in our thinking, attitudes and perceptions, and personality type.

    Values and Beliefs. These are deeply-held philosophies we usually learn in childhood and hold to be absolute. They can be very positive, helping to direct our lives, but at times they may also cause us stress.

    Faith. Our faith can be extremely valuable in helping us cope with life's challenges. It can also be a source of internal stress, particularly if we mistakenly believe we are expected to be perfect and adhere to all the doctrines of our faith without exception. Because we are human, we may find we are not living according to our professed beliefs. This discrepancy is a significant source of internal stress, creating guilt and perhaps a sense of failure. To address this discrepancy, we must change either our belief or our behavior. We might recognize that we can adhere to our faith and yet be human, modifying our expectations. Or, if our expectations are already

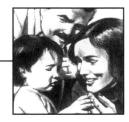

reasonable, we must change our behavior so that it is more in agreement with what we actually believe.

Values. As with our faith, we may cling to values that are demanding or unrealistic. For example, if you say you value nutritious eating yet choose "junk food" at every turn, the discrepancy will make you feel guilty and disapprove of yourself. You must question your values about nutritious eating. Perhaps you can modify it in terms of degree—nutritious eating is important most of the time, or some of the time. However, if you decide that you strongly value nutritious eating, you then need to change your behaviors so your actions reflect your beliefs.

Goals. As children, many of us were taught to "shoot for the moon." Unfortunately, this set us up to establish goals that are sometimes unrealistic. Having overly high expectations sets us up for failure and, therefore, a great deal of internal stress. When we miss targets, we focus on what we have *not* achieved rather than what we have accomplished. Feelings of failure become not only a source of internal stress, but an obstacle to further effort. Setting realistic, achievable goals for success is the real motivator. When you accomplish goals, you affirm your capability and motivate yourself to try for new goals. If you happen to have a goal that is too high to reach immediately, break it into smaller steps so you may experience the sense of success that will motivate your continued efforts.

Self-concept. We all have an image of who we are, and we constantly evaluate that image. People used to think if you talked to yourself you were crazy. That's baloney. We talk to ourselves all the time. We have an internal monologue going in which we evaluate ourselves and everything around us. Often this monologue and our self-evaluations come from comments about us or responses we have received over the years. Unfortunately, we often tend to minimize the positive feedback from others, while magnifying the negative or critical comments. This leaves an internal monologue that's often negative and self-critical: "I never do anything quite right." "I'm worthless, I'm a failure, I don't deserve anything good." These "killer phrases" erode self-esteem and make people less happy, less effective, and less likely to take care of themselves. It's unfortunately true that many of us can say, "One of the worst of *many* faults is that I'm too critical of myself." The problem with this kind of thinking is that it adds a great deal of internal stress and may become a self-fulfilling prophecy. We don't always get what we want in life, but we often get what we expect. If we tell ourselves long enough that we are losers, we may live down to those expectations.

Making The Negative Cycle Positive. The first step in turning this negative cycle around is to listen to your internal monologue. If you hear those killer phrases, stop them and turn them around. Give yourself

325

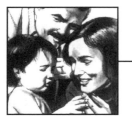

positive affirmations. An affirmation is a strong positive statement: "I am capable." "I do a good job." "I deserve to live well." When you change your internal monologue, you'll begin to live up to your positive expectations. This does not happen overnight, however. It's a choice. Listen to your internal monologue. You can always say, "I may not be totally perfect, but parts of me are excellent."

ERRORS IN THINKING

We all make errors in thinking at one time or another. These errors often become automatic, occurring mostly in stressful situations and intensifying the amount of stress we feel. Here are some of the more common ones.

All-or-Nothing Thinking

This type of black or white thinking is evident in statements such as "If I don't follow my diabetes schedule perfectly, there is no point in doing it at all." The problem is that few things in life are so clearly black or white. In addition, all or nothing thinking sets up unrealistic expectations, because it's nearly impossible to "do it all." When people who think this way fall short of their expectations, they often give up entirely. This leaves them with a huge contrast between their expectation of perfection and their behavior of doing nothing or very little. Such a contrast is the same type of nagging, internal stress discussed earlier. To eliminate stress, we must begin to look at the "gray" zone. Setting more realistic goals can help us achieve this.

Magnification

Magnification involves overestimating the importance of a negative event or overreacting to it. A person may see one high blood glucose reading and panic, thinking "Something terrible must be happening." Magnification can often be identified by words such as "awful, horrible, or terrible." While those words are appropriate in some situations, we often use them in situations in which they clearly don't belong, such as being late, being stuck in traffic, and being criticized. When we tell ourselves that a situation is awful, horrible, or terrible we add a great deal of internal stress. Eliminating those words when they are not appropriate can reduce the stress we feel.

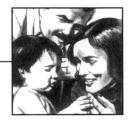

Overgeneralization

Overgeneralization involves seeing a single negative event as a pattern of defeat. For example, a person may get one high blood glucose reading and say, "I can never stay in good control!" Few things are always or never. In truth, it may happen frequently or sometimes. Always and never are power words that can add a great deal of stress for people who constantly use them. Becoming more realistic will reduce that stress.

"Should" Statements

Many people attempt to motivate themselves or other people with "shoulds" or "oughts." You may find yourself feeling guilty thinking "I should test four times a day, exercise routinely, and follow my meal plan exactly."

People often mistakenly believe that shoulds are motivating, that if you tell yourself you *should* do something long enough, you will finally do it. In reality, we just build up an enormous list of shoulds. It may be interesting to write a list of those things you tell yourself you should do. We then find ourselves looking at a huge list, not knowing where to start. Unfortunately, we often become overwhelmed and don't start. We're left then with a long list of shoulds and no action. This discrepancy produces a significant source of internal stress.

What we can do is begin. Choose one item on your list, perhaps the one that's most important to you. Make sure it's realistic, then change the way you say it. Instead of "I should do..." say "I choose to do...," or "I will do...." Changing "shoulds" to "choose" or "will" turns all of the procrastination and excuses into action. With the rest of the list, remember this phrase: "THOU SHALT NOT SHOULD ON THYSELF!"

ATTITUDES AND PERCEPTIONS

Attitudes and perceptions have to do with the way we view the world. While there is a "real world" out there, we all see it a little differently. An example of this is the half-filled glass of water. Is it half-full or half-empty? Attitudes and perceptions are important because they often affect what the world becomes for us.

Typically people believe that events cause feelings. Horror movies make us scared, comedies make us laugh, traffic makes us angry. Actually this is not the case. Dr. Albert Ellis, a psychologist who founded Rational Emotive Therapy, suggests it's what we believe, or what we tell ourselves

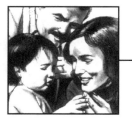

about an event, that creates our feelings. This is important because we can change those labels and, as a result, change how we feel and respond. For example, let's say you miss an exercise session because of a meeting. If you say to yourself, "I'll never be able to exercise regularly" (overgeneralization), you may feel frustrated. But if you say instead, "I'll plan to exercise tomorrow before work," you'll feel confident. All that changed was your response to the event.

Imagine getting up too late for work. This is a stressful situation for almost everyone. But keep in mind that you have a choice about how much additional stress you will add. Telling yourself "This is horrible, this is awful, this is going to be a terrible day" is likely to start a negative pattern of extra stress and ensure that you indeed have a terrible day. Instead, thinking "this is not the worst thing in the world, I'll call in and let them know I'll be delayed and make up my work later" can reduce the stress you feel and start you off toward a much better day. The choice is yours. Listen to the messages you give yourself and the labels you apply to situations. Changing those labels or self-messages can drastically reduce the amount of stress you feel.

PERSONALITY TYPE

Finally, your personality type may be a source of internal stress. Many of you are familiar with the personality types A and B. Type A personalities are often characterized as driven, aggressive, perfectionists whose hostility is easily aroused. They are the go-getters, often in a hurry. Type Bs, on the other hand, are more laid-back, easygoing, and mellow. Many of us are not pure Type A or B but fall somewhere between the two. If you are uncertain where you fall, answer these questions yes or no:

1. I always move, walk, and eat rapidly.
2. I become enraged when a car ahead of me travels at a pace I consider too slow.
3. I find it anguishing to wait in line.
4. I frequently try to think about or do two or more things at once.
5. I try to schedule more and more into less and less time.
6. I am always rushed.

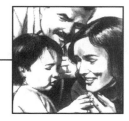

If you answered yes to most of those questions, you may be Type A; if you answered no, you may be more Type B. While there is no right or wrong personality Type, research has shown conclusively that Type A behavior adds stress and, therefore, can exact a toll on a person's health.

What can you do? While it may not be realistic to go from being Type A all the way to Type B, you can move toward it. If you identify yourself as Type A, you can work on reducing your perfectionism, urgency, and hostility. This is a choice. Type A behavior is learned and can be unlearned. Remember that in addition to creating stress for yourself, your behavior is also a model for your children. Any benefits you derive from changing your behavior will also extend to them.

THE NEGATIVE PROGRESSION

We have discussed different *life events* (external stressors) that add stress to our lives. We have also discussed how our *perceptions* (internal stressors) can add stress.

Emotional arousal refers to the feelings you may have when under stress. Some people describe anger, sadness, or fear when they experience stress. You may feel a wide range of emotions. Attending to these feelings may help you discover what is causing stress for you.

Physical arousal refers to the signals your body gives you when you're experiencing stress. Some people feel their muscles tighten (for example, in their shoulders or necks), others have headaches, stomach problems, rashes or hives, or maybe grind their teeth at night. These signals, like the emotions you may feel, can raise your awareness of the stress you're experiencing.

If you ignore these signals, things can get worse. Many *illnesses or diseases* have been found to be related to stress. Stress may contribute to or make worse high blood pressure, coronary artery disease, insomnia, asthma, ulcers, colitis, and most recently identified, cancer and arthritis. (Remember that all of these problems may be caused by other agents as well.) While it has never been conclusively shown that diabetes is caused by stress, stress may play a part in the timing of diagnosis and, as discussed earlier, in blood glucose control after diagnosis.

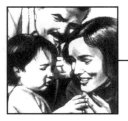

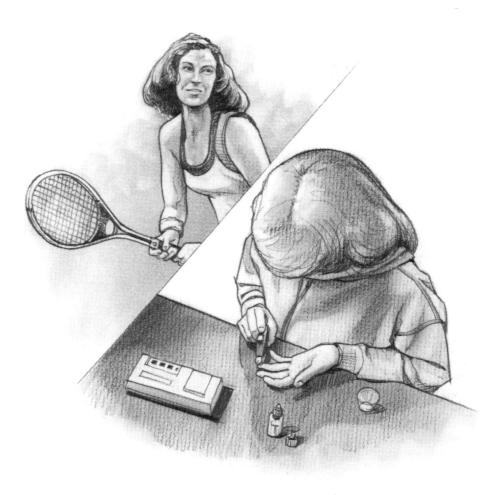

STRESS BREAKERS

What we must find, then, are stress breakers; ways of interrupting this
negative progression all the way along the line.

Change the Situation

One of the first things we can sometimes do is change the situation. While
this may initially seem impossible, stepping back from a situation may

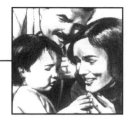

provide some objectivity to help you identify what aspects you could realistically change. You may be familiar with the Serenity Prayer:

"God grant me the serenity to accept things I cannot change,
The strength to change the things I can,
And the wisdom to distinguish between the two."

Think about a stressful situation in your life and brainstorm a number of alternatives to change the situation.

Change Your Perception

Some situations cannot be changed or are too difficult to change. In that case, you can change your perceptions, or the way you think about the situation. While you may not go from a negative to a positive, changing what you say to yourself from a negative to a neutral may be enough to reduce much of the stress you're experiencing.

Relaxation

Remember the hypothalamus—the master gland of emotion that controls the stress response as well as the relaxation response? The problem is that while the stress response is automatic—it just happens—the relaxation response must be learned. There are a number of excellent relaxation techniques, such as meditation, yoga, biofeedback, self-hypnosis, and progressive muscle relaxation. Any of these techniques can help you learn what your body feels like under stress and how to relax. If you're intimidated by these formal relaxation techniques, try one of the others that is available to all of us every day. Daydreaming, praying, taking naps, walking, listening to music, laughing, deep breathing, doing a hobby, or sitting and thinking tranquil thoughts are all relaxation techniques that can be easily applied when we feel stressed.

Another very promising technique is imagery. Imagery involves using your imagination to take yourself from a stressful situation to an imagined place that is safe, peaceful, calm and *yours*. You might also imagine yourself living well in the future: healthy, competent, and happy. While using any of the relaxation techniques, including imagery, we are particularly receptive to positive affirmations. Therefore, combining relaxation and affirmations may be especially helpful in reducing stress.

Exercise

Exercise is a uniquely positive form of stress management because it's similar to the fight or flight response. Our bodies are prepared for action, and exercise gives it that action. Exercise does not have to mean jogging 10 miles a day or participating in strenuous aerobics. Taking a walk is a wonderful form of exercise. If you're unable to do that, even stretching or range-of-motion exercises can be helpful.

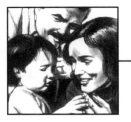

SUMMARY

Rather than trying to manage stress in just one way, see that you have a variety of stress management strategies. Change the situation one time, change your perception of the situation another time, and use some relaxation or exercise yet another time. Remember to set realistic goals for adding stress management techniques to your life.

And hang on to your sense of humor. Humor is not telling good jokes or stories; it's an approach to life. Many things happen that we cannot change, and when we can't, we may do well to laugh at them. The author Robert Louis Stevenson, who had tuberculosis, was credited with saying, "Life is not a matter of getting a good hand, but of playing a poor hand well." Humor can be a valuable aspect in helping you play your cards, whatever they are.

But you can't do it alone. Along with humor we need support. Family, friends, the health care team, support groups, and mental health professionals are all a part of the support net that can help you to manage your stress and live well with diabetes.

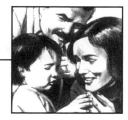

CHAPTER 24

Dean E. Goldberg, PharmD, CDE

Medications:
How They Can
Affect Diabetes

How do medications affect blood glucose levels?
Why do some nonprescription drugs warn against using them
if you have diabetes?

Do I need to use sugar-free medications?

Medications, or drugs, are used to treat many medical conditions.
They help us live longer, more productive lives. Without drugs, it
would be difficult for us to live well with conditions such as high
blood pressure, headaches, or diabetes.

However, medications can have many different effects on diabetes.
Some may increase or decrease blood glucose levels. Others may
cause or worsen complications of diabetes such as kidney disease, eye
disease, the inability to function sexually (impotency), and high blood
pressure. Some drugs may interact with the insulin or oral agents
(diabetes pills) you take to control your diabetes, causing inappropriate
rises or drops in blood glucose levels. This chapter reviews many
commonly used medications, both prescription and nonprescription,
and outlines some of the many ways they can affect diabetes.

333

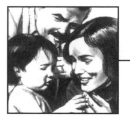

Drugs (or medications, the two words are usually used interchangeably) are defined as substances that have an effect on the human body. In some cases this effect may provide a great benefit, whereas in other cases the effect may be undesirable. For example, you may take aspirin to relieve a headache, but it may also upset your stomach.

MEDICATION GUIDELINES FOR PERSONS WITH DIABETES

Although it's difficult to remember how individual drugs can affect diabetes, there are three things to remember whenever you buy a prescription or nonprescription drug.

1. Tell your doctor and pharmacist that you have diabetes whenever you begin taking a new medication. This applies for when your doctor gives you a prescription as well as when you purchase nonprescription drugs (sometimes called over-the-counter, or OTC, drugs) such as aspirin, Tylenol, cough syrup, or products to relieve symptoms of a cold.

2. Ask your doctor or pharmacist if the drug can affect your diabetes or any complications you may have.

3. Monitor your blood glucose levels before and after starting any prescription or nonprescription medication to see how it affects your control. If you notice a difference in blood glucose control after starting a new medication, contact your doctor immediately. He or she may change the dose of the drug, prescribe a different drug, or instruct you to modify your diabetes therapy.

DRUGS THAT CAUSE HYPERGLYCEMIA

Drugs may cause blood glucose levels to increase in several ways. They may decrease the release of insulin from the pancreas, decrease the action of insulin, or cause the liver to release stored glucose.

Medications that cause blood glucose levels to increase are listed in the following chart. It's important to note that not every person taking these drugs experiences increases in their blood glucose levels. If you're taking

334

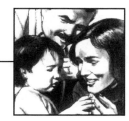

one of these medications, you may find that your blood glucose level does not increase at all.

Because these medications are known to increase blood glucose levels in some people, it's important that you check your blood glucose levels closely if you begin or discontinue taking one of them. That way, you'll be able to see their effect on your blood glucose levels. Notice that things like caffeine, nicotine, and niacin are included in this list. We don't always think of these as drugs, but they are because they have an effect on our bodies when we take them.

It usually takes large amounts of caffeine, nicotine, or niacin to increase your blood glucose. However, consider the fact that caffeine, in some persons, can also increase blood pressure. If you have high blood pressure, caffeine may cause it to go higher and may cause the drugs you use to control your blood pressure to not work. When you consider that high blood pressure and diabetes are both risk factors for developing heart, blood vessel, and kidney disease, it is important to control your blood pressure. Thus, it's important for some people with diabetes to minimize the amount of caffeine they take. Remember, caffeine is not only found in coffee and tea but in many foods, soft drinks, and over-the-counter (OTC) medications as well.

Commonly Cause Increases

thiazide diuretics (Diuril, Dyazide, Esidrix, HydroDIURIL, Maxzide, others)
corticosteroids (Decadron, Medrol, Deltasone, Cortef, others)
glucagon
estrogen (Norinyl; conjugated estrogens such as Premarin; others)
phenytoin (Dilantin)

May Cause Increases

calcium channel blockers (Adalat, Procardia, Cardizem, Calan, Isoptin)
cyclosporine (Sandimmune)
encainide (Enkaid)
caffeine—large doses
cold preparations with decongestants
medications containing sugar
nicotine
niacin (nicotinic acid)—large doses

This is not a complete list. Check with your doctor or pharmacist for other drugs that increase blood glusose levels.

DRUGS THAT INCREASE BLOOD GLUCOSE LEVELS

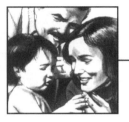

Nicotine is found in cigarettes and can increase your blood glucose in several ways. In addition, smoking also increases the risk of developing heart and blood vessel disease.

It's difficult to predict how each of these drugs will act in your body, but self blood glucose monitoring will help you know.

DRUGS THAT DECREASE BLOOD GLUCOSE LEVELS

insulin
oral agents/sulfonylureas (Diabeta, Micronase, Diabenese, Glucotrol, others)
ethanol (alcohol)
beta blockers (Inderal, Tenormin, Lopressor, Visken)
anabolic steroids (Maxibolin, Durabolin, Deca-Durabolin, others)
salicylates (Anacin, Ascriptin, Bayer, Bufferin, Emperin, others)
monoamine oxidase inhibitors (Parnate, Nardil, Marplan)

This is not a complete list. Check with your doctor or pharmacist for other drugs that increase blood glucose levels.

DRUGS THAT CAUSE HYPOGLYCEMIA

Very few drugs cause blood glucose levels to decrease by themselves (see chart above for those that do). Drugs may cause low blood glucose when food intake is decreased, when too much insulin or oral agent is taken, or when drugs interact with oral agents.

People usually don't think of alcohol as a drug but, according to the definition of a drug, it is. Alcohol may lower blood glucose levels when taken on an empty stomach, which can be a real problem when a person with diabetes becomes hypoglycemic. Because alcohol leaves an odor on the breath, hypoglycemia may be mistaken for drunkenness and treatment may be delayed. This is one of many reasons why it's important to wear visible identification that tells others of your diabetes. Alcohol may also increase blood glucose levels if taken in excess, or with sweet mixers.

If you have Type II diabetes, you may be taking an oral agent to control your blood glucose (see Chapter 12). Some drugs may interact with oral agents to increase their blood glucose-lowering effect (see the following chart for a list). If you're taking an oral agent and are prescribed one of these medications, you must do two things. First, remind your doctor and pharmacist that you have diabetes and are taking an oral agent.

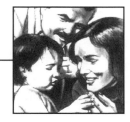

This will alert them to look for drug interactions and tell you of any other possible ways the drug could affect your diabetes. Second, monitor your blood glucose level carefully to determine how the drug affects it. Notify your health care team as soon as you notice a significant change.

phenylbutazone (Butazolidin)
sulfinpyrazone (Anturane)
clofibrate (Atromid-S)
sulfonamide antibiotics (Gantrisin, Gantanol, Septra, Bactrim)
coumadin (Warfarin)
salicylates (aspirin)—large doses
allopurinol (Zyloprim)

DRUGS THAT INCREASE THE EFFECT OF ORAL AGENTS

NONPRESCRIPTION (OVER-THE-COUNTER OR OTC) MEDICATIONS

When you go to a drugstore to buy something for that headache, runny nose, nagging cough, or sore back, you may not realize all the important decisions you face. Of the medications available to treat these and other conditions, many can be purchased without a prescription.

When you buy a prescription drug, your pharmacist makes sure the drug, dose, and dosing interval are all appropriate. He or she checks this drug against others you may be taking to look for possible interactions. The pharmacist makes sure the drug does not interfere in any significant way with any medical conditions you may have. He or she also provides any necessary instructions about taking the drug.

When you buy a nonprescription medication, the person at the counter may not know you have diabetes. Your doctor and pharmacist won't be able to do any of the usual safety checks to assure that the drug is safe for you to use. Yet you may buy a drug that may have a significant influence on your blood glucose level or that may cause or worsen complications of diabetes (see charts on pages 339 and 340).

The labels of some OTC drugs warn patients with high blood pressure, diabetes, and thyroid and other disorders to take these medications only under their doctor's direction. This is because use of these drugs may sometimes lead to serious consequences when taken by persons with these

337

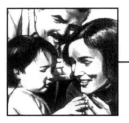
conditions. Selecting a nonprescription medication that will meet your needs and not interfere with your other medications, or your diabetes control, is a big responsibility.

To assure that you make the right decision in buying an OTC drug, it's critical that you openly communicate with your pharmacist and/or doctor. Tell them you have diabetes. Let them know of any other medical conditions you may have, such as high blood pressure, retinopathy, nephropathy, neuropathy, or heart disease. Mention all of the medications you're currently taking to control each of these conditions. This way, your pharmacist and doctor will be able to provide you with important recommendations about the OTC drug you want to buy.

Some OTC medications, such as cough syrups, contain sugar. If you follow the directions on the label and use according to the manufacturer's directions, they don't provide a significant amount of sugar and shouldn't affect your blood glucose levels. Cough drops, throat discs, or throat lozenges also contain sugar. If taken more often than recommended by the manufacturer, they could potentially increase blood glucose levels.

SUMMARY

Drugs can affect diabetes by raising or lowering blood glucose levels. In addition, they may worsen existing complications of diabetes or cause new ones. Drug interactions also may affect how the medication you use to control your diabetes works.

Always tell your doctor and pharmacist that you have diabetes whenever you begin taking a new medication. Ask if the drug may affect your diabetes in any way. And remember to always monitor your blood glucose levels before and after starting any prescription or nonprescription medication to see how it affects your blood glucose levels. Contact your doctor immediately if you notice a change in your blood glucose control. Now that you know how drugs affect diabetes, you can play an important role in assuring that they do not adversely affect your diabetes.

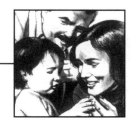

	Examples	Use	Effects
Aspirin	Anacin, Excedrin, Bufferin, Bayer, generics	Relieve inflammation, pain, and reduce fever	• May increase the effect of oral agents if taken in large doses • May worsen kidney function in patients with nephropathy • May cause false-positive urine glucose test
Ibuprofen	Advil, Nuprin, CoAdvil, others	Relieve inflammation, pain, and reduce fever	• May worsen kidney function in patients with nephropathy • Available in prescription strength as Motrin, others
Decongestants	Sudafed (many products on the market)	Relieve nasal congestion	• Contain pseudoephedrine, phenylpropanolamine, phenylepherine • Usually in available in combination with antihistamines • May increase blood glucose and blood pressure • May worsen retinopathy, heart disease • May make you feel "jittery" like you are having an insulin reaction
Antihistamines	Chlor-Trimeton	Relieve the runny nose, watery eyes, and itching seen in allergy and colds	• Contain chlorpheniramine, brompheniramine, doxylamine, pheniramine • May cause you to become drowsy, less alert; may cause you to forget to take medication, eat, or monitor blood glucose at the appropriate time • Can increase the sedative effects of alcohol and other CNS depressants • May cause confusion in older persons • May worsen some types of glaucoma • May cause urinary retention, dry mouth, constipation

EFFECTS OF OVER-THE-COUNTER DRUGS ON DIABETES AND ITS COMPLICATIONS

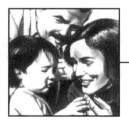

EFFECTS OF OVER-THE-COUNTER DRUGS ON DIABETES AND ITS COMPLICATIONS (CONTINUED)

	Examples	Use	Effects
Cough Preparations	Benylin, Cheracol, Formula 44, Robitussin, Triaminic	Stop coughing in nonproductive coughs	• Contain dextromethorphan, diphenhydramine, others • Many contain alcohol; may cause you to become drowsy, less alert; may cause you to forget to take medication, eat, or monitor blood glucose at the appropriate time • Can increase the sedative effects of alcohol and other CNS depressants • Many contain sugar. May not influence blood glucose significantly if taken according to manufacturer directions.
Combination Cough, Cold, and Pain Medications	Actifed, Chlor-Trimeton Decongestant, Contac, Co-Tylenol, CoAdvil, Dimetane, NyQuil, Sudafed Plus, Triaminic, Triaminicin	Combinations of several medications to stop cough, and relieve runny nose, congestion, inflammation, and reduce fever	• Most cough and cold medications contain combinations of products. • Read the label carefully to determine which medications are contained in these preparations. Ask your pharmacist or physician how these may effect your diabetes.
Diet Aids	Dexatrim, Dex-A-Diet, Acutrim, Appedrine, Grapefruit Diet Plan with Diadax	Diet aids (help suppress appetite and control weight)	• Contain phenylpropanolamine, caffeine • May increase blood pressure • May worsen retinopathy, nephropathy, heart disease • May make you feel "jittery" like you are having an insulin reaction • Some contain significant amounts of fructose, sucrose, dextrose, corn syrup, and vegetable oils. These may influence blood glucose control and cholesterol levels.
Stimulants, Sleep Aids	Nytol, Sominex, Compoz, Unisom, Quiet World		• Stimulants cause same effects as diet aids and decongestants • Sleep aids cause same effects as antihistamines

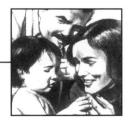

CHAPTER 25

Priscilla M. Hollander, MD

Insulin Intensification:
Fine-Tuning Blood Glucose Control

What is insulin intensification?

Who should use insulin intensification?

How do I know if it would work for me?

More and more evidence shows that blood glucose control plays a role in whether or not people with diabetes develop long-term problems, such as eye, kidney and heart disease. Since maintaining good blood glucose control can lower a person's risk for developing these problems, health professionals are looking for ways to help people with diabetes achieve the very best blood glucose control possible.

This chapter discusses insulin intensification, a treatment program that uses three to four injections of insulin a day or an insulin pump to help you achieve normal or near normal blood glucose control. But insulin intensification is more than just insulin delivery. It is an entire diabetes management program.

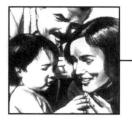

In an ideal world, people with diabetes would be able to achieve blood glucose levels in the normal or close to normal range using one or two insulin injections a day (the conventional treatment plan). Because in the past it was difficult to achieve such excellent blood glucose control with a conventional treatment plan, attention turned to finding improved insulin programs that could more appropriately copy the action of a normal pancreas.

With a normal pancreas, insulin levels in the blood are generally low except for a one to two hour period after a meal. To duplicate this in someone with diabetes, you need a way to deliver a low background amount of insulin (basal) most of the day and then an extra amount of insulin (bolus) at each meal or snack.

This can best be accomplished by using multiple insulin injections (three or four a day). At least one of these injections should be a background intermediate or long-acting insulin. The other injections would be short-acting (Regular) insulin given before each meal. The same effect can be achieved using an ambulatory insulin pump, which is discussed later in the chapter.

Although the goal of insulin intensification is to achieve and maintain near normal blood glucose levels, it should also allow more scheduling flexibility for food and exercise.

Insulin intensification has much to offer different groups of people. If one of the following descriptions fits you, insulin intensification might be just the ticket.

- You monitor your blood glucose levels routinely and use the results for pattern control, follow a meal plan, and exercise regularly, yet you still don't have the blood glucose control you'd like.
- You have good blood glucose control but want a more flexible schedule.
- Your blood glucose control is erratic (frequent unpredictable low or high blood glucose levels).
- You're interested in better control so you can become pregnant and deliver a healthy baby.

Now that we've emphasized the positives of this treatment program, what about the negatives? Studies show that hypoglycemia occurs more often with insulin intensification programs than in people on conventional insulin programs. Insulin intensification also requires more education, more time, more blood glucose testing, and more shots. But not everyone would consider this negative. You have to decide for yourself if the results are worth the extra effort.

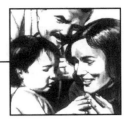

ELEMENTS OF AN INTENSIFICATION PROGRAM

The first thing to know is that this is not a diabetes treatment program you can simply do on your own. You need the help of a health care team to do it safely. If you decide you'd like to start an insulin intensification program, discuss it with your health care team.

Insulin intensification requires *self-adjustment* of insulin. Since your pancreas can't automatically adjust your insulin in response to exercise, food, or blood glucose levels, you must do this job yourself. Insulin *algorithms* (guidelines) that tell you how much insulin to take are the key to self-adjustment of insulin. These guidelines will help you make daily insulin choices based on blood glucose levels and planned daily schedules, food intake, and exercise.

Insulin intensification would not be possible without certain technological advances made in the past ten years. For instance, self monitoring blood of glucose is essential for success. You must measure your blood glucose at least four times a day, if not more. These tests are especially important before meals. You need the information to correctly adjust your insulin.

BLOOD GLUCOSE GOALS AND ASSESSMENT

One of the first steps in starting an insulin intensification program is to set *target blood glucose goals*. We talked about achieving blood glucose levels that are as near equal as possible to those in people without diabetes (70 to 120 mg/dl before meals and up to 140 to 180 mg/dl an hour after a meal). But these are ideal goals and may not be right for everyone. Your blood glucose goals may vary depending on what particular blood glucose problems you may have. For instance, if the problem is too many low blood glucose levels, you may only need to stabilize your blood glucose levels at a more reasonable range and not attempt to achieve normal blood glucose levels. Discuss your glucose goals with members of your health care team. They can help decide the appropriate goals for you.

Starting an insulin intensification program takes time. First you'll need to know the basics of insulin action (Chapter 5) and pattern control (Chapter 10). The next step may be an actual change in your insulin program,

343

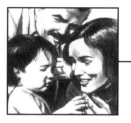

perhaps just a very simple one. Changes in insulin dosage should be made slowly and in small steps, one to two units at a time. Depending on how much you need to change your present insulin program, it may take a number of weeks to several months before you reach your goals.

COMPENSATORY INSULIN ADJUSTMENTS

Once you've mastered pattern control and understand your insulin program, you can start making *compensatory insulin adjustments*. Compensatory insulin adjustments involve increasing or decreasing your Regular insulin dose to *compensate* for or correct a special situation. For instance, you occasionally may have a high or low blood glucose value for no apparent reason. You could also have a high blood glucose value caused by overeating, stress, or lack of exercise. Or your blood glucose may be low from skipping a snack or increased activity. You can take care of the situation with compensatory adjustments. Understanding this level of insulin use brings you one step closer to mastering insulin intensification.

The chart below is a general guide to compensating for high or low blood glucose values. It's really a starting point for changing insulin doses. Work with your health care team to individualize the chart as you identify and determine your individual needs.

ALGORITHMS FOR BREAKFAST, LUNCH, AND SUPPER*

*Do not use these algorithms at bedtime. Your physician may give you individualized algorithms.

Blood Glucose Below 70:	Reduce Regular insulin by 1–2 units
Blood Glucose 71–120:	Take prescribed Regular insulin
Blood Glucose 121–150:	Increase Regular by 1 unit
Blood Glucose 151–200:	Increase Regular by 2 units
Blood Glucose 201–250:	Increase Regular by 3 units
Blood Glucose over 250:	Increase Regular by 4 units

Do not use any of these algorithms unless your physician reviews and agrees with them. You may need algorithms individualized for you.

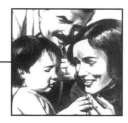

The following practice example shows compensatory adjustments for blood glucose readings outside the target range of 70 to 120 mg/dl. Remember that compensatory adjustments differ from pattern control and that you subtract or add Regular bolus insulin before meals. To avoid confusion between adjustment doses and primary doses, write the adjustment dose in the smaller box.

Month	Night-Time	Break-fast		Insulin		Notes	Lunch		Insul.		Notes	Supper		Insulin		Notes	Evening Snack		Insulin		Comments
Date	BG	BG	K	R	N/L/UL		BG	K	R			BG	K	R	N/L/UL		BG	K	R	N/L/UL	
June 1		134		*1* 4	8N		117					162	5				110		16N		
2		89		4	8N		102					152 *2*	5				89		16N		
3		59		*-1* 3	8N		112					98	5				106		16N		

ANTICIPATORY INSULIN ADJUSTMENTS

It's also possible to *anticipate*, or plan, changes in food and exercise and adjust insulin accordingly. These are called *anticipatory insulin adjustments*. Adjusting insulin for extra (or less) food is generally based on personal experience and on specific nutrition guidelines. For more information on nutrition, see the section on Intensified Insulin Therapy in Chapter 8. The chart on the next page is an example of an individualized guide for making insulin adjustments when you anticipate changes in exercise or food intake. Work with your health care team to come up with a chart that fits your needs.

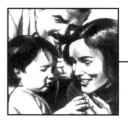

SAMPLE VARIABLE INSULIN DOSE SCHEDULE*

Each person should have an individualized schedule.

	Breakfast Regular 6		Lunch Regular 5		Supper Regular 7		Evening Snack Insulin
If blood glucose is:	If Active	If not Active	If Active	If not Active	If Active	If not Active	
0–50	-2	-1	-2	-1	-2	-1	
51–70	-2	-1	-2	-1	-2	-1	
71–120	-1	6	-1	5	-1	7	
121–150	6	+1	5	+1	7	+1	
151–180	6	2	5	+2	7	+2	
181–210	+1	+3	+1	+3	+1	+2	
211–240	+2	+4	+3	+4	+3	+3	
241–300	+3	+4	+3	+4	+3	+3	
301 & over	+3	+4	+3	+4	+3	+4	

Basal: NPH 16 at Evening Snack

INSULIN PUMPS

The *ambulatory insulin pump*, or continuous subcutaneous insulin infusion (CSII), is another method of insulin delivery used with intensification programs. The insulin pump is a small device about the size of a deck of cards. It contains an insulin reservoir, a pump mechanism, and a small computer to direct the pump. A length of tubing with a needle is connected to the pump. This needle can be inserted into the skin of the abdomen for continuous insulin delivery.

The insulin pump can be set to deliver a small amount of Regular insulin slowly, over time (basal), or a burst of Regular insulin over a few seconds before meals (bolus). The delivery of a constant background level of Regular insulin works better for some people than the injection of an intermediate insulin like NPH or a long-acting insulin like Ultralente. It's thought that some people have problems absorbing and dispersing the intermediate and long-acting insulins, which could contribute to unexpected ups and downs in blood glucose levels.

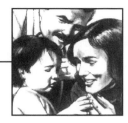

Some people have one basal rate for the entire day. Others may have a lower basal rate during the day and a higher basal rate at night. In some pumps, the change in basal rates can actually be preprogrammed to occur automatically. This can be especially helpful for people who may need more basal insulin between 3 and 6 AM to cover the blood glucose surge that may occur around those particular hours in some individuals.

The pump method for adjusting bolus insulin is very similar to that used with multiple insulin injections. The same anticipatory and compensatory adjustment ranges can be used. Even finer adjustments are possible with the pump, such as a change of 1/2 unit rather than one unit.

SUMMARY

If you're interested in insulin intensification and feel it may be helpful for you, discuss it with your health care team. Also, read the IDC's workbook *Intensified Insulin Management For You: A Personal Program For Advanced Diabetes Self Care* (see the back of the manual for more information).

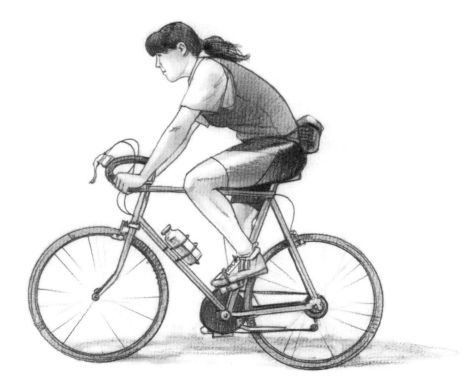

CHAPTER 26

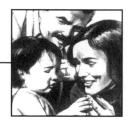

Priscilla M. Hollander, MD
Leslie Pratt, MD

Pregnancy and Diabetes:
Careful Planning and Control

Can I get pregnant?

What will I have to do during pregnancy in order to have a healthy baby?

Will my baby have diabetes?

The decision to have a child is a major step for any woman, but if you have diabetes it takes on a special significance. Not too long ago pregnancy was considered a risky proposition for women with diabetes. But within the past ten years, new discoveries and technologies have made it possible for women with diabetes to have safe pregnancies and healthy babies, just like other women.

This chapter presents these discoveries and technologies to help you understand the importance of careful pre-pregnancy planning and strict diabetes control. It also discusses how you can work with your health care team to protect your health and that of your baby.

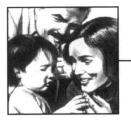

The use of advanced techniques in obstetrical care has also helped women with diabetes to have safe pregnancies and healthy babies. But it's the developments in diabetes care, such as self monitoring of blood glucose, that really made a difference. The importance of strict blood glucose control before and during pregnancy can't be stressed enough. Fortunately, technology is available today so women are able to achieve and maintain excellent blood glucose control during their pregnancies.

PLANNING IS IMPORTANT

Pregnancy for a woman with diabetes must be given careful consideration and planning by both prospective parents. A pregnancy complicated by diabetes requires more time, effort, and expense. Extra costs may include frequent doctor visits and more laboratory tests. If a problem develops, hospitalization may be necessary. Occasionally women are asked to be less active during the last months of pregnancy. They then may need help with housekeeping and child care. If they work outside of the home, they may have to take extra time off.

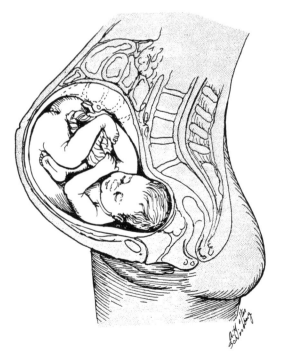

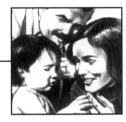

Once you've made the decision to have a child, you must understand the importance of strict blood glucose control both before and during pregnancy. Although the chances for a successful pregnancy are excellent, the incidence of birth defects is still higher for infants of women with diabetes than the general population. Most birth defects originate during the first months of pregnancy, so tight blood glucose control during this period is important. Since most women do not yet know that they are pregnant during the first month, strict blood glucose control must be maintained whenever there is a chance you might become pregnant.

For this reason, it's important that women with diabetes who are sexually active but don't want to become pregnant get advice on birth control from their doctors. There is no *one* best method of contraception for every woman, so the choice should be made carefully with your doctor. Contraception is discussed later in this chapter.

BLOOD GLUCOSE CONTROL

A successful pregnancy depends on your ability to achieve and maintain strict blood glucose control before conception and throughout the pregnancy. This requires a close working relationship with a health care team that is knowledgeable about diabetes and pregnancy. You are the most important member of this team, which should include a diabetes specialist, obstetrician, pediatrician, dietitian, and diabetes nurse specialist. Each has an important role in caring for you and your child, both before and after your baby is born.

Strict blood glucose control means keeping blood glucose levels as near normal as possible. During pregnancy, blood glucose levels are lower, even in women who do not have diabetes. Blood glucose levels rarely go higher than 100 mg/dl, 60 to 80 mg/dl fasting (before breakfast) or before other meals, and 120 mg/dl or lower after meals. For pregnant women with diabetes, the goal is to keep blood glucose levels between 65 and 95 mg/dl fasting and before meals and less than 120 mg/dl 1 1/2 hours after finishing a meal.

Achieving strict blood glucose control during pregnancy depends on three things: blood glucose monitoring, the right insulin program, and close communication with your health care team.

Blood glucose monitoring. The ability to reliably check blood glucose levels at any time has improved the care of pregnant women with diabetes. Blood glucose levels are checked anywhere from four to seven times per

351

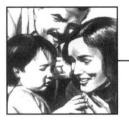

day. Testing should be done before breakfast, lunch, dinner, and bedtime. If blood glucose control is not optimal, you may be asked to test blood glucose 1 1/2 hours after finishing a meal and possibly at 3 AM.

Insulin program. The right insulin program is essential to achieving strict blood glucose control during pregnancy. This doesn't mean all women must have identical insulin programs. All good insulin programs have several common elements. Most women will be able to get the best blood glucose control by using an insulin intensification program (see Chapter 25). Intensified insulin programs use multiple insulin injections (three to four shots per day) and insulin algorithms (adding or subtracting Regular insulin from the usual dose, depending on the blood glucose level). The program of three to four shots per day most often includes Regular insulin before meals supplemented by a background insulin (NPH, Lente, or Ultralente) once or twice a day. Insulin algorithms are guides that help you adjust your insulin daily. These guides allow you to adjust the amount of Regular insulin you take based on blood glucose results, anticipated food intake, and anticipated physical activity.

Health care team. Close communication with members of your health team ensures that you're managing your pregnancy properly. They'll help you to set up an evaluated, individualized insulin schedule and meal plan. They'll provide guidelines and teach you how to make insulin adjustments independently at home. They'll also evaluate your diabetes control at each health care visit by looking at your blood glucose testing records. In addition, they'll do a glycosylated hemoglobin test at two weeks to monthly intervals to help monitor your overall blood glucose control.

NUTRITION DURING PREGNANCY

The meal plan for a pregnant woman must take into account not only her nutritional needs but also those of the developing baby. An individualized meal plan also plays a crucial role in helping keep blood glucose levels under strict control.

For women who are of normal weight before pregnancy, a total weight gain of 25 to 35 pounds is recommended. A 28- to 40-pound gain is recommended for underweight women and a 15- to 25-pound gain is recommended for women who are above their desirable weight. However, a gradual pattern of weight gain is more important than the total amount gained.

The caloric requirements of pregnancy can usually be met by adding 300 calories per day to your regular meal plan. This is done at the

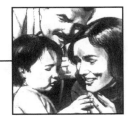

beginning of the second trimester (fourth month). Many women find they don't need or want this many extra calories. In that case, an extra 150 to 200 calories per day may be sufficient. The best way to determine a meal plan is to find out how much food you're comfortable eating and the amount that satisfies your appetite. If your weight gain is appropriate, you can assume the amount of food you're eating is fine. Extra calories can be supplied by drinking two more glasses of skim milk and/or by eating an extra 50 grams of carbohydrate (two starch/bread and/or fruit exchanges). The meal plan should contain approximately 1,800 to 2,500 calories a day.

Your caloric needs may drop during the first three months of pregnancy because of a decrease in appetite and nausea. Insulin needs may also drop slightly during this time. As appetite improves, usually toward the beginning of the second trimester, the extra calories can be added and insulin requirements should be reevaluated.

The importance of maintaining a regular schedule of meals and snacks during pregnancy cannot be overemphasized. Caloric intake should be divided into three meals and two to three snacks per day. The evening snack is particularly important to help prevent hypoglycemia during the night. Your baby continues to feed 24 hours a day, even when you are sleeping. Some women find they need to drink an extra glass of milk and eat some crackers in the middle of the night to prevent hypoglycemia.

Frequent appointments with your health care team will help you continually modify your insulin schedule and meal plan as needed throughout your pregnancy. You should have telephone access to your health care team at all times in case you have a problem or question.

QUESTIONS WOMEN HAVE ABOUT PREGNANCY

Will my diabetes be more difficult to manage during and/or after my pregnancy?

Pregnancy obviously causes changes in your body. Some of these changes can increase the need for insulin. For instance, during pregnancy the placenta produces hormones that resist the actions of insulin and increase production of glucose by the liver. The increased levels of estrogen, progesterone, and human placental lactogen (a hormone secreted by the placenta) are needed to support and maintain a healthy baby.

353

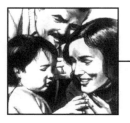

The weight you may gain during pregnancy, which includes the weight of the baby and the placenta, also increases your need for insulin. This means that your insulin requirements will increase as your pregnancy progresses. Often insulin requirements may actually double or triple by the end of a pregnancy. As your pregnancy progresses, expect that your individual insulin dose may increase. This does not mean that the pregnancy has made your diabetes worse. The amount of increase may vary from woman to woman. Your health care team will work closely with you to make sure that correct insulin adjustments and increases are made. Once the pregnancy is over, insulin requirements generally return to what they were before pregnancy. In fact, sometimes during the first day or two after delivery some women may need no insulin at all.

Will pregnancy increase my risk for developing complications of diabetes?

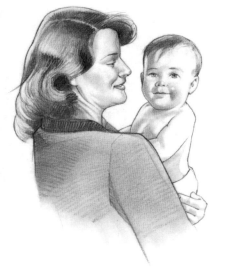

In general, studies have shown that pregnancy does not appear to promote the development of complications nor make existing complications worse. Women with eye, nerve, or mild kidney damage can all have successful pregnancies. However, pregnant women with eye disease (retinopathy) should be closely followed by an eye specialist because there have been some concerns about the effect of pregnancy on retinopathy. Although not all the evidence is in yet on this particular question, studies tend to show that if eye problems develop during pregnancy, they probably would have occurred anyway. Pregnancy is not advised for women with uncontrolled high blood pressure, advanced kidney failure, and/or heart problems. These problems make pregnancy dangerous for both the mother and the baby.

What effect does hypoglycemia or ketoacidosis have on my baby?

Ketoacidosis may be harmful to both the baby and the mother. Ketoacidosis is more likely to occur when blood glucose control is poor. It could also occur if problems develop that put extra stress on the body and increase insulin needs. The best examples would be an illness, such as the flu, or a bladder infection. Both increase insulin needs and can lead to ketoacidosis. Pregnant women with diabetes must be aware of the problems that infections can pose and be familiar with how to manage diabetes during illness. Don't hesitate to call your health care team as soon as an illness or infection is suspected. Early treatment of these problems can reduce their effect on diabetes control and prevent ketoacidosis.

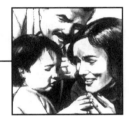

Mild hypoglycemia may occur occasionally whenever people with diabetes have strict blood glucose control. Studies have shown that mild hypoglycemia does not appear to hurt the pregnancy or the health of the baby. This doesn't mean that hypoglycemia is encouraged. The rare, severe episode of hypoglycemia should most definitely be avoided. But dangers to the success of pregnancy come more from high blood glucose levels and ketones than from the occasional episode of mild or moderate low blood glucose levels. Ideally, blood glucose control will be stable during the pregnancy, with no prolonged periods of high or low blood glucose.

Will diabetes affect my ability to become pregnant?

Most women with diabetes have no trouble getting pregnant. This is true whether or not the woman's diabetes is well controlled. However, women who are in very poor control, with frequent bouts of ketoacidosis, may have some trouble conceiving. Before insulin, it was very rare for a woman with insulin-dependent diabetes to become pregnant.

Will my baby have diabetes?

The risk is really fairly low: if a woman has Type I diabetes, the chance of her child developing the disease is about 2%. Interestingly enough, the chance is greater (4%) if the father has Type I diabetes. If both parents have Type I diabetes, the child's chances for developing it become greater—about 25 to 30%.

OBSTETRICAL CARE FOR WOMEN WITH DIABETES

Both your obstetrician and diabetes specialist should see you before you become pregnant to discuss possible problems and cautions. Your first visits after you become pregnant will allow the obstetrician to determine due date, rule out medical problems other than diabetes, and do routine laboratory blood tests to determine your blood type, hemoglobin level, immunity to rubella (German measles), and evaluate your kidney function.

A schedule of routine visits will be set up for the rest of your pregnancy. Women with diabetes are usually seen every two weeks for the first 28 weeks, weekly from 28 to 34 weeks, and every three to seven days from 34 weeks to delivery.

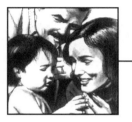

Some of the obstetrical problems that may develop during the first half of pregnancy include:

- **Infections,** especially bladder infections. Your urine will be checked for signs of bladder infection at each visit.

- **Miscarriage,** although if blood glucose control is good, the risk of miscarriage is no greater for women with diabetes than for those in the general population (about one in five pregnancies ends in miscarriage).

In the second half of pregnancy, problems may arise with preeclampsia (toxemia—a buildup of waste products in the blood), which may cause high blood pressure, edema, and decreased kidney function. Other potential problems include premature labor, excessive weight gain by you or your baby, extra fluid in the uterus (which can increase the risk of premature labor), and problems with the function of the placenta in delivering nutrients to your baby.

If you have blood vessel disease, which can occur as a result of diabetes, the blood vessels in the uterus and placenta may be affected. This may cause a decreased supply of nutrients to your baby and result in low birth weight. In extreme cases this may result in the baby dying in the uterus (stillbirth). In the past, there was a much higher rate of stillbirth among women with diabetes, but with improved blood glucose control and close monitoring of the fetus in the last two months of pregnancy, the stillbirth rate is now close to that of pregnancies in the general population.

Several tests and procedures have been developed that greatly increase doctors' and nurses' ability to closely monitor the fetus during pregnancy.

- **Nonstress test.** This test uses a fetal monitor to compare the baby's movement with its heart rate. Acceleration of your baby's heart rate at time of activity suggests that the baby is healthy. This test is painless and is usually started at 30 weeks and performed weekly thereafter.

- **Stress test.** This test involves injecting a medication into a vein to cause mild contractions. It allows the function of the placenta to be evaluated by watching the baby's heart-rate monitor to see how the baby reacts to the contractions.

- **Ultrasound.** This tests uses very low frequency sound waves to measure the size and rate of the baby's growth and its movements within the uterus.

- **Kick counts.** These measure the movements or kicks you feel from your baby and are an important indicator of your baby's health. You may be asked to count the number of times you feel your baby move during a particular time of the day. Your health care team will explain how to do this and how to recognize problems.

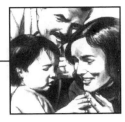

DELIVERY

The best time for delivery is decided by the results of the above tests, the maturity of the baby (especially the lungs), and the mother's condition. Premature babies may have severe problems with breathing, called *respiratory distress syndrome (RDS)*. RDS occurs more frequently in babies born to women with diabetes. A test called *amniocentesis*, which involves withdrawing and examining fluid from around the baby, can help determine the maturity of the baby's lungs and allow a decision to be made on when to deliver the baby.

In the last month of pregnancy, if all the tests are normal and the pregnancy is proceeding normally, deciding on a time for delivery may mean simply waiting for labor to begin. If early delivery is necessary, the amniocentesis will help evaluate if there is any risk to the baby.

Women with diabetes are not allowed to go beyond their due date, because the function of the placenta decreases at this time and increases the risk for stillbirth. Approximately 50% of pregnant women who have diabetes have cesarean section deliveries. This is higher than the general population rate. Cesarean sections may be done if the baby is large, if there is toxemia or problems with the placenta, or if previous deliveries were by cesarean section.

Babies born to women with diabetes have more of a risk for birth defects than those born to women who don't have diabetes. It's believed that poor diabetes control, especially early in the pregnancy, is at least partly responsible for these birth defects. High blood glucose levels and ketones can affect the baby and increase the chances for birth defects.

High blood glucose levels also cause the baby to get fat. The mother's high blood glucose crosses the placenta and raises the baby's blood glucose level. Because the baby does not have diabetes, its pancreas produces extra insulin to lower the blood glucose levels. As a result, the baby grows bigger and fatter than normal. This is called *macrosomia*.

This production of too much insulin can cause another problem. After birth, the glucose from the mother is no longer available to the baby but the extra insulin is. As a result, the baby's blood glucose levels can drop dangerously low (hypoglycemia), which can cause serious problems for the baby. If hypoglycemia occurs, the baby is given glucose and needs to be watched very carefully.

Jaundice is common among all newborns, but it's more common in babies born to women with diabetes. Jaundice is a yellowing of the skin caused by broken-down red blood cells or pigments called bilirubin. It's

357

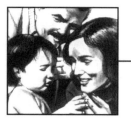
treated by exposing the baby to special lights that help break down and get rid of the bilirubin.

None of these conditions is fatal, and they can all be corrected. However, it's important that your baby be closely monitored during its first 24 to 48 hours of life.

AFTER DELIVERY

Breast-feeding can be a healthy and gratifying experience. There is no reason why an otherwise healthy woman with diabetes should not breast-feed her baby. In general, if you breast-feed your baby, your insulin requirements will be less.

Before you leave the hospital, discuss with your doctor the type of birth control you will use. Breast-feeding women should not use birth control pills. Also discuss your diabetes control; you'll have to adjust your insulin and meal plan as your body adjusts to not being pregnant.

Stay in touch with your health care team after you go home, and feel free to ask for help with any of the concerns and adjustments that new parents have. Maintaining the good diabetes control you achieved during your pregnancy will prepare you for a full life as an active and proud parent!

BIRTH CONTROL OPTIONS FOR WOMEN WITH DIABETES

An important aspect of sexuality for any woman is the ability to feel secure in making the decision to have a baby. Many women with diabetes have concerns about the safety of various methods of contraception, the advantages and disadvantages of each, and whether one method is better than another. One of the most important aspects of family planning is choosing the right method of birth control. Several methods are available, and no one method is appropriate for all women. One exciting new form of contraception, Norplant System, involves implanting six soft capsules under the skin of a woman's upper arm. The Norplant System provides continuous contraception for five years and is reversible.

Perhaps the best known and one of the most frequently used methods is the *oral contraceptive*, known as the Pill. The greatest advantage of this

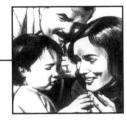

method is its reliability; it is 99% effective when taken correctly. The Pill contains a combination of estrogen and progesterone, two female hormones that are important for the menstrual cycle. Taking the Pill for 21 days out of the usual 28-day cycle prevents release of the egg cell (ovulation). Today research has shown that any short-term risks of taking the Pill are slight, if any. However, some questions may still exist about taking the Pill for longer periods. If you have any complications from diabetes, you need to discuss with your doctor your specific risks for using the Pill. Birth control pills may cause an increase in blood glucose levels. So if you take the Pill, you may have to increase the amount of insulin you take.

The *diaphragm* is another method that, when used correctly, can be up to 95% effective in preventing pregnancy. The diaphragm is a rubber cap that a woman lubricates with a spermicidal gel and inserts into her vagina before intercourse. It's called a "barrier method" because it fits over the cervix and acts as a barrier to prevent sperm from entering the cervix and passing to the uterus. The uterus is where the eggs are fertilized by the sperm. Some women express concern that a diaphragm is awkward and difficult to use. They feel it affects the spontaneity of their relationship. This need not be true, because the diaphragm can be inserted as much as one hour before intercourse. Any woman who chooses this method must see her doctor to be fitted for the diaphragm and be instructed on its use.

Another barrier method is the *condom*, a thin membrane sheath that fits over the man's penis. It can be effective by itself but is even more effective when the woman uses a sperm-killing foam or gel suppository. Statistics indicate that the condom and foam or gel can be up to 85% effective in preventing pregnancy. Using sperm-killing foam or gel alone is much less effective and should not be relied upon by a woman with diabetes.

A newer barrier method is the *sponge*. This small, porous, sponge-like object holds sperm-killing gel and is placed in the vagina before intercourse. Researchers have not determined how reliable the sponge is in preventing pregnancy. Therefore, the sponge is not recommended for women with diabetes.

The *intrauterine device (IUD)* is a small plastic device that is placed inside the uterus by a doctor. Some IUDs were suspected to cause pelvic infections and were taken off the market. Because they have been linked to infections, IUDs are not generally recommended for women with diabetes.

The least effective method of contraception, which really cannot be recommended for the woman with diabetes, is the *rhythm method*. This is one of the oldest methods of contraception, and it requires the most motivation. It's based on avoiding intercourse over a three- to four-day period around the time of ovulation, which occurs during the middle of the

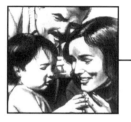

menstrual cycle. Because menstrual cycles can be irregular, it may be very difficult to determine the exact time of ovulation. The best (but not foolproof) method is to measure your temperature in the early morning before getting out of bed. Body temperature increases slightly during ovulation. A fair amount of planning is required to make the rhythm method even remotely successful, and its riskiness makes it a poor choice for women with diabetes.

Sterilization can be considered another form of contraception. The most common form of sterilization for women is a tubal ligation. This involves surgically blocking the fallopian tubes, two tube-like structures through which the egg must pass from the ovaries to the uterus. If these tubes are blocked, the egg cannot pass to the uterus and be fertilized. It may be possible to reverse a tubal ligation if a woman later wishes to attempt pregnancy, but this surgical procedure is not always successful.

Sterilization may be appropriate for women who choose not to have children or who feel they have completed their families, or for women who have serious complications of diabetes. If a woman with severe complications of diabetes becomes pregnant, the pregnancy can be a very serious threat to her life. In these cases, abortion may be a legitimate consideration for the woman.

An effective method of male contraception is a vasectomy. This minor surgical procedure closes the tubes by which sperm travel to reach semen. When these tubes are blocked the semen is still ejaculated, but it will not contain any sperm and therefore cannot cause pregnancy.

Keep in mind that pregnancy can still occur soon after giving birth. Even if you haven't had a menstrual period, you still may ovulate. Breast-feeding your baby will not prevent you from becoming pregnant.

Several methods of contraception are available to couples, and a number of new methods are on the horizon that may be helpful in the future. Talk to your health-care team and then decide what is best for you.

GESTATIONAL DIABETES

Approximately 1 to 3% of all women who become pregnant develop a type of diabetes during pregnancy called *gestational* (during pregnancy) *diabetes*. It's now recommended that all women be tested for gestational diabetes by their 28th week of pregnancy. As discussed previously, pregnancy increases insulin needs for all women. In some women without diabetes, the pancreas cannot always meet this increased need for insulin. This problem usually becomes apparent somewhere after the 24th to 26th week of

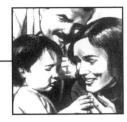

pregnancy. The usual screening test for gestational diabetes is called a *glucose tolerance test*. The woman takes an oral dose of glucose and has her blood glucose level checked one hour later. If the blood glucose level is 140 mg/dl or higher, she may have gestational diabetes. To confirm the finding, a three-hour glucose tolerance test is done. If this test is positive, a diagnosis of gestational diabetes is made.

Treatment for gestational diabetes can vary, but it usually depends on returning blood glucose levels to normal. All patients should be taught to do self blood glucose monitoring. Generally a fairly strict schedule is recommended, with six blood glucose tests daily—before each meal and 1 1/2 hours after finishing each meal. Treatment with a meal plan and mild exercise may often be enough to control blood glucose levels. However, some women who develop gestational diabetes need insulin injections to maintain normal blood glucose control during the remainder of their pregnancy. Good blood glucose control is as important in gestational diabetes as it is for women who have diabetes before becoming pregnant.

In most cases, blood glucose levels return to normal after delivery. It's recommended that women have a follow-up oral glucose tolerance test six weeks after delivery. Having gestational diabetes does increase a woman's risk for developing diabetes in the future. Over time, it has been shown that approximately 34% of women who have had gestational diabetes develop diabetes later on in life. Keeping body weight reasonable is very important in preventing diabetes from developing. At one time it was thought that most women would develop Type II diabetes, but recent studies have shown that a number of these women go on to develop Type I as well.

To learn more about gestational diabetes read the IDC's booklet *Gestational Diabetes: Guidelines for a Safe Pregnancy and a Healthy Baby* (see the back of the manual for more information).

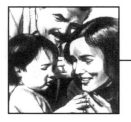
SUMMARY

This chapter will help you think about and plan your pregnancy. Remember, how you care for yourself before pregnancy can be almost as important as how you care for yourself during pregnancy. The nine months of pregnancy will be challenging but rewarding; perhaps it is more rewarding in some ways than a routine pregnancy because you will have a very special role in making it all happen.

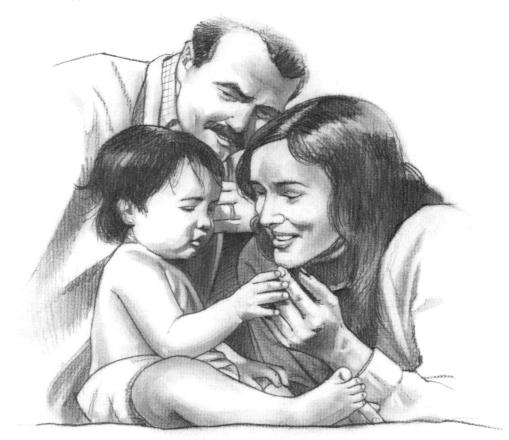

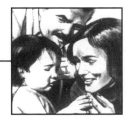

CHAPTER 27

Marion J. Franz, MS, RD, CDE
Jane Norstrom, MA

Athletes:
Juggling Insulin, Food, and Activity

Can you have diabetes and still be an athlete?

How do you adjust insulin for athletic events?

What kind of food should I eat?

Are sports drinks okay to use?

Sports and exercise are an important part of a healthful lifestyle, and all athletes vary in their response to these activities. If you have diabetes, participating in sports and/or exercise means you must continually juggle insulin, food, and activity in order to perform to the best of your ability and training level. This chapter provides suggestions and guidelines to help you do that. With the right knowledge and training, you'll be better able to safely enjoy the thrill of victory or the agony of defeat.

363

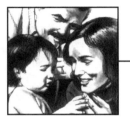

Each athlete's response to exercise is highly individual and depends on many factors during training and competition. We can only provide general advice for managing your diabetes during these times. The best way to determine insulin and food adjustments is to monitor your blood glucose and keep records of all variables and their effects during training. These records can help you evaluate your progress and improve your performance during competition.

BLOOD GLUCOSE MONITORING AND RECORD KEEPING

Blood glucose monitoring has expanded the opportunity for athletes with diabetes to enjoy sports and exercise. It has allowed athletes to learn about their own response to different activities and has helped many to safely challenge the limits of their athletic abilities.

With regular physical training, your body's ability to use insulin improves. Once you develop a plan that works well, it's essential to continue monitoring your blood glucose and be alert to the need for adjustments. As your fitness improves, you'll continually need to make adjustments in your diabetes management plan. Frequent blood glucose monitoring will give you and your health care team the information needed to adapt your insulin schedule to your sports or training schedule.

An exercise diary is a good tool to help make decisions about insulin, food, and activity. Record your usual injection times, insulin dosages, and blood glucose testing results, but add a column where you can record what exercise or training you performed, how long it lasted, and how you felt. Include any changes you made in your daily routine, meal plan, or diabetes management to accommodate the activity. Also, keep track of insulin reactions, the time they occurred, and how much food was needed to treat them.

Start by testing your blood glucose at the beginning of your training activity. Every hour (sometimes you may need to do this more often) during the activity, stop and test your blood glucose again. If it's falling near 100 mg/dl or less, drink or eat 10 to 15 grams of carbohydrate.

After exercise continue to test your blood glucose every two hours for the next 12 hours to evaluate how your body reacts to activity. Repeat this process whenever you make a major change in the intensity or duration of your training pattern or whenever you begin a new sport or activity.

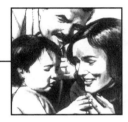

Most athletes find if they gradually begin training and extend it over time, their bodies adapt physically as well as metabolically. As a result, there can be gradual adjustments (usually decreases) in insulin, and food intake can be adapted. By training gradually and making the right decreases in insulin, you'll be less likely to have an insulin reaction or, if one does occur, to treat it by overeating.

INSULIN ADJUSTMENTS

As you become better trained, you'll probably find you need less insulin. You may need to reduce daily insulin dosages or change your injection schedule to allow for the glucose-lowering effect of exercise.

When training for more than 60 minutes at a time, you may need to reduce your daily insulin dose even further. Start by reducing by 10% the dose of insulin that will be acting during the time you're exercising. For activities of very long duration (especially activity not performed regularly, such as a long training run), try reducing the dose by 15 to 30%. On days of a long competitive event, reduce insulin dosages as you think necessary— perhaps 20 to 50%. Remember that only blood glucose monitoring can help you and your health care team determine the changes you need to make in your insulin dosages and the effects these changes will have.

If you plan to exercise immediately after doing your injection, use injection sites that will not be involved when exercising. For example, if you play tennis or racquetball, avoid injecting into your arms. If you jog or cycle, use the abdomen instead of the thighs. If you're not exercising immediately after your injection, don't be concerned about the injection site.

TRAINING

Choose a time of day to train when blood glucose is slightly elevated (180 to 200 mg/dl). An hour or two after a regularly scheduled meal is a good time. Try to train at the same time each day. If this isn't possible, you may have to make different adjustments in your insulin and food, depending on your training times.

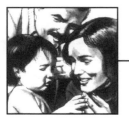

EXERCISE AND CARBOHYDRATE REPLACEMENT

An exercising body uses carbohydrate as its main fuel source. Carbohydrate stored in the liver as glycogen breaks down and circulates in the bloodstream as blood glucose. Athletes who don't have diabetes have enough stored carbohydrate, or glycogen, to exercise intensely for about 90 to 120 minutes. For them, carbohydrate replacement is needed only when exercise exceeds 90 minutes or more at moderate to high intensity. Up to that point, plain water is probably the best replacement beverage. If you have diabetes, you may need carbohydrate replacement after an hour to prevent hypoglycemia, especially if your blood glucose was in the normal range before exercise. Even athletes who don't have diabetes can benefit from eating some carbohydrate during events lasting an hour or more. This can delay the onset of fatigue by slowing depletion of glycogen stores.

If blood glucose is in the normal range before exercise, consume only water and your usual snack before exercise or events lasting less than one hour. For exercise lasting longer than an hour, drink water and eat extra carbohydrate—and be especially aware of possible symptoms of low blood glucose.

Fruit juices or other beverages that contain glucose are good sources of carbohydrate and fluid. Juices should be diluted with about the same amount of water (1/2 cup juice, 1/2 cup water) so they can be absorbed more quickly. Try to consume 10 to 15 grams of carbohydrate every hour during a long event. For very intense or competitive activities, such as marathons, athletes may need 10 to 15 grams of carbohydrate every 30 minutes.

FLUID REPLACEMENT

Athletes with diabetes often become so preoccupied with replacing carbohydrate they forget the most important nutrient needed during regular exercise: water. Drink plenty of fluids before, during, and after practice or athletic events.

Large amounts of water can be lost during exercise and, if not replaced, can cause the body to become dehydrated and unable to cool itself. The result can be a very dangerous condition called heat stroke, in

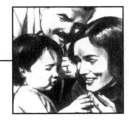

which body temperature can rise so high that the brain or other body systems are damaged.

Dehydration is especially likely in hot, humid weather, but large amounts of body water can be lost in any weather. Thirst is not a good indication of how much fluid to drink, because thirst will be satisfied long before the body's fluid needs are met. You need to replace fluids according to a schedule, not in response to thirst. The following guidelines will help you maintain adequate body fluid during exercise and sports of long duration:

- Drink eight 8-oz glasses of fluid the day before an athletic event or exercise session lasting several hours.
- Drink three or four glasses of fluid about 2 hours before the event.
- Drink one or two glasses of water 5 to 10 minutes before beginning the event.
- Drink 3 to 6 oz (1/2 cup) every 10 to 15 minutes to replace sweat losses. This is especially important in hot and/or humid weather.
- If you're exercising regularly for long periods or in hot, humid weather, weigh yourself before each session to make sure you've replaced fluid weight loss. Don't rely on thirst. You need to drink approximately two cups of water to replace each pound of body weight lost during exercise. Drink water if you're exercising for an hour or less. Cold drinks empty more rapidly from the stomach than warm drinks. For exercise longer than an hour, use a fruit juice and water drink or a sports beverage or drink.

SPORTS DRINKS

Several sports drinks are now on the market that may also be helpful if you have diabetes. They contain water, sucrose or glucose, sodium, chloride, potassium, and phosphorus in varying amounts. Sugar content may range from 2 to 10%.

These drinks have two purposes: to supply carbohydrate to working muscles and to replace fluid and electrolytes (salts) lost through sweat. They use glucose polymers as the source of carbohydrate. Glucose polymers are made by breaking down cornstarch into small glucose chains (polymers).

Several glucose polymer drinks are currently available, such as Exceed, Bodyfuel 450, and MAX. Gatorade is another sugar drink. The following table compares sports drinks and their carbohydrate content.

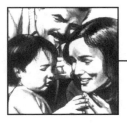

SPORTS DRINKS

Sports Drink	Main Ingredients	CHO Concentration	Calories (1 8-oz Cup)	Grams CHO/Cup
Body Fuel 450	Maltodextrin Fructose	4.2%	40	10
Carb. Plus	Glucose polymers	16.0%	170	42
Exceed: Fluid Replacement & Energy Drink	Glucose polymers Fructose	7.2%	68	17
Fruit Juice	High fructose corn syrup/sucrose	11–15%	120–180	30–45
Gatorade Thirst Quencher	Sucrose Glucose	6.0%	50	12
Gatorade Light	Glucose	2.5%	25	65
Gookinaid E.R.G.	Glucose	5.7%	45	11
Max	Glucose polymers	7.5%	70	17
Mountain Dew® Sport	High fructose corn syrup/sucrose	10%	100	25
Pripps Pluss	Sucrose	7.4%	70	17
Soft Drinks	High fructose corn	10.2–11.3%	110–130	27–32
Tour De France Carboplex II	Glucose polymers	5.9%	45	11

Adapted, with permission, from Franz MJ, "Drinks on the run." *Living Well with Diabetes* 1989;4(2): 16.

Sports drinks supply a steady source of carbohydrate to working muscles. As a result, blood glucose levels stay steady and you don't feel tired. However, too much sugar can slow you down. Sports drinks (or any other carbohydrate solution, such as fruit juice or soda pop) that are too concentrated slow the emptying of fluid and glucose from the stomach to the small intestine, where it is absorbed into the bloodstream.

Drinks containing 5 to 10% carbohydrate are absorbed best. Don't drink anything with a carbohydrate concentration greater than 10%. Concentrated drinks that exceed 10% carbohydrate can cause

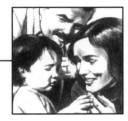

gastrointestinal upset such as cramps, nausea, diarrhea, or bloating. Fruit juices and most regular soda pop contain about 11 to 15% carbohydrate, so they need to be diluted with an equal amount of water to give the right concentration. Practice using sports drinks before a competition or event to make sure your body tolerates them.

Although sports drinks contain sodium, potassium, and chloride that are lost through perspiration, replacing these electrolytes is not necessary unless you're exercising at high intensity for several hours at a time. Following a moderate workout, lost electrolytes can be replaced quickly and easily when you eat your first meal. On the other hand, drinking them isn't harmful either.

EXERCISE AND HYPOGLYCEMIA

Don't wait for symptoms of hypoglycemia, such as loss of coordination, concentration, or tiredness, to develop. Loss of consciousness is not only embarrassing, but it may go unnoticed by others during the excitement of an athletic event. Obviously you want your senses in top condition when competing or participating in athletics.

Athletes should carry some form of carbohydrate with them in case hypoglycemia occurs. Change for a telephone or vending machine can also be useful. This is absolutely essential if you're exercising alone, although you should exercise with a partner whenever possible.

It's wise to do everything possible to prevent an insulin reaction during sports and exercise, but it's also necessary to be prepared in case one occurs. Use the following guidelines to design your insulin reaction game plan. If you feel symptoms of an insulin reaction:

1. STOP your activity immediately—DON'T WAIT.
2. THINK. Use your brain to decide on action. Test blood glucose if possible.
3. EAT the amount of glucose-containing food that experience has taught you is enough to recover.
4. REST. Let your body absorb the glucose.
5. RESUME your activity only when a blood glucose test is above 100 mg/dl and you are sure you can continue without further problems.

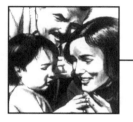

TEAMMATES AND COACHES

Informing teammates and coaches about diabetes and what to do in case of an emergency is important. In general, tell your coach about your diabetes, how you manage it, the possibility of an insulin reaction, and how you plan to avoid insulin reactions. Explain to your coaches how they can help you, and make them feel comfortable with, rather than fearful of, your situation.

Show coaches and teammates where you keep your supply of carbohydrate-containing foods to use during practices and athletic events. Emphasize their importance so teammates don't snack on these foods.

Arrange an "insulin reaction signal" with your coach so you can remove yourself from the action to treat it. Tell your coaches and teammates how to recognize and treat insulin reactions so they can help you, if necessary. Discuss with them what to do in case of an accident or emergency. Even with the best of planning, reactions can happen during a practice or game. Always have a source of simple sugar readily available. Glucose tablets or gels are easy to carry with you and are quickly absorbed. Avoid high-fat snacks such as chocolate candy bars, because they are absorbed slowly and are therefore not helpful for treating reactions.

Your coaches, teammates, or exercise partners should be able to:

- Recognize the signal you give them when you need to treat an insulin reaction.
- Detect the symptoms preceding a reaction.
- Supply carbohydrate-containing foods to you.
- Know emergency telephone numbers.
- Help you decide if you have recovered from a reaction.
- Be supportive but not too protective.
- Allow you to handle your diabetes as you choose.

SNACKS

Contrary to the popular belief that some snacks, such as candy bars, are a source of "quick energy," high-sugar foods should be avoided before exercise. Quick energy is already stored in the liver and muscles as glycogen and is available as fuel for exercise—as long as enough insulin is available.

To prevent an insulin reaction when glycogen stores become low, it's helpful to eat slowly absorbed carbohydrate foods before exercising.

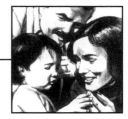

Suggestions for pre-exercise snacks are found on page 150 in Chapter 9. These snacks can also be eaten after exercise to prevent post-exercise hypoglycemia. After exercise, a bigger snack, such as a sandwich with milk or fruit, is often needed.

EATING FOR COMPETITION OR ENDURANCE EVENTS

On the day of competition, eat a light breakfast and lunch. Toast, juice or fruit, and cereal with skim milk are good breakfast selections. A turkey sandwich, skim milk, and fruit make a good lunch.

A lighter pre-event meal should be eaten one to two hours before the starting time. This meal should contain mostly carbohydrate and some protein, but a minimal amount of fat. The menu could include lean meat (fish or poultry without the skin), potatoes without gravy, vegetables, bread with no butter, salad without dressing, fruit, and skim milk. If you have diabetes, additional snacks as well as additional carbohydrate may be needed about 20 minutes before a long endurance event.

SUPPLEMENTS

Although research has shown that most persons do not need vitamin or mineral supplements, some athletes psychologically feel better if they do use them. In that case, a multivitamin with iron that does NOT exceed 100% of the Recommended Daily Allowance (RDA) is your best choice. The RDA is any amount of a vitamin or mineral recommended for all healthy persons, and a large margin of safety is figured in.

An athlete's vitamin requirements are not significantly greater than those of a sedentary person. Usually enough vitamins and minerals can be obtained from the meal plan. Although vitamin and mineral deficiency could impair performance, it would be very unusual for athletes with diabetes to have such deficiencies. They usually eat better than the general population. As a result, they meet their needs for vitamins and minerals.

Likewise, supplements of liquid protein, amino acids, wheat germ, and bee pollen have no proven benefit in building muscles or improving performance. Use of extremely high protein supplements places an additional load on the kidneys and has been shown to be harmful.

371

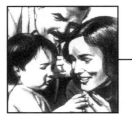

NUTRIENTS AND EXERCISE

In general, the percentages of carbohydrate, protein, and fat needed by an active person are similar to those recommended for everyone else:

50 to 60% carbohydrate

15 to 20% protein

25 to 30% fat

The difference is that an active person needs more calories to maintain weight. Total caloric needs depend on the type and duration of activity. Most of the additional calories should come from carbohydrate foods, meaning that the active person will be eating closer to 60% carbohydrate and 25% fat. If weight loss is desired, daily caloric intake can be reduced slightly. The easiest way to do this is by eating less high-calorie, high-fat food.

Athletes who want to lose or maintain weight, such as wrestlers and gymnasts, should do so gradually with the assistance of a dietitian and doctor. This may require insulin adjustments along with changes in your meal plan.

Because regular exercise requires frequent replenishing of stored carbohydrate, more carbohydrate is also needed in the meal plan. This should come primarily from naturally occurring sugars, starches, and fiber-containing foods rather than refined sugar foods, which supply only calories without other nutrients. There is no need for an increase in fat or protein intake. In fact, excessive protein intake can make it harder for the body to use its most efficient fuel—carbohydrate. Foods high in fat contain large amounts of calories, so they will contribute to excessive body fat, which is both unhealthy and an unnecessary burden for athletes.

SUMMARY

The suggestions in this chapter will not automatically result in a problem-free athletic event or training session. Just as practicing athletic skills and building endurance levels lead to better performance, learning your insulin and food needs and your response to exercise is a major part of reaching your athletic potential. Building up gradually to competitive activity levels while learning how to keep your blood glucose in control will help prevent unpleasant surprises in sports and exercise.

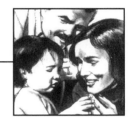

Although guidelines to help you get started can be helpful, remember that you're an individual. All athletes vary in their response to training and physical stress. Adjustments that work for one person with diabetes may not work for you! Be aware of signals your body gives you; all good athletes become experts at interpreting these signals. With proper preparation, training, and attention to your body's needs, you can enjoy the thrill of becoming physically fit and athletically active to the best of your ability and desire. To learn more about exercise and diabetes, read the IDC's book *Diabetes Actively Staying Healthy (DASH): Your Game Plan For Diabetes and Exercise* (see the back of the manual for more information).

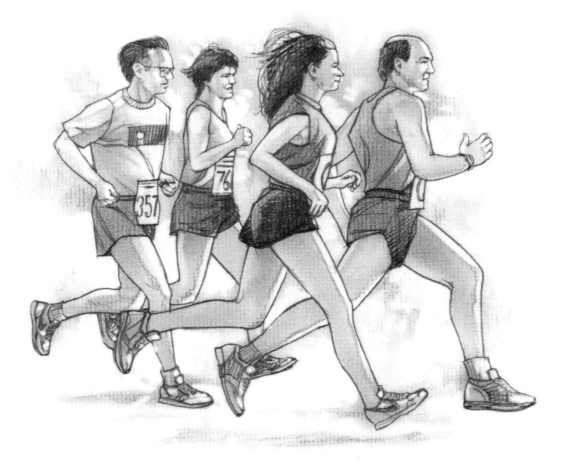

CHAPTER 28

Jan Pearson, RN, BAN, CDE

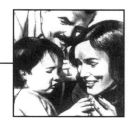

Planning Travel:
Your Ticket to Opportunity

How should I handle my insulin schedule during my trip to London?

What do I need to know to go backpacking at Isle Royale?

What special considerations would be involved in taking a bus tour of the Canadian Rockies?

If I spend three days driving Aunt Violet to Florida, will it throw my diabetes off?

There's no need to have misgivings about traveling with diabetes—go for those opportunities! If you know the basic skills essential to diabetes management and if you learn to plan accordingly, you'll be able to travel safely and with greater confidence. This chapter provides information and practical suggestions for successful trip planning and travel with diabetes.

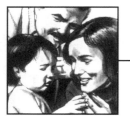

Traveling presents an array of challenges and plenty of opportunity for adventure. Having diabetes is no reason to deny yourself the pleasure of going places and seeing things. Part of the fun of traveling is not always knowing quite what to expect. But the more you know about yourself and your diabetes, the easier it will be to make decisions as new challenges are presented. If you're well-grounded in the basics of diabetes management and confident in your knowledge, you need just one more ingredient for successful travel—planning. Once you learn how to adequately plan and prepare for a trip, you're another step closer to becoming a seasoned traveler.

PLANNING YOUR TRIP

Make this checklist a priority when preparing for a trip.

___ Schedule immunizations early.

___ Have a general health check-up close to departure date.

___ Review your treatment plan. Ask your health care team how to adjust insulin doses when crossing time zones.

___ Discuss guidelines for illness.

___ Get a prescription for nausea and diarrhea medications.

___ Have your health care team write a letter stating that you have diabetes and listing the medications you take.

___ Make a list of your current medications (use generic names).

___ Carry your medications in their original containers.

___ Wear an Identification Aid.

___ Pack comfortable shoes—at least two pair!

___ Pack an extra week's worth of supplies. It's better to have extra than to chance running out. Your travel bag should include:

- supply of food (cheese, crackers, dried fruit, fruit juices, glucose tabs)
- blood glucose meter with an extra battery
- cotton balls or tissues for testing (if needed)
- blood glucose strips
- Ketostix (foil-wrapped are best because they're less affected by extremes in temperature/humidity)
- record book

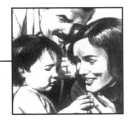

- insulin
- syringes
- insulin storage kit (if you'll be traveling where temperatures are above 86° F or below freezing)
- glucagon
- over-the-counter antibiotic ointment (such as Bacitracin, Neosporin)
- gauze dressing
- paper tape
- sunblocking agent

Be certain to carry your supplies with you. It's one less thing to be worried about if your luggage is lost or arrives after you do! It's also wise to have a travel companion carry an extra set of supplies.

BLOOD GLUCOSE MONITORING: JUST DO IT!

Vacationing with blood glucose monitoring rather than from it is essential to feeling well while traveling. Stock up on supplies before you leave. Then you don't have to spend precious travel time looking for glucose strips, or worse yet, having to switch methods because you can't find the product your meter requires. Protect your supplies from temperature extremes. Temperatures above 86° F or below freezing may produce inaccurate results. If you're going to be in extreme temperatures for a prolonged period, keep supplies in an insulated container.

HYPOGLYCEMIA: KNOW WHAT TO DO

It's always smart to review how you are handling hypoglycemia. Testing your blood glucose level when you feel the jitters coming on will help you know if they're truly caused by low blood glucose or, perhaps, by something else. Who knows, it may be because you are about to walk across a suspension bridge and you're usually shaky when you get on a stepladder! It's always safer to check and see what your blood glucose level actually is.

377

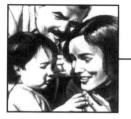

Carry a source of glucose so you can quickly handle a reaction without relying on others. Particularly if language is a problem, you want to eat some fast-acting glucose and not waste energy trying to explain to someone what you need. Teach your travel partner how to use glucagon. The chances of you needing it are quite remote, but it's a great product to have on hand, just in case. The glucagon powder with a prefilled syringe that's now available may be less stressful for someone to use in an emergency. If you weigh more than 50 pounds, you would need the entire amount (1 mg); if you weight less than 50 pounds, take half the amount (0.5 mg).

If you have a severe reaction, be sure you eat something when you wake up. Your blood glucose levels will be low and will need to be replenished. Try sips of regular (not diet) soda pop first, followed by a sandwich. Your blood glucose levels will probably be high the rest of the da,. but that's expected. Don't take Regular insulin to counter it. Just live with the highs for the next 24 hours. Then things should settle down.

OUT AND ABOUT WITH INSULIN

Stock Up. Always travel with an adequate supply of insulin. It's wise to bring extra Regular insulin along for use in case of illness. If you plan to be gone for an extended time, contact your insulin manufacturer to check insulin availability in the country you'll be visiting. A foreign country may have your same insulin but manufacture it under a different name. Also, remember that U-100 insulin is not available in all countries. The same is true for U-100 insulin syringes. For information about insulins and syringes, contact your local diabetes educator.

Storage. It's best to store insulin in the refrigerator (36° to 46° F), since it loses 1.5% of its potency when stored at room temperature for one month. Insulin deteriorates in extreme temperatures (above 86° F [32° C]) or below freezing (32° F [9° C]), so it's best to protect it in some way. Pack insulin in an insulated container, wide-mouth thermos, or cooler. Don't place insulin directly on ice or an ice pack, as it could freeze. Insulin is totally ineffective if frozen and should not be used.

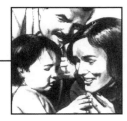

CROSSING TIME ZONES

If you'll be traveling across different time zones, contact your doctor or diabetes educator at least two weeks before departure to help you determine any adjustments you may need to make in your insulin dosage. Various methods are used to determine your dosage. To develop your travel plan, your health care team needs to know:

- your destination
- your usual insulin dosage
- your current meal plan schedule
- your departure and arrival times for both going and returning

In general, when you lose hours from your day (for example, traveling east from the United States to Europe), you may need a schedule of Regular insulin only and/or a reduction in your mixed dose of insulin. When adding hours to your day (for example, traveling west from Europe to the United States), you may need an extra dose of Regular insulin. Consult your health care team well in advance of travel for an individualized food and insulin schedule.

During active vacations, such as backpacking, it's likely you will see a big change in blood glucose levels. Discuss plans for such vacations with your health care team, since your insulin dose may need to be decreased (possibly as much as 10 to 30%). It's important to know your insulin action times when making these decisions.

EXERCISE

Spending several hours driving or traveling in a tour group may wreak havoc with glucose control. If you're able to move around, do so every one to two hours. Walk the aisles if you are traveling by plane. When your bus stops at rest areas, take advantage of the time and do some walking. When driving, stop every two hours and get some exercise. It's important to do anything you can to improve circulation, such as moving your toes and feet, when sitting for prolonged periods.

When activities increase, plan ahead by eating more or taking less insulin. See guidelines for making food adjustments for exercise or adjusting insulin for extended activity in Chapter 27.

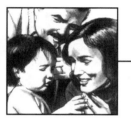
FOOT CARE

Once you arrive, you're going to want to see the sights. Comfortable, well-fitting shoes (at least two pair) are a must. Be certain to break them in before the trip. Wearing different shoes each day reduces your risks for developing foot problems. Make sure you wear sandals or shoes on the beach to protect your feet from sharp objects or burns.

Check your feet each day and watch for any signs of redness. If a blister should pop up, wash the area with mild soap and water and keep it covered with a plastic adhesive strip to lessen further irritation. If the blister should break, wash the area with soap and water, dry well and apply an over-the-counter antibiotic ointment. Cover the area with a light gauze dressing fastened with paper tape. This should be done twice a day until the area is healed.

COPING WITH BEING SICK

Feeling crummy and being away from home are not a good twosome. Plan ahead so you're prepared to cope. Ask your doctor for a prescription in case of upset stomach, nausea and vomiting, or diarrhea, and fill it before you leave. Some people have found it helpful to use antibiotics (Vibramycin or Septra) as a preventive medication against some of the diarrhea-causing organisms. Discuss this with your doctor. If you need a doctor while traveling, contact the American Embassy in the country you are visiting for names of English-speaking doctors.

Testing your blood glucose four times a day (before meals and bedtime snack) and checking for ketones are a must when you are ill. If your blood glucose levels are above 240 mg/dl and your tests show moderate to large ketones in the urine, call a doctor. Besides needing extra Regular insulin, you may have some kind of infection that needs to be treated as well. A general guideline is to take 10% of your total insulin dose in Regular insulin every four to six hours when blood glucose levels are high and ketones are moderate to large. This is in addition to your normal insulin dose. Continue supplementing with Regular insulin until blood glucose level is under *240 mg/dl* and/or ketone levels are less than moderate.

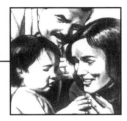

SUMMARY

Adequate planning and knowledge about your diabetes management are the two ingredients needed for a successful trip. Investment in both will be returned in the confidence you feel as you set out on your venture. Your health care team is there to assist you as you plan—don't hesitate to contact them. Happy traveling!

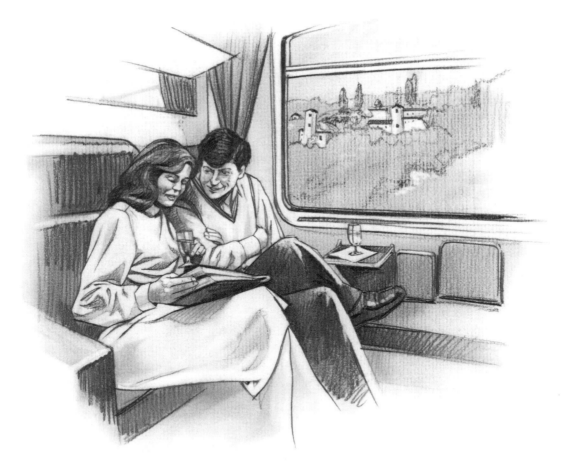

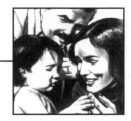

CHAPTER 29

Helen Bowlin, RN, BSN, CDE

Healthful Habits:
Strategies for Living Well

■ Why is it important to be concerned about healthy teeth and gums?

What is the relationship of infections to diabetes?

Why should I carry food in my car?

How do I communicate with my doctor or diabetes educator?

Good health care for people with diabetes requires more than just food, insulin, and activity. This chapter provides guidelines and suggestions for maintaining other aspects of good health.

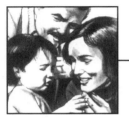

Good health habits are important for everyone. Your desire to live well with diabetes may be the motivation you need to make positive decisions about your health. Using your knowledge, your judgment, and the advice of your health care team, you'll be able to assess your state of health and maintain it at the best possible level.

DENTAL CARE

Careful care of your teeth and mouth is necessary to prevent tooth decay and mouth infections. Infections are caused by germs that live in our mouths. Regular use of dental floss and frequent brushing help prevent infections and cavities. It also helps prevent buildup of a substance called plaque. If plaque is not removed it hardens to form calculus, which can grow underneath the teeth and into the gums and cause pain and infection.

If you have diabetes, poor blood glucose control increases your risks for developing gum disease. This means that proper dental care should be an important part of your health care plan.

Your dentist is an important member of your health care team who needs to be informed that you have diabetes. Your diabetes should be noted on your dental chart. Time your appointments so your meal schedules are not interrupted. Be prepared to test your blood glucose levels if your appointment takes longer than expected. Make certain that food is available to you if you need it. If you need dental surgery, your dentist and doctor need to work together to help you regulate your diabetes.

Follow these dental habits to maintain healthy teeth and gums.

1. Brush after each meal, using a soft toothbrush and fluoride toothpaste.

2. Floss daily, getting between each tooth gently.

3. Visit your dentist every six months.

4. Plan the timing of your dental appointments to avoid insulin reactions.

5. Make sure your dentist knows you have diabetes. Your dentist must be able to recognize and treat an insulin reaction.

6. Make sure your doctor and dentist are working together, especially when anesthesia is needed for dental work or oral surgery. If you must miss meals because of dental work, consult your doctor or diabetes educator. Consult them before the procedure so they may advise you on insulin and food adjustments.

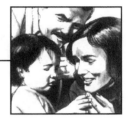

PREVENTING INFECTIONS

It's especially important for people with diabetes to avoid infections. If you have an infection, your body needs more energy to fight it and you may need more insulin.

High blood glucose levels decrease your resistance to infection. Good blood glucose control helps you to prevent infections. If you do have an infection and your blood glucose is high, test every four hours for ketones. Ketones in your urine may be an early warning that ketoacidosis is developing.

You can avoid infections by following some good health practices.

1. Bathe or shower frequently to keep your skin clean. Use a lanolin lotion if your skin is dry. If you are obese, carefully dry all areas of overlapping skin and powder with cornstarch. Don't allow the cornstarch to adhere to skin creases. This may cause irritation.

2. Promptly treat all cuts or broken skin. Wash with soap and water, cover with a clean bandage, and watch for warmth, swelling, or redness until the area has healed.

3. Use caution while shaving, and be careful not to break the skin. Use an electric razor if you shave your legs. A sharp-edged razor is more likely to cause cuts, which may become infected. Other hair-removing methods, such as chemicals, waxing, and electrolysis, may also irritate the skin.

4. Contact your doctor if pimples show redness, warmth, or swelling or become painful.

5. Watch for bladder infections, which may be a problem for people with diabetes. The symptoms are frequent and urgent urination, a burning sensation when urinating, blood in the urine, and back pain. You may also have a fever with chills. You can help prevent urinary tract infections by:

    - drinking fluids often and urinating every three to four hours
    - wearing cotton underwear to absorb moisture
    - washing daily around the rectum and vagina

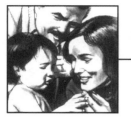

PREVENTING INJURY

To avoid burns:

- Always wear sunscreen, which helps prevent sunburn. Expose your skin to the sun only for short periods.
- Always cover your feet when walking on sand—it may be hot.
- Test bathwater temperature with your wrist rather than your feet.
- Don't use hot water bottles or heating pads because they may cause burns.

To avoid circulation problems:

- Don't wear stockings that are tight at the top.
- Don't cross your legs while sitting.
- If your feet or ankles tend to swell, elevate them several times a day.
- Don't smoke. Smoking constricts blood vessels, which impairs circulation.

TIPS FOR DRIVING

Having an insulin reaction while driving could cause severe injury to the driver, passengers, and others. To prevent accidents, follow these guidelines.

1. Check your blood glucose before driving. If it's 80 mg/dl or less, eat 15 grams of carbohydrates (such as 1/2 cup orange juice, 1/2 cup regular soda, a small box of raisins, or 6 LifeSavers). Wait 15 minutes and re-check your blood glucose before driving.

2. If you're unable to check your blood glucose and two hours have passed since your last meal or snack, eat 15 grams of carbohydrate before you begin driving.

3. If you feel even minor symptoms of low blood glucose, pull over to the side of the road and eat 15 grams of carbohydrate. Don't drive until your symptoms are gone.

4. Always keep a supply of carbohydrates in the car.

5. Don't drive after drinking alcohol. Alcohol has a hypoglycemic effect and may impair your driving skill.

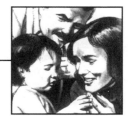

ALCOHOL, TOBACCO, AND DRUGS

Having a healthful lifestyle includes making wise choices about the use of mood-altering substances. These can range from the use of legal drugs such as alcohol and tobacco, to the abuse of prescribed drugs, such as tranquilizers, sedatives and diet pills, to the use of illegal drugs, such as marijuana, crack/cocaine, and other street drugs. How these substances affect people varies, as does their effect on diabetes.

Alcohol and Tobacco

- Alcohol can lower blood glucose levels in persons using insulin.
- Alcohol can contribute to obesity and may cause unpleasant reactions in some persons who take diabetes pills.
- Tobacco is a major health hazard that causes lung cancer and damages blood vessels. Nicotine, a tobacco ingredient, can cause blood vessels to narrow, which results in reduced blood flow to the heart, the brain, the kidneys, and other parts of the body. This contributes to the development of retinopathy, kidney disease, nerve damage and foot problems. Inhaling other people's smoke is also hazardous to your health. Be assertive in your right to breathe clean air!

Prescription and Nonprescription Drugs

Everyone who takes a medication should be aware of why, how, and when to take it as well as its intended action and possible side effects. It's also very important to know what *not* to do while taking a medication. The best source of this information is your doctor or pharmacist.

If you develop a skin rash, pain, or other symptoms after taking a medication, you may be allergic to it. Report such incidents to your doctor immediately. Many medications can interact with diabetes medications to reduce or increase their effects or cause side effects. See Chapter 24 for detailed information on diabetes and drug interactions.

Street Drugs

People with diabetes are as vulnerable as anyone else to the peer pressure, curiosity, or emotional problems that lead people to use street drugs. However, as a person with diabetes, you're working hard to have a healthful life. Street drugs can prevent you from making good decisions about your diabetes and can threaten your emotional and physical health.

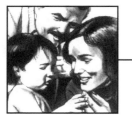

When under the influence of drugs, it's difficult to recognize and treat insulin reactions.

Whether to use street drugs is an individual choice, but the healthy choice is to decide against their use. Your health care team can provide you with the facts. A counselor can be an especially helpful resource for assistance with underlying personal or family problems.

COMMUNICATING WITH YOUR HEALTH CARE TEAM

You are the most important part of your health care team. Nurses, doctors, dietitians, counselors and other health care professionals need your input to help you stay in good health. You are the person who knows just how you feel, physically and emotionally. You know what you can reasonably fit into your lifestyle to help you have a happy, productive life.

Be assertive when discussing problems with your health care team. If answers or directions are not clear, ask that they be repeated or explained. The following suggestions will make discussion with your health care team more rewarding.

1. Before phoning or visiting your health care team, collect all the information you might need. Have your diabetes record book in front of you so you can share important information about your diabetes management plan.

2. Have a written list of questions so you don't forget any important items.

3. If you're not feeling well, take your temperature and record it.

4. List symptoms in the order they happened. Think about your symptoms so you can describe them accurately.

5. Know what medications you take, how much, and how often. If medications are new to you, be sure you understand why you're taking them and what side effects might occur, especially when used in combination with other medications or alcohol.

6. Report any situations of stress that might lead to changes in blood glucose control.

7. Make sure you understand everything the health care team says. Repeat your instructions and write them down, and if you don't understand a medical term, ask that it be explained in words you understand.

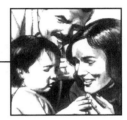

SUMMARY

You are the most important member of your health care team. With the proper information, you can make intelligent decisions about your own state of health. Using your best judgment and your health care team as important resources and partners, you'll be able to make good health decisions.

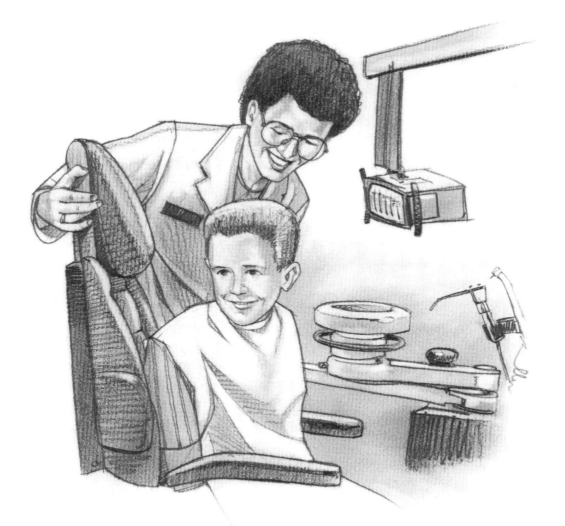

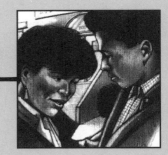

Diabetes
and
Youth

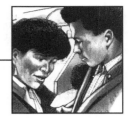

CHAPTER 30

Barbara Balik, RN, MS
Becky Clasen, RN, BA, CDE
Gretchen Kauth, RD, CDE

For Kids:
Taking Care of Me

Note to Parents:

This chapter is meant to be read with your child to explain diabetes in words he or she is able to understand. As you read, you will come across frequent questions. Use them as an opportunity to see your child's view of life and diabetes. Discuss topics honestly. Keep a list of questions you and your child can ask your health care team. If your child asks a question about diabetes, ask what she or he thinks first. There are lots of thoughts behind children's questions. Don't expect to answer all the questions. If you don't know, say so. It's OK to not know everything.

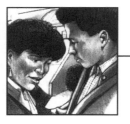

What children can manage by themselves varies. Remember, children need your support and involvement even as they gain greater independence. Staying involved while letting go is a tricky balance. You must listen to and communicate with your child. Both are skills that take time to learn.

Communication is important for all families, but diabetes requires that family members communicate especially well. If families have problems with communication, talking about diabetes becomes a source of constant friction. Diabetes can become the focus of an entire family. We hope your family will focus on health and love and fun and communication. In that environment, diabetes will be managed best. Children who grow up feeling good about themselves will be more likely to succeed at self-management and living well.

TAKING CARE OF ME—CHRIS' STORY

My name is Chris and I have diabetes. I got diabetes about three years ago. My grandma had diabetes but I didn't think kids got it. I didn't know I had diabetes at first. My mom thought I was acting tired all the time. I was drinking lots of water and I had to go to the bathroom a lot. A couple of nights, I even wet the bed. I hadn't done that since I was a really little kid. My doctor said those were signs of diabetes.

How did you feel when you got diabetes? Write the signs you had or draw a picture of how you felt.

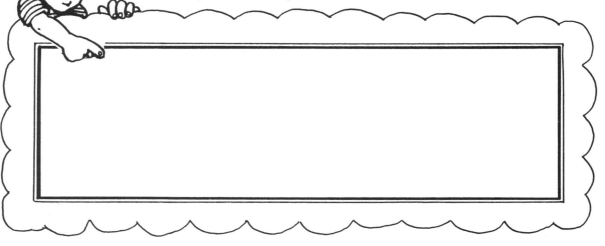

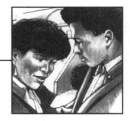

I wanted to know why I got diabetes and how long it would last. Do you want to know what I learned at my diabetes clinic and my special diabetes class?

First: I didn't do anything to make me get diabetes.

Second: There was nothing I or anyone else could have done to keep me from getting diabetes.

Third: Right now, no one knows how to make diabetes go away.

But I still didn't know what diabetes is or why I got it. Why do you think you got diabetes? Write or draw what you think.

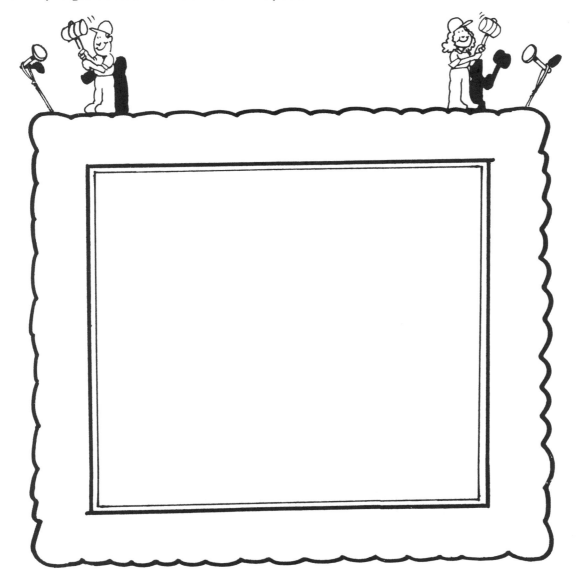

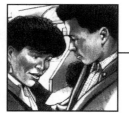

Here is what I learned from the people who help take care of my diabetes: Inside my body are lots of things. There's my stomach and my lungs. Can you draw lines to the correct body parts?

**Draw lines
to the correct
body parts:**

PANCREAS

KIDNEYS

STOMACH

BLADDER

HEART

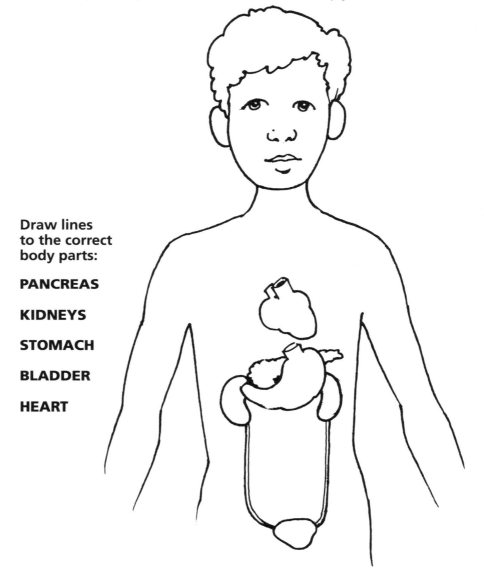

One of the things inside my body is my *pancreas*. Can you find your pancreas in the drawing? The pancreas does lots of things to help my body. One part of the pancreas makes *insulin*. Insulin helps your body use the food you eat. Diabetes means your body doesn't make enough insulin. What happens if your body doesn't have enough insulin?

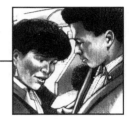

Do you turn green? No!

Do you fly like a bird? No!

Do you grow four extra hands? No!

So a person with diabetes doesn't look different.

What does happen is that when there's not enough insulin, your body can't use the food you eat. Food makes us strong and helps us grow and gives us energy to play. The food changes to a kind of sugar called *glucose*. Your body needs insulin to help use this glucose for energy. If you have diabetes you don't have enough insulin, so your body can't use the glucose. Too much of this sugar stays in your blood and urine. That's why my friend Ann thought you got diabetes because you ate too much sugar. She was wrong! You get diabetes because you don't have enough insulin to help food make you strong and help you grow. Instead, you feel tired and go to the bathroom a lot and drink a lot. If your body can't use glucose for energy, it will use fat. When the body uses fat for energy, *ketones* are made. Ketones show up in your urine when you go to the bathroom.

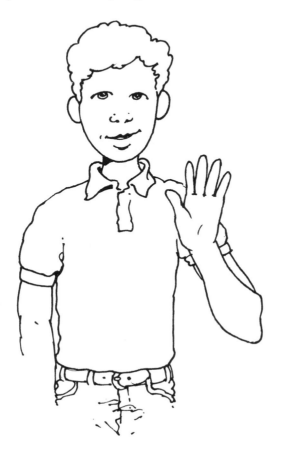

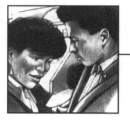

I wanted to know why part of my pancreas stopped working.

I found out that dietitians and nurses and doctors aren't sure why kids get diabetes. Here are some of the reasons why they think it happens.

- You are born with differences in your pancreas that later make the pancreas stop making insulin.
- You get sick and sometimes that makes your pancreas not work.

But most of all, they don't know why kids get diabetes. Just remember, there was nothing you or your mom and dad could have done to keep you from getting diabetes. You didn't do anything to make yourself get diabetes.

So I have diabetes. What happens now?

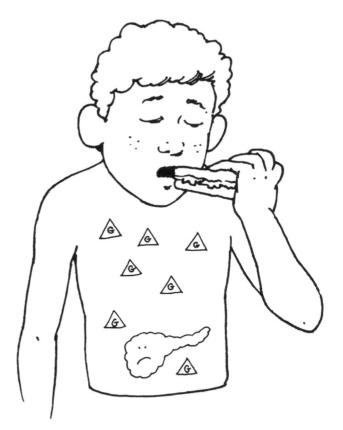

NO INSULIN

NO ENERGY

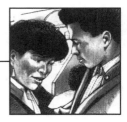

Remember when you first got diabetes? Write a story about what happened.

_____

_____

_____

_____

_____

_____

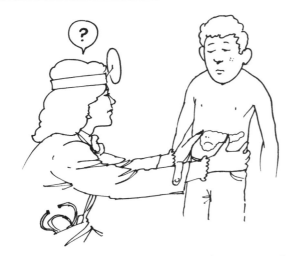

Some kids get sick, like my friend Jamie. She went to the hospital and stayed four days. Some kids are not very sick when they get diabetes, like me. My mom and dad took me to the clinic. The doctor knew I had diabetes when they checked my blood for glucose and my urine for ketones. Then my mom and dad and I talked to a dietitian and a doctor and a nurse and a family counselor to learn how to take care of my diabetes. Mom and dad called the clinic a lot. They had bunches of questions. We can always call the clinic with questions. My mom and dad also looked worried and tired. They were worried about learning all about diabetes and helping me take care of it.

At the clinic I learned lots of things. They told us that since my pancreas doesn't make insulin, we have to learn to do some of the things my pancreas used to do.

First I learned that insulin won't work if you take it in a pill, so it has to be a shot. I also learned that I had to give myself a shot. When I heard

399

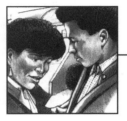

that, I said, "A shot! NO WAY!!" But the nurse helped me and mom and dad to learn. It wasn't that hard and I felt proud that I could do it!

Next I learned to check my blood glucose. Checking your blood glucose levels helps you know if you are getting enough insulin and food. Blood glucose values are not good or bad. They just let us know what's going on inside our bodies. Your doctor will tell you what range your blood glucose should be in. Write your goal range here:

It's important to always do your blood glucose test the way your nurse taught you so you know you're getting the right information. Draw a picture of how you check your blood glucose.

ORANGE II

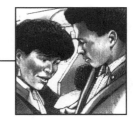

I use a machine called a *meter* to check my blood glucose. I learned it's important to clean my meter and use control solutions regularly so it is working okay. I also take it to the doctor's office so they can check it with their meters. One time my meter didn't work so I had to match the color on my blood glucose strip with a chart on the bottle. I am lucky I know how to do my blood glucose tests both ways. When I go camping I don't take my meter because I might lose it or drop it.

Another test that's important is checking my urine for ketones. I do this whenever my blood glucose is over 240 mg/dl or when I'm sick. My nurse taught me how to do this and told me it's important to call my doctor if the test shows there are ketones in my urine.

The dietitian helped us learn about food. I thought I already knew how to eat pretty well but we learned a whole lot more! My mom said because I had diabetes, the whole family was going to eat so much better. She said it was a chance for us to eat smart. We learned to balance my food and insulin and activity (like swimming, running, riding my bike, or just playing). I learned that I had to eat at the same time for breakfast, lunch, dinner, and snacks because I had taken my insulin. It was already working and ready for my food.

Draw a picture or write three of your favorite foods.

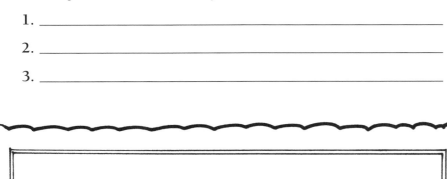

1. _____

2. _____

3. _____

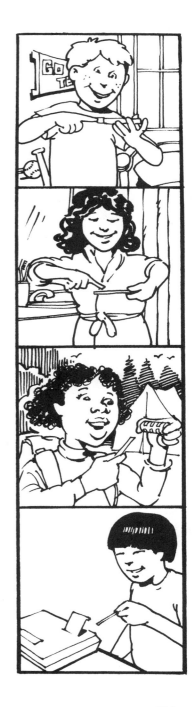

401

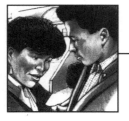

I wanted to know why I couldn't eat all I wanted of foods like candy bars and ice cream sundaes or pie. The dietitian said that foods with lots of sugar can make your blood glucose go way up. Eating smart means eating lots of different kinds of foods in the right amounts at the right times. Can you draw a picture of a smart food for your body?

When I see my dietitian I get a card that looks like this. Fill in your meal plan.

Name _____		Date _____
Total Calories _____ **Carbohydrate** _____ gm. **Protein** _____ gm. **Fat** _____ gm.		
_____ % _____ % _____ %		
BREAKFAST time: _____	**LUNCH** time: _____	**DINNER:** time: _____
Starch/bread _____	Starch/bread _____	Starch/bread _____
Meat _____	Meat _____	Meat _____
Fruit _____	Vegetable _____	Vegetable _____
Milk _____	Fruit _____	Fruit _____
Fat _____	Milk _____	Milk _____
	Fat _____	Fat _____
Morning Snack time: _____	**Afternoon Snack** time: _____	**Bedtime Snack** time: _____

International Diabetes Center

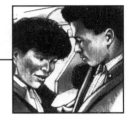

What you just marked on the pages is special for you. No one else has a meal plan exactly like yours! Following your meal plan will help you control your blood glucose levels and grow well.

Some foods are made by nature and some are manmade. Look at the chart below. Do you know which foods are better for you?

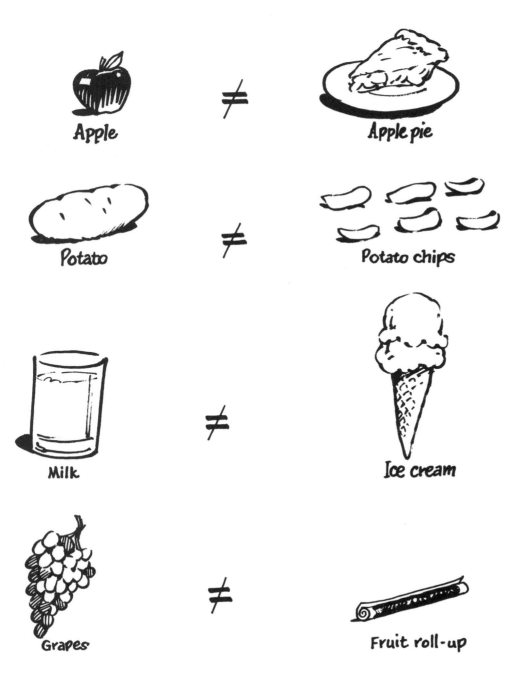

403

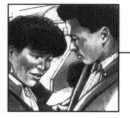

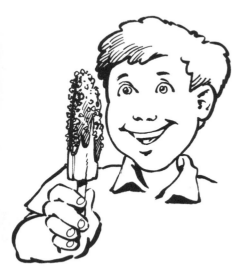

The foods made by nature are better because they don't have any added sugar, fat, or salt.

My favorite snack is a "Banana Cycle." I cut one large banana in half and put a Popsicle stick in one end. Then I dip it in low-fat plain yogurt and then roll it in wheat germ. Yum Yum! This is one fruit exchange. What's your favorite snack?

If I'm active and play, my body uses insulin better. My doctor, nurse, and dietitian at the clinic call it exercise—I call it fun.

For a healthy body, exercise is real important. Everyone should try to exercise every day. Exercise could be going for a walk, gym class, riding a bike, or sports practice after school. What do you like to do for exercise?

_____

_____

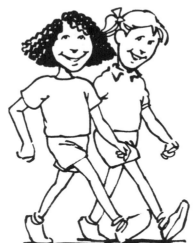

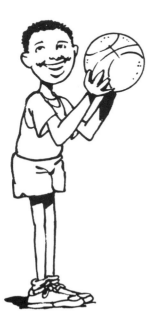

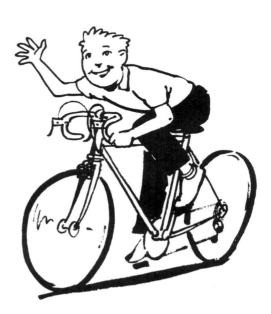

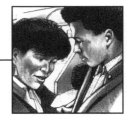

Sometimes it's hard to balance my food and insulin and exercise. Sometimes my blood glucose is high and sometimes it's low and sometimes it's in the middle. If my blood glucose levels is too low that's called a reaction. I get reactions if:

- I didn't eat all my meal or snack.
- I ate my meal or snack late. My insulin is already working and ready for the food and the didn't show up.
- I played real hard. Sometimes when I play real hard, I need an extra snack. Remember, exercise helps your body use the insulin better.

Sometimes I have a reaction and can't really figure out why it happened—it just did.

So a reaction means not enough blood glucose. How do I know if I don't have enough blood glucose? There are some signs. I may have a headache or feel:

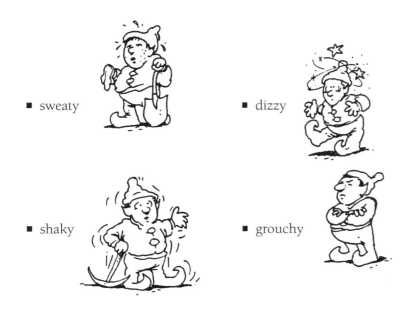

- sweaty
- dizzy
- shaky
- grouchy

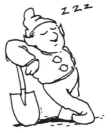

- sleepy

Sometimes I feel one of those things, other times I feel a lot of them. Sometimes I don't feel any of them, but my mom and dad usually notice that I'm acting different.

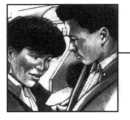

To make a reaction stop, I eat something right away. That makes my blood glucose go up. Then in 10 or 15 minutes, the signs of a reaction usually go away. Some foods you can eat are:

- 1/2 cup of fruit juice
- 1 cup of milk
- 1/2 cup of regular soda pop
- 2 to 3 glucose tablets
- 1 small box of raisins
- 6 or 7 LifeSavers
- 5 small sugar cubes
- 2 big sugar cubes

If you don't feel better in 10 to 15 minutes, eat the same amount of food again.

I also learned about too much blood glucose. It happens if:

- I don't take enough insulin
- I'm sick
- I watch TV or just sit around all the time
- I eat extra food or I don't eat smart food
- I forget my insulin shot
- I get real worried or scared or excited about something

Feelings can make your blood glucose go up or down. Sometimes my blood glucose level is high and there doesn't seem to be any reason except that I have diabetes.

When I have too much blood glucose, I may:

- not feel any different
- drink a lot
- go to the bathroom a lot
- have a stomachache
- have urine ketones

When people with diabetes get sick, their blood glucose can go either up or down. Usually the blood glucose goes up because the body is under stress. I learned that it's important to check my blood glucose more often and my urine for ketones when I'm sick.

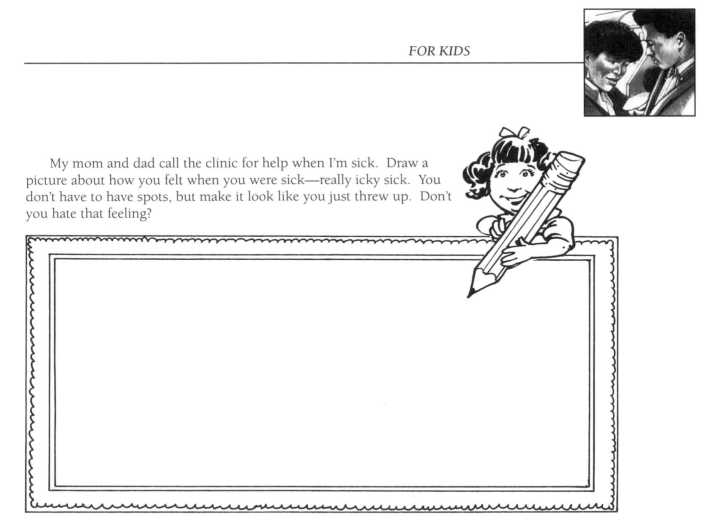

My mom and dad call the clinic for help when I'm sick. Draw a picture about how you felt when you were sick—really icky sick. You don't have to have spots, but make it look like you just threw up. Don't you hate that feeling?

I still need to take my insulin when I'm sick, even if I don't feel like eating my meal plan. If I cannot eat my usual meals and snacks, I need to eat or drink one of these foods slowly over 45 to 60 minutes.

FOODS TO EAT WHEN YOU'RE SICK

Food	How Much
regular soda pop	3/4 cup
orange juice	1/2 cup
ice cream *(Hurray! But stick to vanilla, or else you might throw up again.)*	1/2 cup
sherbet	1/4 cup
soup	1 cup
toast	1 slice
soda crackers	6 crackers

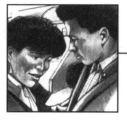

Can you write your name?

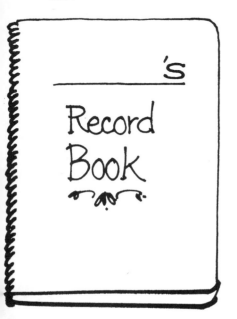

_____'s

Record Book

I try to check my blood glucose level three or four times a day before I eat. Then I write the blood glucose level and how much insulin I took in my record book.

If I check my urine for ketones I also write that down. I try to remember to write if something different happened that day, like a long bike ride or if I was sick. I don't have to draw it for them though.

My mom and dad and I look at the record book once or twice a week and talk about if we need to change anything like my insulin or food or exercise to help my blood glucose levels or to make my numbers fit in my goal range.

Sometimes, we need to call the clinic to get help. We work on things together. Then every three months we go to the clinic. They check my height and weight and we talk about diabetes. My mom and dad and I learn more about diabetes. Sometimes it's boring to go to the clinic and sometimes it's fun. What do you do when you go to the clinic?

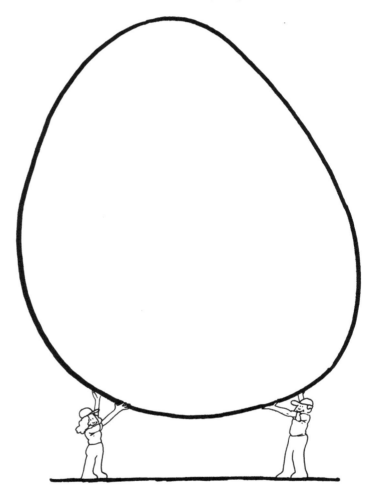

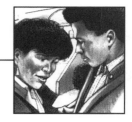

My mom and dad and I also went to a week-long class about diabetes. There were other kids with diabetes and their brothers and sisters in the class. We had fun.

Sometimes I don't want to do things like clean my room or take a bath or test my blood. But some things you just have to do. That's when I tell my mom and dad or friend about my feelings.

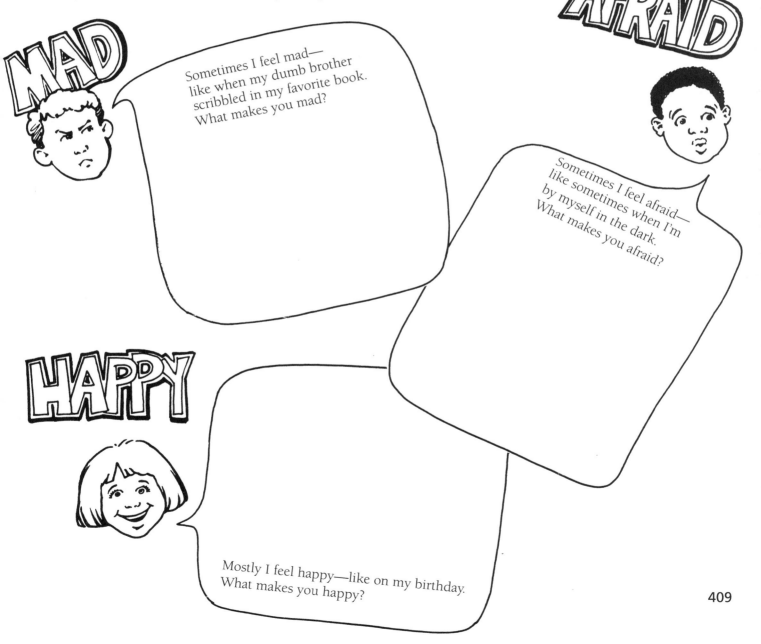

Sometimes I feel mad—like when my dumb brother scribbled in my favorite book. What makes you mad?

Sometimes I feel afraid—like sometimes when I'm by myself in the dark. What makes you afraid?

Mostly I feel happy—like on my birthday. What makes you happy?

409

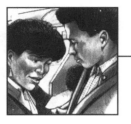

I have feelings about my diabetes too. Sometimes it doesn't seem fair that I got diabetes. Sometimes I want to pretend I don't have diabetes—but I know I do! It helps to talk about my feelings. I talk to my parents or my friend Jason. Who can you talk to about your diabetes?

I used to need help:

- getting dressed
- tying my shoes
- riding my bike

But now I can do them by myself. I just need some help sometimes, like getting a tight shirt over my head.

Now I do new things because I have diabetes. I check my blood glucose. My mom and dad help me sometimes. I get a shot twice a day. Last year I started helping with my shots. Pretty soon I'll be able to do my shots all by myself. What things do you do because you have diabetes?

1. _____

2. _____

3. _____

4. _____

Sometimes I need a grown-up to help me.

- A grown-up needs to drive a car.
- A grown-up needs to help fix some things.
- A grown-up sometimes needs to help check my blood glucose levels or give me my insulin.
- A grown-up needs to help if I have a reaction that won't go away.

Grown-up help is nice to have when you need it.

I'm in charge of some things.

- I get my shot on time.
- I eat what I'm supposed to.
- I tell my friends I have diabetes.
- I make sure my teachers know I have diabetes.
- I take something to eat with me in case I have a reaction.
- I ask grown-ups if I need help.

When I get bigger, I'll be in charge of more things. What do you tell your friends about diabetes?

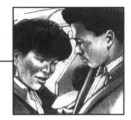

SUMMARY

So that's what I learned about diabetes. I can do lots of things. I can take care of diabetes, like give my insulin shots, eat smart, test my blood glucose, check my urine for ketones, and get lots of exercise.

Then, I can do all the really important things I want to do! Like be a professional ball player someday or invent new Lego toys, or go camping next week, or take a trip to Disneyland without my parents but just Aunt Sally (she's great!).

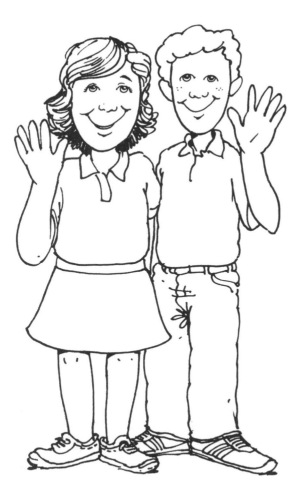

CHAPTER 31

Patricia M. Moynihan, RN, MPH

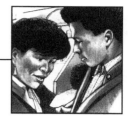

For Parents:
What You Should Know About Normal Growth and Development

Should children with diabetes be treated differently than their brothers or sisters?

At what age can a child with diabetes accept some of the responsibilities of diabetes management?

What should I tell my child's school personnel about diabetes?

When Adam developed diabetes at the age of two, he became the terror of the household. His mother excused his actions and blamed everything on the diabetes. The rest of the family was told they would have to put up with Adam's behavior and give him whatever he wanted so he wouldn't get overexcited. When Adam was five, he was still an undisciplined terror "because of his diabetes." His father gave up trying to reason with him, and his brothers and sister stayed away from him as much as possible so they wouldn't get blamed for causing his tantrums.

Now Adam is a teenager, and even his mother has given up hope, forcing herself to realize that "diabetes was just too much for poor Adam to handle." There is a great deal of tension within the family and

413

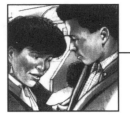

they never really talk to each other anymore. Adam's diabetes is in very poor control and he spends most of his time alone; he never really made any friends because he and his family let his diabetes prevent him from playing with the other kids and participating in activities at school.

A ridiculous, unnecessary situation? Certainly, but unfortunately it happens all too often because families don't realize that boys or girls with diabetes are more like other children than different. When a child has diabetes, it's common for everyone to focus on the disease—on how to control the diabetes—and forget to look at the broader picture. Expectations of our children must take into consideration the broader issues of growth and development. Children change physically, intellectually, and emotionally, and what works to help control diabetes when they are six will not work when they are sixteen.

For this reason, parents should understand the growth and development stages every child goes through and how these normal behaviors may be affected by diabetes. This chapter will help you better predict changes, encourage independence in your child at the right times, and avoid feeling guilty that his or her behavior is not always what you think it should be.

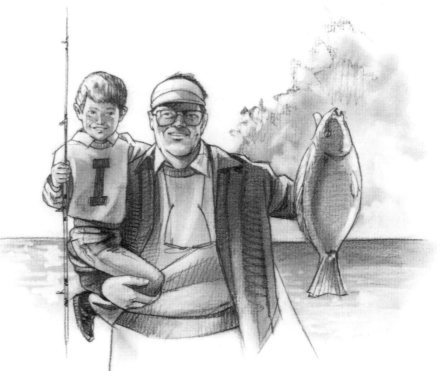

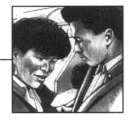

We'll discuss normal childhood development in five stages: infant (birth to 1 year), toddler (1 year to 2 1/2 years), preschool (2 1/2 to 5 years), school-age (6 to 12 years), and teenage (13 to 19 years). Within each stage the physical, intellectual, and social needs of children with diabetes are explored along with some ideas about expectations based on these needs.

INFANTS: YOUR BABY
FROM BIRTH TO 1 YEAR

Your child grows faster during the first year than at any other period in life. Birth weight generally doubles by the age of five months and triples by one year. During the first year, an infant's length increases about 50% and the large muscles begin to work together, helping the child control and direct movement.

If your child develops diabetes during this time, careful observation is necessary. Babies have limited means of communication, so daily blood glucose testing is extremely important to monitor insulin and food requirements. Generally, a minimum of two to four blood glucose tests per day is required to measure diabetes control. More frequent testing should be done when you suspect hypoglycemia or when your infant refuses food or is ill.

Blood samples can be obtained by poking the fingertips, toes, and heels. As with injections, it's important to be honest with yourself about your own fears and resistance to poking your infant for blood glucose testing. Babies quickly learn to be fearful and/or upset about daily testing if they sense you are.

Blood glucose goals for infants are usually between 100 to 200 mg/dl throughout the day and night. Since infants can't tell you when they are having reactions, it's safer to not try for blood glucose levels less then 100 mg/dl. Grouchiness, irritability, and unexplained crying may be the only warning signs of low blood glucose level.

Be prepared to treat hypoglycemia if you notice any behaviors that may be warning signs. A simple blood test is a quick and easy way to know if it's hypoglycemia or just irritable behavior. Treat blood glucose levels less than 80 mg/dl with two to four ounces of fruit juice or milk. Stay away from hard candies or sugar tablets because they may be difficult or impossible for your baby to suck or swallow. Don't be afraid to use glucagon (see Chapter 11) for reactions that seem more serious (such as

415

unconsciousness or seizures) or for milder reactions that are not improving after one or two treatment attempts and a wait for results. The usual dose of glucagon for infants is 0.5 mg (50 units on an insulin syringe), or half the amount in the vial. Follow up with juice and a call to your health care team to discuss the cause and obtain reassurance.

Insulin requirements may be very low, sometimes less than one unit, which hardly seems worth the needle poke. But blood glucose levels will rise if insulin is not given. Some infants do well on just a long- or intermediate-acting insulin. If it's difficult to measure small doses, ask your health care team or pharmacist about diluting the insulin to a lower concentration.

Testing urine for ketones is very important when blood glucose levels are high (greater than 240 mg/dl) and when your infant is ill. Infants can become ill quickly and may develop ketoacidosis in a matter of hours. You can easily test a baby's urine by pressing a urine ketone strip into a wet diaper, waiting the appropriate length of time, and comparing the color change on the reagent pad to the color chart on the product's can or bottle. When urine tests are positive for more than four hours, call your health care team for advice.

A regular schedule of mealtimes and bedtimes is important during the first year. Children need this, because it comforts them to know what to expect and when to expect it. Consistency will make your job as a parent easier.

Listen to the words you use to describe injections, finger pokes, and food items. Make sure they have positive meanings whenever possible. There is discomfort with shots and blood glucose testing, but it's quickly forgotten if you give a message of reassurance.

You're not expected to be an expert parent the first year of your baby's life, or for the next twenty years for that matter! Be patient with your learning and your baby's. There is a great deal to learn and incorporate into your lives, especially with diabetes. It does not come all at once.

TODDLERS: YOUR CHILD FROM AGES 1 TO 2 1/2

Growth slows during the toddler stage. Between 1 and 2 1/2 years, children gain about five to six pounds and grow four to six inches. All primary teeth are present by 2 1/2 to 3 years and appetite becomes much more variable. You and your health care team must watch for weight and

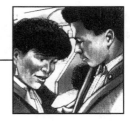

length gains consistent with your child's potential, comparing them with growth charts for most children of the same age.

As much as possible, model your toddler's eating schedule after the family's mealtimes. Avoid constant snacking as a substitute for regularly scheduled meals. Don't force-feed children. There will be times when they refuse food because of decreased need or desire. When this happens, you may need to reduce insulin to keep blood glucose levels in a safe range. Be sure to discuss this with your health care team.

Blood glucose goals are not strict for toddlers with diabetes. Aim for levels between 100 to 200 mg/dl throughout the day and for absence of hypoglycemia. Test blood glucose at least four times a day and also when you suspect hypoglycemia or when the toddler refuses food or is ill.

Blood glucose control is most easily obtained by twice-daily insulin injections (before breakfast and before the evening meal). Insulin requirements may remain very low. Children this age can be sensitive to fast-acting insulins, so often very small dosages are needed.

Hypoglycemia can be difficult to identify in toddlers. You'll most likely notice decreases in activity, pale skin, or temper tantrums that seem totally out of line for your child's normal behavior. Hypoglycemia may cause seizures. A simple blood test is an easy way to determine if the problem is hypoglycemia or just irritable, toddler-like behavior. Be prepared to treat any behaviors you think are hypoglycemia. To treat blood glucose levels less than 80 mg/dl, follow the guidelines given for infants.

All adults and older teenagers in the family should learn and try to be comfortable with the daily diabetes care routine. Sometimes toddlers may express a definite preference for one parent. This results from a need to control and has nothing to do with the skills of either parent. Let your child choose a parent for a specific task, such as injections. However, both should be competent with handling the details of diabetes care. Insist on following the care routine. You must determine what is safe or dangerous for your child, yet let the toddler play, experiment, discover, and learn within limits you set.

Design daily routines so there are fair but firm limits on the range of your child's choices. For example, decide that insulin shots will be given at specific times, then allow the child to choose the injection site. The injection itself is not negotiable. Or allow the child to choose between two vegetables at mealtimes. If you allow too many choices, you'll spend all your time as a short-order cook.

This principle also applies to health care visits. If your toddler suddenly cries when you bring him or her in for a check-up, don't overreact by rescheduling the appointment or avoiding treatment. Instead, try to associate the visit with something fun, such as a follow-up trip to the

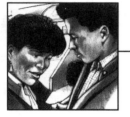

park for play. Be firm about your basic expectations. Your toddler's feelings are real, but they will adjust if you don't give in. Try not to reinforce your child's anxiety with your own.

Be careful not to place "good" or "bad" values on the results of medical tests and lab procedures. With diabetes, blood glucose numbers are high or low, but children are not good or bad because of those numbers. It's natural to feel frustrated when results are outside the goals you're working to achieve. Look back briefly on possible reasons for not meeting those goals, but don't get hung up on this. It's more important to look ahead and define the changes you need to make.

Expect your toddler to conform to the family routine and schedules as much as possible—not vice versa. Yes, you could let the child sleep late and then fix a separate breakfast. In the long run, however, it will be easier—and more healthy for your child—to eat on the family schedule. Remember, if the whole family would benefit from changes in the routine, this is an excellent opportunity to make those changes.

A healthy, supportive relationship between you and your toddler is one that takes both of your needs into account. Balance your child's needs with the needs of everyone in the household, including parents, brothers, and sisters. As parents, you need time away from the child and the chronic illness. Use this time to nurture your relationship. Schedule some time to be alone—weekly if possible. Moreover, treat private time as you would a business or medical appointment—cancel only when absolutely necessary.

Teach other important people in your child's life—babysitters, relatives, close friends—about your child's care routine. Doing so can help you build a reservoir of competent help—people who can care for your child and give you some relief.

PRESCHOOLERS: YOUR CHILD FROM AGES 2 1/2 TO 5

Michael's worst time of the day was in the morning when it came time for his shot. He would scream and hide and eventually upset the entire family before breakfast could begin. His parents tried a different approach every day, searching for the way to satisfy and quiet Michael. What they didn't know was that by changing their approach each day—a different family member giving the shot, sometimes before and sometimes after breakfast— they were acting as their own worst enemies. Michael needed one routine

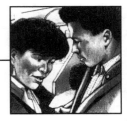

done firmly and matter-of-factly, so he could understand and accept that this was the way he could count on things happening each day. Shortly after a regular structure was developed for the family's mornings, everyone, including Michael, stopped reacting to each other's frustrations and breakfast once again became a calm and enjoyable family gathering.

Preschoolers usually have improved bladder and bowel control and have mastered toilet training. Urination is more frequent when blood glucose levels are high, so increased difficulty with toilet training may tip you off to a problem with your child's diabetes control. It's important not to make your child feel guilty when he or she has an accident during these times. Illness normally increases children's dependence and causes changes in behavior. Illness is also a time of higher blood glucose levels, so toilet accidents may be more frequent.

Blood testing for glucose and urine testing for ketones should be part of your child's regular management routine. It's important to allow the child to participate in this care so he or she begins to understand and not be fearful of it.

A preschooler's ability to tell others of an insulin reaction is unpredictable. Many three- to four- year olds cannot identify their own signs of a reaction, so it's important that those who care for the child know how to identify one and how to treat it. After a child has had a reaction and is feeling better, it's important to explain in simple terms what happened and why. This helps lessen fear of reactions and helps your child begin to make an association between shakiness and ill feelings and not eating enough food.

Preschoolers begin to develop a sense of time and an understanding that things and events happen in a sequence. Routines throughout the day are important to children because they provide a sense of predictability and control of the world. Children need routines in their day so that they know what they can count on. The morning routine of insulin injection, blood glucose testing, and eating is more successful if done in a short time and if the time, place, equipment, and people are usually the same rather than always changing and chaotic.

Finally, preschool is a time to prepare yourself and your child for the separation that occurs when school starts. Any parent may be anxious about this separation, but parents of a child with diabetes may be even more anxious about entrusting someone else with the responsibilities for their child's daily care. A successful separation requires three things: trusting your child to take care of himself or herself, being confident in your abilities to prepare your child and yourself for the separation, and good planning with specific school personnel about the basic management of your child's diabetes.

SCHOOL-AGE: YOUR CHILD FROM AGES 6 TO 12

At the fall school conference, Erin's parents told the counselor and school nurse that Erin is an inactive girl who would rather play video games than anything else. What they didn't mention was that her inactivity was caused mostly by their fear and overprotectiveness in trying to prevent insulin reactions. They didn't want Erin to participate in any rigorous activity at school and didn't allow her to play active games with her friends at home. What Erin's parents needed to learn—painful and frightening as it may be at first—was that Erin and her school needed to be, and could be, trusted to handle reactions. Preventing her from participating in exercise activities was hurting her more than helping her in the long run.

As children grow, so does their world and the number of people they know. These physical and emotional changes are accompanied by changing needs for diabetes care.

Basic physical coordination in both large and small muscles improves tremendously during the early school years. Your child's interest and ability in physical activity should increase. Sports and athletic events for both boys and girls should be encouraged if the child shows interest. Having diabetes is not a reason to avoid activity.

Because the small muscles and fine motor coordination are developing during these years, and your child's need for independence is increasing, it's a good time to teach him or her how to do insulin injections and test blood glucose and urine ketones. Children this age can add numbers, compare colors, and print and write increasingly better. They also want and need to control more situations. This is the prime time to teach a child about diabetes management.

The world of school is a big step for all children and parents. Children with diabetes make this transition and progress through the school years as well as any other child, but the family must take a few additional steps. You must tell the school your child has diabetes, and you must inform the school personnel (teacher, coach, bus driver, cook) how best to help your child take care of himself or herself.

It's neither necessary nor realistic to tell the school everything you know about diabetes. But, some basic topics need to be discussed regularly. These include:

- describing your child's usual symptoms of an insulin reaction

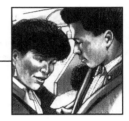

- providing foods that should be readily available to treat reactions. Make these foods available to the school and check the supply several times throughout the school year.

- indicating times when your child may be likely to experience a reaction, such as during unplanned physical activity, when snacks are missed, and during times of emotional stress.

- preventing reactions by simply planning ahead. Teachers and coaches most commonly fear that a child with diabetes will have a reaction and the teacher won't know what to do. Reassure the teacher that most reactions can be prevented and that your child is capable of treating most of his or her reactions (if this is true).

- reviewing your child's method for testing blood glucose during the school day and discussing the amount of supervision required. Provide all necessary supplies and check the supply regularly. School personnel may not be expected to interpret the results of the testing, but they should be told when to notify you about unusual results.

- discussing with school personnel a reasonable length of time and place for your child to test and eat snacks. This time should not be used by your child as a way to avoid other activities. The less these routines disturb the child's school day, the better.

- discussing the school lunch system, especially any food alternatives that are necessary to meet your child's meal plan. Children with diabetes can eat the school lunch, or they may prefer to bring a lunch to school. Either option can work well, but the lunches must be planned.

- planning for parties and special school events. This helps your child participate and not feel left out because of food restrictions. You can suggest kinds of party snacks your child may have, or you may want to provide them for special occasions.

- telling school personnel the information you need to know about your child's handling of diabetes (such as the occurrence and severity of reactions). Ongoing communication between you and the school will make everyone feel more comfortable.

During the school years, children develop and mature in how they understand diabetes and how they feel about having it. Children tend to compare themselves to friends. Your child may learn that no other children in the class or school have diabetes, which can make him or her feel different. The truth is that your child is different because of the diabetes, but he or she must learn that all children are different and have things that set them apart. This is a time to talk about these feelings of being different and discuss how being different can be a strength.

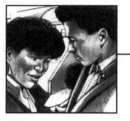

School-age children are better able to deal with present reality than with the abstract future. They're ready for a deeper explanation of diabetes and what it means, but they aren't ready to understand diabetes in the same way you do. Although they can gain some understanding of what causes reactions and how to prevent them, long-range complications and their prevention have little meaning to children at this age. Children vary in their readiness to take over responsibilities for their care, but most, with parental support in problem-solving, can do injections and testing (with recording) by the age of 12. They will feel more independent and ready to start their teen years if encouraged to do so.

The school years experiences—the successes and the failures—will affect how your child enters adolescence. Each year, as your child matures and as interests and social contacts increase, there are new opportunities for growth. These should not be limited by diabetes.

TEENAGERS: YOUR CHILD FROM AGES 13 TO 17

When Bob's doctor told him and his parents he had diabetes, he thought it was the most unfair and cruel thing imaginable. He had worked hard in school, had always respected his parents and teachers, and was looking forward to playing varsity hockey. Was this how he was being rewarded for all his hard work and energy? Why should he bother to do anything now, least of all follow the diabetes tasks that were being "shoved down his throat"?

In his first year with diabetes, Bob learned he had built all the resources he would need to do the things he had planned. His self-discipline and motivation would carry over to allow him to control his diabetes, enjoy his teen years, and become a productive and responsible adult.

Increased physical growth and maturity and the onset of puberty mark the entry to the teenage years. The rate of physical growth is faster during these years than at any other time in a child's life, except for the first twelve months.

This rapid growth affects your teenager's sleep patterns, eating, and activity. As growth increases so does food intake, and insulin requirements reflect this increase. There is usually a slow but steady increase in blood glucose levels. This is normal and not a sign that diabetes is worsening. It simply shows that the body's needs are changing, and these changes are best matched by increasing the insulin dosage.

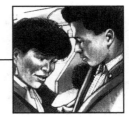

As growth slows in the mid- to late-teen years, insulin requirements need to be reevaluated. When growth is complete, insulin dosages may even be decreased. Insulin can stimulate the appetite, so if requirements are not reevaluated at this time, obesity can become a concern.

Intellectually, teenagers' abilities to think and reason become more adult-like. They begin to think logically and understand the consequences of their own behavior and that of others. Your child now has the ability to look not only at the past and present, but also at the future. Interest and concern for the future will extend from your child to the outside world. It's important to understand that although your teenager has the ability to do these things, he or she does not do them automatically or consistently. It's common for teenagers to fluctuate between thinking like adults and thinking like children. This is an important time to make certain they understand the nature of diabetes and its management. It is a good time to have them attend education classes.

You must continue to set reasonable rules and expectations. These provide the guidance and reassurance that is needed and wanted, although seldom asked for. Rules and expectations result in a sense of values that are important for your teenager and your whole family to understand. Because teenagers now understand that there are several consequences to any specific behavior and many different opinions on a subject, they are likely to question values and what they stand for. They may even question the value you place on their health and diabetes control.

The teen years are a time of experimentation to discover what is real and what is not. As teenagers experiment, the strength of values is tested. This experimentation may involve diabetes. The questions "How serious is my diabetes?" and "Does it really matter if I take care of myself?" surface and are explored with new insights.

Because teenagers are now capable of understanding the future, they may begin to realize that diabetes is a serious, chronic disease that does not go away. This realization may be too much to handle all at once, so they may choose to deny that diabetes exists. Such denial actually allows time for teenagers to get comfortable with the reality they know will follow. But prolonged denial can become destructive. Even though the teenager is denying diabetes, it's important that parents and family do not. Continue to voice an interest in diabetes management and support the value that your teenager's health is important. Not all teenagers go through this denial period, but if they do, it's important that you understand its purpose and remember that it usually passes. When it does, your teenager will have a clearer understanding and better acceptance of his or her diabetes.

Teenagers face new interests and opportunities. A driver's license is a symbol of independence. Teenagers need to understand that there are no

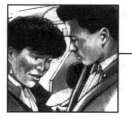

restrictions to getting a driver's license, but they must state that they have diabetes at the time of application. A medical form also must be completed regularly by a doctor, who evaluates if the diabetes is under reasonable control. Its purpose is to protect the safety of the driver and others. Because hypoglycemia can cause drivers to have a traffic accident, all people with diabetes who drive should have food in the car for easy access, if needed.

Finally, you and your teenager must deal with the issue of intimate relationships and the development of a sexual identity. Many teens have "street smarts" about sexual development, but they are often misinformed. Additionally, teenagers with diabetes have many questions about their changing bodies, their feelings, and how diabetes may affect all of this. You can help your son or daughter learn accurate information on these important subjects by expecting and discussing their concerns and helping them ask the right questions of their health care team. See Chapter 33 for an in-depth discussion on sexuality issues for teens.

SUMMARY

It's important to remember that "growing up" is a process that takes more than just time to complete. Your child with diabetes will move through this process at a different rate than your other children—not because of diabetes, but simply because each child is different. The amount of attention your family places on diabetes will affect the growing-up process. Each family must determine the right amount of attention. Listen to your child and family; they will give you cues. And include your health care team in the decision process. They can provide suggestions based on experience and impartial but concerned interest. The final outcome is what parenting is all about!

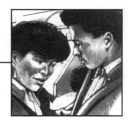

For more information about the growth and development of children with diabetes and suggestions for parenting, you may want to read the IDC's book *Whole Parent, Whole Child: A Parent's Guide to Raising a Child With a Chronic Illness* (see the back of the manual for details).

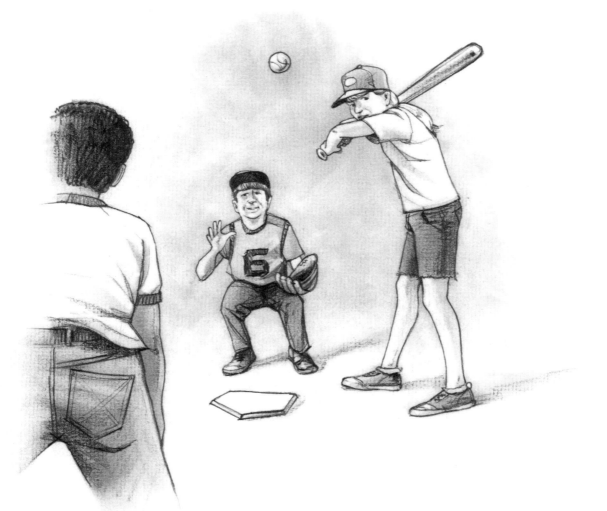

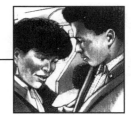

CHAPTER 32

Broatch Haig, RD, CDE
Marion Franz, MS, RD, CDE

For Parents:
Meals, Not Military Maneuvers

How do you feed the finicky eater?

What should you do when your child doesn't eat the entire meal or snack?

How can you live by meal plan recommendations—and still avoid power struggles?

To grow normally, children need adequate nutrition. The unpredictability of children's eating habits only increases a parent's anxiety about proper nutrition and its role in diabetes management.

Children are born without food prejudices—eating habits are learned. So it's important for parents to set a good example with their own eating habits. This makes you an essential role model, whether you want the responsibility or not. Children quickly learn which foods are desirable by observing which foods their parents and brothers and sisters relish most.

This chapter discusses eating habits of children and teenagers, common eating problems, and tips for making changes in eating habits and handling eating problems—especially for a child who has diabetes.

The nutrition and exercise recommendations for anyone with diabetes are part of a healthy lifestyle. Expecting a child to make major changes while the rest of the family continues to eat inappropriately is certain to cause problems. Parents should not feel guilty or feel they are depriving other family members, especially if there are no longer as many "sweets" and high-fat snacks around the home. Even lean teenagers need to learn good eating and exercise habits. We know of one family who celebrated the anniversary of "their" diabetes diagnosis because they were thankful for the positive changes in the family's lifestyle.

KNOW WHAT TO EXPECT

As parents, you need to understand normal eating patterns for children. Knowing what to expect can help you anticipate problems and find creative and workable solutions for eating problems you may face with a child who has diabetes.

Children's appetites change frequently for no apparent reason. They go through whimsical phases of alternately liking and disliking certain foods. They may want the same food for a long time and then abruptly refuse it. Try not to overreact—assume the food fancy will soon pass.

Children's appetites also wax and wane with growth rates. Periods of rapid growth are usually accompanied by increases in appetite. Sometimes the increased appetite and weight will precede the growth spurt. Don't immediately assume it's the beginning of obesity—watch carefully and wait awhile before curbing portions.

Youngsters usually have larger appetites during the summer when they are more active physically. Not only do appetites vary by season, they vary daily as well. This makes attempts at consistent eating for children with diabetes all the more challenging.

Children do not eat foods in the same order as adults. Youngsters often eat one food at a time, which is perfectly acceptable. Try to look at meals as children see them. A large plate with a mass of food can be overwhelming to those little eyes. Scale your portions down to their size.

All children thrive on regularity and routine in daily activities. They need to have meals served at approximately the same times, otherwise they'll be hungry and irritable. Planning meals for a child with diabetes results in a regular meal schedule for the whole family.

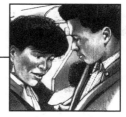

Children, like adults, occasionally have off days when they are irritable and don't feel like eating. Accept this as gracefully as possible! If you're concerned about injected insulin, try offering smaller and more frequent snacks.

WHAT PARENTS CAN DO

Knowing what to expect is the first step, but parents can do other things to make nutritional management of diabetes easier. Mealtime atmosphere has a significant influence on how the whole family enjoys a meal. If mealtimes are a tense battleground, children often rebel by refusing to eat anything. This sets up a vicious cycle. Children who feel they are under constant scrutiny at the table lose their appetite in a hurry. A relaxed atmosphere at meals helps children eat better.

Children are good judges of the *amount* of food they need, but it's up to parents to provide the right *kinds* of foods. Wise food purchases are most often the result of factual nutrition information, planned menus, and unhurried selection. If only appropriate, nutritious foods are available in your cupboards and refrigerator, good eating habits are encouraged. Other family members not following a meal plan can snack on what they wish away from home.

Varied and interesting menus introduce the pleasure of variety. Children who taste new foods each time they are served learn to know and enjoy many different foods. But don't be disappointed when foods are not a hit the first time around. It's important to introduce only one new item at a meal, perhaps along with a favorite food. Offer unfamiliar foods when children are hungry and in good health—never when they're ill, cross, or tired. Serve very small portions of new foods and be sure to compliment, even when only one bite is eaten. Establish a rule that all foods must be tasted—a "no-thank-you bite"—before having a second serving of preferred foods or returning to play. This can increase food acceptance over time.

Whenever possible, allow children to have a choice. "You have a fruit exchange—what would you like?" Or offer a choice between a cooked or a raw vegetable. Allowing children to choose between two foods gives them a feeling of control over which foods they eat.

Families who share meal preparation tasks find that children who are given simple cooking tasks are better eaters. They will eat foods they prepare and most often are fair about tasting meals others prepare.

Don't play games or employ trickery to encourage eating. Inform the child—after about 15 or 30 minutes at the table, whatever seems

429

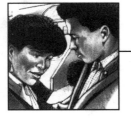

reasonable in your family—that there will be no more food until the next planned snack or meal is served. Let the child decide whether to eat or go without. If the child still shows no interest, remove the food without further comment. Follow through with your plan or you defeat the purpose. If a reaction occurs, treat it appropriately, but without a lot of fuss or attention or "I told you so." Remember, it's not uncommon for children to rebel when forced to eat. Rejecting food is a way to assert independence.

In a situation where appetite just isn't hearty and it's not a behavior problem, the child should eat as much of the planned meal as possible. Take note of what is left and offer an equivalent amount of food (such as juice and crackers) an hour or so later. This is especially important if blood glucose levels have been in the normal range.

Consistent timing and spacing of meals and snacks are essential for the child with diabetes. Insulin injections must be given at the same time each day, which makes it important to eat at set times. If necessary, you can divide food intake into smaller snacks or meals without causing low blood glucose levels, but don't delay meals. If meals must be delayed—such as when eating out in restaurants or traveling—a fruit, bread, or milk exchange should be eaten at the usual mealtime to prevent low blood glucose levels. This should allow the meal to be delayed by about one hour.

Snacks should be eaten at least 1 1/2 hours before mealtimes. If children don't eat well at meals, it may be that snacks are too large or are eaten too close to mealtime. A pattern of too much food for the child's appetite is a signal that the meal plan needs reevaluation. Children should not feel either hungry or "stuffed" continually.

Children with diabetes need the same amount of food as those without diabetes. Do not delete food from a young child's meal plan because of high blood glucose levels. Young children need all of their planned food. If blood glucose levels show a pattern of elevation, adjust the insulin acting at that time of day.

It's important to keep meal plans updated. If the meal plan is reviewed at every quarterly check-up, it will be easier to keep current with the child's growth and appetite. Spring and fall are good times to update meal plans, since these are natural breaks in the child's routine.

SOLVING FEEDING PROBLEMS

In the real world, feeding problems develop in many children. These problems seem to be magnified when a child has diabetes, because eating is

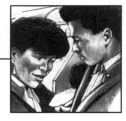

such an important part of the management plan. What can parents do when an eating behavior becomes a problem?

First, serve meals and snacks of appropriate portion sizes on a regular schedule and set a good example by the foods you eat. The next step is behavior modification. To begin changing an established behavior, clearly define what behavior is expected and then reward it. Common sense tells us that when an act is followed by a reward it tends to occur more frequently. Ignore undesirable behavior, or at least don't overreact to it. And although it may be difficult, avoid criticizing. Criticism is a common means of trying to change a child's behavior, but it's a form of attention, and attention of any kind often acts like a reward. Verbal praise from parents or brothers and sisters for eating good meals can encourage and reinforce a child's eating behavior and serve as a reward.

"Star charts" can be used effectively as a reward plan for children. A star on a chart can be an immediate award for finishing a meal. It usually works best if stars are used for only one meal—breakfast, lunch, or dinner. The habit of finishing a meal or changing any behavior tends to carry over to other meals or similar situations. The task for which the stars are given should be simple and easily achievable. When a certain number of stars have been received, they can then be exchanged for a prize—playing a game, going to a movie, buying something special, or allowing the child to act as chief cook and menu planner for a whole meal! Don't overdo this reward business, though. A toddler who is rewarded with toys or food fast learns to anticipate a lifetime of bigger and better rewards.

Because snacks are essential in diabetes management, you may need to use some snacks because of their convenience, even if there are more ideal ones. For example, granola bars are convenient because they are individually wrapped and can be carried in a purse or pocket. One plain granola bar (not dipped or coated in chocolate) usually equals one starch/bread and one fat exchange. Check labels for the number of calories. Purchase bars that are 130 calories or less. Treats such as ice milk, frozen low-fat yogurt, cookies, or cake can be used occasionally as bread/starch exchanges, but try not to overuse them.

Resist interference from grandparents, other relatives, and neighbors. The more people who are involved, the larger and more complex the problems become. Also, a problem child need not and should not know of the parents' concern. Food is a great battleground, and the less the child views it as a weapon, the better.

Remember that progress takes time. It takes children a while to make the connection that eating right makes them feel better. Sometimes children need to experience a reaction to realize that finishing meals is important. You can't always prevent a child's hypoglycemia, but you can keep meals on schedule and stick to the meal plan as much as possible. Don't let your child skip snacks or meals entirely and, if needed, provide extra food to compensate for extra exercise.

THE IMPORTANCE OF EDUCATION

Being well informed about diabetes management is essential. Education increases parents' confidence in the decisions they must make. Correct information is a vital support for good, consistent parenting skills. It also helps determine priorities.

Education also helps parents understand realistic expectations of children at various ages (see Chapter 31 for more information on normal growth and development). With very young children, you can't expect tight blood glucose control. But even for the very young child, it's important to have a meal plan and to establish appropriate eating habits. If a child develops diabetes at age two or three but is not introduced to an appropriate meal plan until age six or seven, it will be difficult to convince him or her that a meal plan is necessary. It's easier to start changing and improving eating habits as soon as diabetes is diagnosed. But be realistic in your expectations. Realize that many changes will be gradual.

The amount of insulin needed by each child is individual. There is no "magical" insulin dosage, and an increased dosage does not signal that diabetes is worsening. Higher blood glucose levels aren't a sign that the child is "bad," nor are they always preventable or a result of "cheating."

Rearing children requires good judgment and firm but loving discipline. It requires the parents to be adults and works best in the form of a benign dictatorship. When children have diabetes, it's easy to want to give in to their every desire to make up for it. Don't do it! You need to treat food and meals as part of a very normal and accepted routine. Backing positive eating habits with a supportive family that treats diabetes matter of factly is the best way to give a child confidence and pride!

Children can learn about nutrition, exchanges, and their meal plan by playing different games. One family dealt out cards that satisfied their child's snack plan choices. The cards could be returned for food at snack time. It was fun and helped the child more easily memorize the snack allotment.

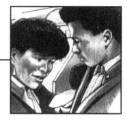

HOLIDAYS AND SPECIAL TREATS

Holidays such as Halloween pose special challenges for children with diabetes. Some families have been successful with creative problem-solving.

- Visit a hospital and give candy to children who are hospitalized there; praise your child for being generous. Then suggest a special occasion —play, sports event, or museum trip—as a treat for your child.
- Collect money for UNICEF and encourage your child to become pen pals with children in other countries.
- Divide collected candy with friends, brothers, and sisters.
- Have your child take treats to school for other kids. It's a good feeling to be the giver of special treats.
- Plan additional physical activity to teach children how to balance moderate increases in calories with exercise.

Easter can be another problem. Try using small gifts, such as coloring books, small toys, or jewelry in Easter baskets rather than candy. Sugar-free gum and hard candy can also be used. Ask grandparents to bring treats other than foods. Things like books, small toys, jewelry, records, and puzzles can be enjoyed by kids just as much as sweet treats.

Sugar-free hard candies can be used for treats. Chocolate dietetic candies are high in fat and calories and are not good choices. A "dietetic" label doesn't always mean the food is a good choice for people with diabetes. Dietetic food products such as chocolate candies, cakes, ice cream, and cookies usually contain as many, if not more, calories than the foods they are replacing and are not recommended.

FEEDING THE INFANT
WHO HAS DIABETES

Diabetes is not frequently diagnosed in children under one year of age, but it does happen. Guidelines for breast-feeding or adding formula and solid foods do not differ for infants with diabetes.

Breast-feeding or giving formula every three to four hours for the first four to six months is generally sufficient. Solid foods two or three times a day are often added at about six months. Keeping feedings fairly consistent and on schedule is an important aspect of your child's health care plan.

433

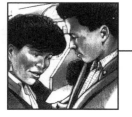

Amounts, however, cannot usually be controlled. Expecting an infant to eat or drink a precisely weighed or measured meal is unrealistic. Spreading a well-balanced meal plan over six to eight feedings daily is more feasible. Discuss the meal plan carefully with your health care team at scheduled visits. Weight and length gains that follow a normal growth curve are proof that a child is eating the right amount.

Since a baby's brain is still developing, it's more susceptible to damage from repeated severe hypoglycemia. For this reason, blood glucose goals are higher than for older children. Make every attempt to avoid hypoglycemia. If it does occur, it certainly should be treated promptly.

When feeding infants, two things apply to nearly all parents. First, a baby's natural appetite is dependable and controls how much he or she is going to eat. While daily intake may vary, things usually average out over a day or week. Second, to comfort and reward your infant, try holding, cuddling, and using a pacifier. Don't use juices or food to comfort, and avoid giving your infant a bottle in bed. Try to hold your baby during feedings.

The following general guidelines are for feeding infants with diabetes. Your health care team will give you specifics for your child.

Birth to Four Months. Breast milk or formula contains twenty calories per ounce and is usually all the baby needs. Insulin adjustment is easier on a consistent feeding schedule versus demand feeding. Offer water between feedings if the baby is fussy. Test blood glucose three to four times a day—just before feedings and at least two hours after the last feeding.

Four to Six Months. Iron-fortified baby cereal is usually the first solid food added to breast milk or formula. It provides ten calories per tablespoon. Check for insulin adjustments with additions of solids. If Regular insulin is part of the insulin schedule, it should be given *before* eating. A baby can usually eat two to three tablespoons of food two to three times a day.

Six Months to Nine Months. During this time, one new pureed food at a time can be added. Use each new food for four to five days until your baby gets used to it. Feed the child from a baby food jar only if you expect the entire amount to be eaten. Opened jars of baby food should be used within two to three days or thrown out. Food should be offered at room temperature or lukewarm.

At this time babies start drinking juice from a cup. Remember to buy fruit juice rather than "drinks" or "ades." Orange juice, although a good source of vitamin C, is not usually used until after twelve months of age. Exchange values for infant foods are listed in Appendix C.

Let your baby's appetite be your guide. As teeth erupt, finely ground foods and safe finger foods may be added. Babies can usually eat six to seven tablespoons of various solid foods at each of three or four feedings.

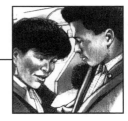

Nine to Twelve Months. During this time your baby starts to drink whole fluid milk from a cup. Use 2% or whole milk until the child is two years old. After that switch to skim milk.

Your baby can now easily eat finely chopped foods. They love finger foods and love to make a mess. Enjoy it, they don't stay babies long.

At ten to twelve months babies start to walk and become more interested in the world around them. By the end of the first year, appetites plateau and growth slows. With all these variables, pay close attention to insulin dose changes.

FEEDING YOUR PRESCHOOLER

For preschoolers, physical growth begins to slow. It's important to monitor your child's height and weight and have it plotted on a growth chart to compare to other children of the same age and sex. Slowed physical growth usually has an effect on appetite and food intake.

This is a time when your child may become very "picky" and show strong food likes and dislikes. Fortunately, this passes with increasing age. Natural hunger helps the appetite of your child and assures that overall food intake is sufficient. The attention span of children this age is short—15 to 20 minutes—so long meals are usually not productive. Shortened mealtimes with small snacks throughout the day are usually more successful.

FEEDING THE SCHOOL-AGE CHILD

The physical growth of a school-age child is slow but steady. Caloric requirements reflect this and should show slow increases over the years. To match this, insulin requirements will also slowly increase. Food requirements will begin to increase significantly when the physical growth spurt of adolescence begins, but this is not until the age of 10 or 11 for girls and 11 and 12 for boys.

Until then, appetite may naturally be slow and children with increasingly active lives tend to forget to eat. You may need to remind your child to eat consistent meals and snacks. Children can become bored with the same food ideas, and they usually begin to prefer more variety and convenience in their food selection.

FEEDING TEENS

Teenagers may have wide emotional swings. Nutritional habits to manage diabetes imply long-term or difficult lifetime changes. Persistence and acceptance are needed. It's easier to do this when life seems rosy, but food modifications may take too much energy when anger, despair, or boredom get in the way. At the same time, the teenage years are a nutritionally vulnerable time.

A teenager's friends are important. What they do sets the norm and what they think (or what the teenager thinks they think) is important. Being different is difficult for teenagers, and being on a meal plan for diabetes suggests they are different. They don't want to seem odd or sick or be singled out for attention.

Changes need to be made gradually. Diabetes education helps provide facts teens need to know and may want to know to better understand diabetes. Once you're confident they really understand the necessity of a meal plan and know their allowance of food, assure them of your confidence in their judgment and your love and support. Then let go. Expect that there will be times when they do not totally follow the meal plan. All the nagging in the world will not change this.

Teens don't need to know every detail about nutrition, but they do need skills to help them change eating behaviors. For example, teens need to know how to refuse family or peer pressure to eat inappropriate but tempting foods. They also need the opportunity to practice and experience success in safe situations. They will not always succeed—nor do we. Threats of chronic complications are more likely to make them feel hopeless and encourage them to ignore the rules and enjoy life "while they can!"

If teens are willing to accept your support, help them by teaching assertiveness skills. A polite refusal has two parts: 1) a thank you for the offer or a compliment to the person making the offer, and 2) a refusal, and perhaps the reason for refusing ("Thanks Mrs. Smith, that cake looks wonderful, but I'm already full"). If people continue to be insistent, continue to refuse politely. No one needs to eat because someone else thinks they should!

Involve teenagers in problem-solving. Help them learn how to analyze and solve meal planning problems. Start by brainstorming. Come up with as many solutions as possible to a problem. Role-playing situations with adolescents in groups is helpful. Once all the ideas are exhausted, select a solution and plan how to use and evaluate it.

Don't give up hope if teenagers seem to rebel against the "diet" for awhile. High blood glucose levels cause fatigue and emotional lows. Many

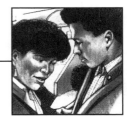

teens will gradually equate feeling good with more normal blood glucose and will choose to stick more or less closely to a consistent, well-designed meal plan. Teenagers need to know that it's their choice to make appropriate changes.

SUMMARY

Problems in children's eating habits become magnified when diabetes enters the picture. How well your family copes with this situation depends on parents' attitude and ability. Parents should be willing to make the necessary changes so eating becomes part of a healthy lifestyle for the child with diabetes as well as the rest of the family. Parents should also be able to make substitutions within a child's meal plan to control diabetes while keeping meals and snacks fun and enjoyable. Look for all the help you can get—from cookbooks, other parents, a dietitian, and so on. See a dietitian at least twice a year to make sure your child is receiving the right amount and kinds of food so essential to good health and control. The tables on the following pages may be helpful in solving specific eating problems.

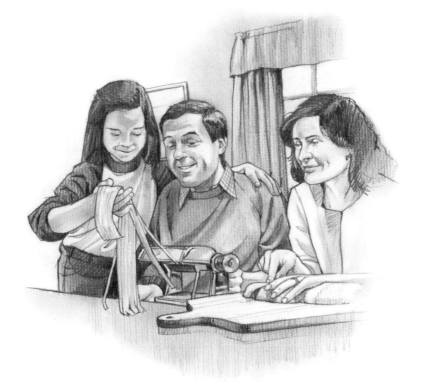

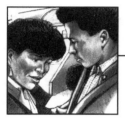

SUGGESTIONS FOR SOLVING CHILDREN'S EATING PROBLEMS

Ages 1 to 5

Problem	Reason(s)	Solutions
"Roller coaster" appetite (desire for food changes daily)	Changes in physical growth. Amount of physical activity varies from day to day.	Monitor blood glucose to adjust insulin needs to appetite changes. Offer choices between two foods. Offer more snacks and smaller meals. Understand child's response to food while encouraging sound food habits. Offer half portions, praise, then offer other half portion.
"Food jags" (eating only certain foods for a time)	Child may be trying to establish independence or attract attention.	Ask child to take a "no-thank-you bite." Don't overreact; offer a substitute but don't become a short-order cook. Go along with it; it can be helpful if it aids in consistency for a time. Establish a variety of foods to choose from early on. Understand that "food jags" are a normal part of a child's development. Express optimism that it will change later.
Refusal of vegetables and foods with a sharp taste	Children have an acute sense of taste and smell and usually prefer mild or non-seasoned foods.	Plan accordingly. Children enjoy foods that are crunchy, chewy, crackly, and smooth. They dislike foods that are lumpy, mushy, slimy or stringy. Serve vegetables raw with low-calorie dip. Cook strongly flavored vegetables with more water and for a shorter time to decrease flavors. (Make soup with the cooking water.) Serve vegetables in taco shells or pita bread. Introduce new vegetables gradually in small amounts. Understand that tastes will change and don't worry too much about it.

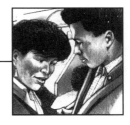

Problem	Reason(s)	Solutions
Can't finish meal	Children have small stomachs and need to eat often.	Plan five to six meals. Make sure snacks contribute to nutrition.
		Try serving smaller meals and snacks.
	Fatigue can overwhelm appetite.	Divide foods into more frequent feedings, but don't skip or delay meals or snacks.
	May have had too much juice or milk.	Look at meal plan if there is routinely too much food left over. Perhaps food needs to be reduced for a time.
Dislike of certain foods	Children assert independence by rejecting things they don't like.	Serve food cut in fun shapes.
		Set a good example. Children often imitate what they see parents, brothers, sisters, and teachers do.
		Assume tastes will change. Offer food again at different meal with another favorite food.
		Don't push. The chance that a child will refuse food increases in direct proportion to your efforts to provide it, or your insistance that it be eaten.
Refuses new foods	Children are curious but distrustful of the unknown.	Introduce only one new food at a time. Offer a very small amount at the beginning of a meal. Finish meal plan with foods child already is familiar with and likes.
		Don't offer new foods when child isn't feeling well.
		Study how foods are grown, color pictures, grow new foods in own small garden.
		Plan meals with new foods to try each month.

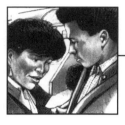

SUGGESTIONS FOR SOLVING CHILDREN'S EATING PROBLEMS

Ages 1 to 5 (continued)

Problem	Reason(s)	Solutions
Refuses to eat	May be asserting independence or may actually not feel like eating for some reason.	Simply remove the food without making any bribes or punishment. Don't let food become a weapon against parents. On a scale of eat versus independence, independence will win.
		Make sure children are at the table long enough (and deprived of other activities) to know they're hungry.
		Monitor blood glucose levels or watch for symptoms of hypoglycemia, and treat accordingly.
Dawdling or playing with food	May be trying to attract attention or may not be hungry.	Wait a reasonable time and then remove food. Watch for symptoms of hypoglycemia.
	May be drinking too much milk.	Treat milk like food; offer water for thirst.
		Offer help if needed.
		Offer more food at next snack or meal.
		Make sure child is getting enough exercise. Limit TV watching time.
Wants to feed self	Eating is a way to be independent.	Offer as many choices as possible that child can handle (finger foods such as raw vegetables, strips of fruit, bite-size sandwiches, and so on).
		Offer food in utensils and dishes that are easy to handle.
		Encourage independence.

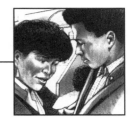

Problem	Reason(s)	Solutions
Wants to eat what other kids may be eating (junk foods)	Need for peer acceptance. Children need to feel that they belong and are accepted by classmates and friends.	Help child learn that uncontrolled blood glucose means not feeling good.
		Point out that all children have differences.
		Know that most children will try forbidden foods. Don't forbid, work toward the positives of other ways of eating.
		Make special treats just for your child, and whole family gets to share it, too.
		Realize that you control the environment by your selection of groceries. Take an interest and spend time preparing tasty, nutritious dishes. Take a proactive approach—you are interested in healthy vs. eating avoidance.
Typically eats four to five times a day	Growing children need to eat more frequently.	May prefer to prepare own snacks after school.
		Encourage independence.
		Use situations to encourage consistency.
Accepts more foods but may still reject vegetables and casseroles	Food likes and dislikes change rapidly during middle years.	Keep offering food with positive expectations for change.
		Encourage child to try new foods and help in food preparation and menu planning.
Television seems to be a big influence on food choices	Children look to parents, teachers, and other media as authorities on many things, including foods.	Make it clear that parents buy the groceries, parents make the choices.
		Set a good example, not just right after diagnosis, but always.
		Make a house rule to not have sugared cereals—not because of diabetes but for the well-being of the whole family.

SUGGESTIONS FOR SOLVING CHILDREN'S EATING PROBLEMS

Ages 6 to 12

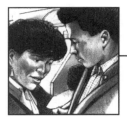

SUGGESTIONS FOR SOLVING CHILDREN'S EATING PROBLEMS

Adolescents: Ages 13 to 20

Problem	Reason(s)	Solutions
Resists attempts to encourage good eating habits	Environment is important; teens will often eat anything that's available.	Deal with weight control and fitness, not diabetes (positive vs. illness). Post cartoons on the refrigerator to help. Post charts and graphs that support positive change.
Sabotaging statements about the kinds or amounts of foods to be eaten	Friends are major influence on teens.	Identify family member or friends who will be supportive or who might help if asked. Discuss thoughts that create problems and foster progress. Don't threaten with talk about complications of diabetes.
Emotional problems related to food	Our society (ads, TV, books, movies) is filled with confusing information about food and eating.	Discuss thoughts that create problems and foster progress. Identify emotions associated with inappropriate eating and those that help the teen stick to his or her dietary goals.
Poor food habits	Teen may exert independence by displaying poor food habits.	Support teen's values, such as physical appearance. Good nutritional habits help us be the most attractive we can be. Discuss whether eating can really make someone popular. Catch them being "good" and eating wisely.
Frequent snacking	Teens like, and sometimes need, to eat frequently. They're always on the go.	Recognize that it can be helpful if snacks are nutritional. Make sure your teen understands the meal plan. Expect teen to act maturely. Let go!

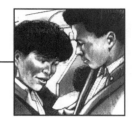

Problem	Reason(s)	Solutions
Trouble complying with meal plan	Teens have hard time focusing on one issue for any length of time.	Look for gradual improvement.
		Consider professional help if necessary.
		Compromise your expectations for a time.
		Support all compliance efforts.
		Applaud self-care measures.
		Encourage testing to monitor control.

SUGGESTIONS FOR SOLVING CHILDREN'S EATING PROBLEMS

Adolescents: Ages 13 to 20 (continued)

CHAPTER 33

Broatch Haig, RD, CDE
Martha L. Spencer, MD

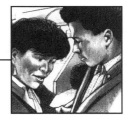

For Teens:
Answers to Your Questions About Health, Growing Up, and Sexuality

"What's the big deal about going to a new camp?"

"What sports can I participate in?"

"Why is a pelvic exam important?"

"Can I have children?"

"What kind of birth control can I use?"

We repeatedly get questions like these, plus so many others, from teenagers. Dealing with diabetes during this most crucial turning point in your life is important. It requires knowledge and understanding on the part of both you and your parents. This chapter is an open letter to you to discuss the questions and concerns you often have about general health, growing up, and sexuality.

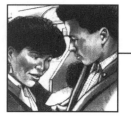

Dear _____:

You have tough work to accomplish during your teenage years. You'll be growing academically, socially, and physically, and you'll be gaining more independence from your folks. Everyone goes through it, but not everyone has diabetes.

Perhaps you've accepted diabetes. You think "so what, I'll do what I must to take care of it and get on with the more important parts of life." If you've taken this attitude, it's likely that all the other growth tasks and decisions you face will be easier to handle. But if you haven't accepted diabetes, you may have daily anger, hassles, and arguments with yourself and everyone else about abusing your body and keeping on track medically. Adding that to the decisions you face about school, dating, relationships, and jobs or careers can make for a pretty unhappy existence. We are writing to you with the hope that we can help you understand the stuff you need to know about dealing with your diabetes and the issues affecting you.

Knowing what's best for your health and doing something about it can be two different things. Sometimes worrying is good for you. The best worrying leads to some action and resolution. You may indeed worry because you're at risk for diabetes complications, but you can do a lot of things to help prevent them—like eat right, exercise, and take care of your body. (You knew we'd talk about the everyday issues first and sex last. If you are properly respectful, you'll read it all and not skip to the end.)

GROWING UP

The teen years can be scary. When you enter junior or senior high it's often a bigger school, with more kids and more competition. It's difficult to cope with all the changes that occur during these years. Height and weight increase dramatically, and you need more sleep, calories, and insulin to keep up with this growth.

School is busy. If you're involved in lots of after-school activities, it takes organization to follow your meal plan. Please get your meal plan adjusted if it doesn't fit your lifestyle. Eating anything and everything means you'll just need more insulin to gain blood glucose control, and pretty soon you're chasing food with insulin and insulin with food.

When it comes to development, at first the girls seem to be beating the boys to adulthood. Some girls worry about baby fat without realizing that

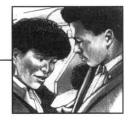

as nature takes its course, the curves will end up in all the right places. However, once you start menstruating (having your period) you don't have much more upward growing to count on, so start taking some steps to make sure you don't continue to grow sideways. But crash dieting isn't the answer. If you have diabetes, you already know more about smart food choices than your friends. You can lead the way and show your friends how to keep from getting fat by eating smart and exercising.

At the same time, know that thinness does not equal beauty and goodness. The models on television are not in reality any more than Barbie dolls. Try not to compare yourself with them. If you or your friends are starving, abusing diet pills or laxatives, binge eating, and becoming obsessed with thinness, talk to your health care team or counselor at school. There are many stressors in your life right now, and destroying your beautiful body is not going to help you cope.

The same is true for boys. While you won't have the curves, you'll be busy building bigger muscles and bones. Rest assured that you will catch up and grow bigger and larger, but you need to follow your meal plan and eat properly to do so.

JUST EATING

Meal scheduling can be difficult when you're a student. In junior high, high school, or college, the trick is to try to get a consistent lunchtime that's not too late. If lunchtime is after noon, you may have to eat a morning snack to prevent your blood glucose from getting too low. Kids with diabetes most often need to eat about every three hours.

In college, the biggest threat seems to be high-fat, high-calorie cafeteria food (fat is cheaper than protein) and the weekend brunch schedules. Brunch saves college food services labor and food costs and at the same time forces you to adapt.

But by now you're getting good at adapting! Most students find it works well to rise within an hour of the usual time, take insulin, eat breakfast from their own refrigerator stashes, and then eat brunch as an early lunch. As with any change, you'll need to *test, test, test* and eat an afternoon snack if necessary. If brunch is quite early, try getting up within an hour of your regular time, taking your insulin, and having some juice or milk. If your blood glucose is below 80 mg/dl, eat a starch/bread exchange. Then at brunch, eat the equivalent of breakfast and lunch. You may need to adjust your insulin for this larger meal unless you are much more physically active on weekends.

447

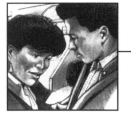

Adapting is also important when it comes to studying habits. All-night studying should be avoided, if possible. When it's unavoidable, plan smart snacks and test your blood glucose often enough to know when you need a snack. You think so much better when your blood glucose levels are not low, so practice prevention versus treatment.

EXERCISE AND SPORTS

Start off right, if you can. Build regular exercise into your schedule. It will help control your blood glucose and prevent the rear-end spread.

Both boys and girls do best in their chosen sports when blood glucose levels are within the goal range. You can't do your best at anything when your blood glucose level is bouncing.

Motor racing and skydiving are out for you. Hypoglycemia in the midst of any of these sports could be fatal. For that same reason, although swimming is fun and great exercise, don't swim alone. You can choose from other activities. Do choose some. Look at your sport and your degree of activity. Are you better off lowering insulin for that daily scrimmage or tennis match? If you're starting to be concerned about your shape, that's probably a smart move. Begin by reducing by 10% the insulin acting hardest at that time. And *test, test, test,* anytime you start a new sport or season (see Chapter 27 for more information on exercise and sports).

If you hate people reminding you all the time about diabetes management tasks, get them off your back by taking care of the situation first. Carry reaction treatment supplies with you so no one else has to be involved in "taking care of you." Certainly your coach or teacher needs to know about your diabetes and to have supplies available too, but if you do it right most often you don't need their help.

Tell your best friends about your diabetes and what they need to know. Let them help you out if the need arises. You'll return the favor in other ways as your friendship grows.

CAMP

Experimenting with independence is part of growing up. Diabetes camp is a great way to meet others, be on your own (in a manner acceptable to your

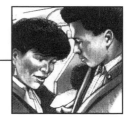

parents), and learn skills so you can camp anywhere, anytime, and feel confident.

Every diabetes camp is different. Some are strong on fairly formal medical education. Some offer a safe place to camp, but work on diabetes in the most subtle way possible. The latter camps emphasize activities, the outdoors, and the support and friendship of other people your age facing the same concerns.

While you're at diabetes camp, ask questions. Find out why changes in insulin are being made. Trust yourself enough to discuss your care. You may find that diabetes camp becomes a refuge, a motivator to get back on your management track. You may enjoy working as a counselor and helping younger children learn the ropes. Being a role model can be great for self-esteem.

Once you're an accomplished diabetes camp veteran, you may choose hockey, basketball, Outward Bound, or any number of other non-diabetes camping experiences. But before you sign up, **tell them you have diabetes** and find out:

- if you'll have ready and flexible access to decent food
- what medical personnel are in residence or how close they are
- what they know about diabetes
- if someone knows how to give glucagon
- if there is access to a phone
- if there is a hospital nearby

If you're satisfied with the answers, be prepared to *test, test, test*. Any change requires more information. If you're not willing to do more testing, you shouldn't be going to a non-diabetes camp. Because of the extra activity, you'll most likely need to reduce your insulin by at least 10% and be particularly careful with before-sleep tests. Be prepared to wake up a couple of nights at 2 AM to test if necessary. It doesn't take much to camp safely, but what it does take is absolutely necessary and worth the effort.

MAKING DECISIONS ABOUT YOUR FUTURE

Are you getting a lot of pressure to decide what you want to be? It's really never too soon to start thinking about your future for several reasons.

1. You spend more than one-third of your life on the job. Better to enjoy it!

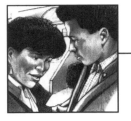

2. The lowest paid work is usually the most dull, dehumanizing work. You need skills for higher pay.

3. Diabetes care costs money. You need to earn enough to take care of yourself.

At the time of this writing some choices are not open to people with Type I diabetes:

- interstate trucker
- pilot
- firefighter
- armed forces

However, other career options are so terrific and so varied that it will take some investigation and self-knowledge to make sure you choose the right one. Ask yourself questions. What do you do well? (Most of us really enjoy what we excel in.) Ask questions of others who are making a decent living. What do they do? What's fun about their careers? Is it a career or just a job? School counselors can help with testing and advice. We recommend three other sources of information:

- *Dictionary of Occupational Titles.* Lists a description of jobs, working conditions, skills, and educational requirements. Check your library.
- *Occupational Outlook Handbook.* Published by the US Department of Labor. Includes employment and earning outlook.
- *State Employment Office.* Check the book that lists civil service employment opportunities. You'll learn all about occupations you never knew existed.

Taking a proactive stance in selecting your life's work can make a big difference. Those who end up in a line of work because "the job was available" when they were looking often feel manipulated by forces and conditions outside of their control. If you visualize and plan your future, you will move closer and closer to your dreams.

STAYING HEALTHY

To get there you have to take care of yourself and stay healthy. Besides doing the basics (eating right, exercising, testing blood glucose, and taking your insulin), you need to lower your risk factors for developing the complications of diabetes (read Section IV for details on complications). You also should know about some other important prevention activities.

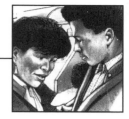

Teeth and Gums. People with diabetes have more gum infections than people without diabetes, and these infections take longer to heal. Long-standing infections may cause loss of teeth, and people with diabetes often have a harder time with dentures. So work to save your teeth and gums.

See a dentist every six months for a check-up. Always tell your dentist you have diabetes. Brush with a soft-bristled toothbrush, using a vibrating motion between your teeth and on your gums. Move the rubber tip on your toothbrush in a circular motion between your teeth. Of course, as you've been told endlessly, floss, floss, floss!

As with everything else in your life, good blood glucose control is important for good dental care. Poorly controlled diabetes can cause gum infections and thrush (that's not a bird, it's a mouth infection that shows up as white patches on the tongue, palate, gums, and other areas).

Any oral surgery or tooth extractions should be delayed until diabetes is under control. Such procedures should be scheduled for early morning, about 1 1/2 hours after breakfast.

Alcohol, Smoking, and Drugs. Alcohol and drugs can affect your diabetes control directly, but they can also affect it indirectly if you are so mellowed or destroyed that you don't take care of yourself. If you use, be prepared for consequences, and there will be consequences!

Tetrahydrocannabinol, or THC, marijuana's principal intoxicating chemical, inhibits the hormone that sets adolescent development in motion. It interferes with learning and may cause cancer and emphysema and affect your heart. Tobacco and marijuana together are a double hazard. Marijuana can also affect your sperm or eggs. Is it worth it?

Self-Examinations. Girls need to examine their breasts for lumps each month beginning around the age of 14. Pelvic examinations and Pap smears are done as part of birth control instruction or are recommended yearly starting at age 18. Boys should examine their testes each month beginning around ages 14 to 16. They should also do monthly breast examinations. These self-examinations can go a long way toward early detection of cancer.

PUBERTY (SEXUAL DEVELOPMENT)

When *puberty* (sexual development) begins depends on family growth patterns and how well your diabetes is controlled. Diabetes and sexual development are interrelated. Poor diabetes control can delay the onset of puberty, prolong its course, and result in poor growth during puberty. High blood glucose levels may cause irregular menstrual cycles and yeast

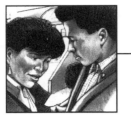

vaginitis. Diabetes can also affect the course of emotional maturation during puberty. Some teenagers find that diabetes delays their efforts in gaining independence from their families.

Boys reach puberty (that is, are able to produce sperm and make a girl pregnant) between ages 12 and 15. Girls reach puberty (that is, are able to produce eggs and become pregnant) earlier—some around ages 10 or 11 but some not until ages 15 or 16.

Hormones bring about breast development, growth of body hair, acne (zits and pimples), and body odor in both boys and girls; growth of the penis and testes in boys; and onset of the menstrual cycle in girls. High levels of these hormones may also cause fluctuations in blood glucose levels. Blood glucose may increase a few days before and during the first few days of menstruation.

The menstrual cycle is a series of hormonal and physical events that determine a woman's fertility. The cycle begins with the first day of menstrual bleeding and ends the day before the menstrual bleeding begins again. Although the average menstrual cycle is described as being twenty-eight days, in reality, women's cycles vary in length. Some are twenty-one days, some last for forty-five days. It's perfectly normal for one person to have variable cycles. Cycle length can also be affected by factors such as hormone activity, fatigue, stress, strenuous exercise, chronic illness, drugs, and body weight. Menstrual cycles in teens tend to be even more irregular. This can last for up to two to three years before settling into a more average rhythm. An irregular cycle also means irregular fertility. Sexually active teens should not rely on so-called "safe" periods during their cycles as a means of birth control.

Sometimes, menstruation is accompanied by some pain (menstrual cramps), particularly the first day. These cramps range in severity and are not usually present until the menstrual cycle is well established. Aspirin and ibuprofen are common drugs used to relieve the pain. Severe cramping may cause vomiting and even more difficulty with metabolic control. The frequency of insulin reactions may increase.

Normally some mucus is discharged from the vagina before menstrual bleeding begins. This is the result of some cells being shed from the lining of the vagina and cervical mucus. You can keep yourself comfortable by wearing cotton panties and loose clothing and practicing good hygiene.

FEELINGS

In addition to the actual physical changes, teens have lots of changing feelings and sensations that are normal. Boys have "wet dreams" and can

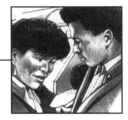

have erections at any time due to emotions or thoughts. Girls, too, have nocturnal sex dreams. Masturbation is common. It's a normal sexual expression for both males and females at any age.

Pretty soon, if not already, you're going to demonstrate an interest in dating, going to parties, and otherwise mixing it up. If you start pairing off with a special person and your friends won't always be there for emergencies, it's time to decide whether this significant other is significant enough to talk to about your diabetes. You may also be wondering if he or she is significant enough to have sexual intercourse with.

To want sexual closeness is normal. Sexual intimacy as a climax to true friendship, love, and shared life goals is one of life's most wonderful experiences. But getting the act right doesn't really take much practice. What does take a lot of practice is the decision about whether to be a sexual partner, when, and why. A lot is at stake, including your health and your future. Ask yourself the following questions when you are considering sexual involvement.

- Is it because of pressure from your friends, or one special person?
- Do you think it will prove your manhood or womanhood?
- Is it because you think virginity is a "burden" to be gotten rid of?
- Do you think it will make you more popular or help you keep your boyfriend or girlfriend?
- Are you planning sex to punish your parents?

None of these are reasons to have sex. The other things you must consider include the risks for pregnancy and sexually transmitted diseases, both of which have long-term effects on your health and your future.

SEXUALLY TRANSMITTED DISEASES

Most sexually transmitted diseases (known as venereal diseases, or VD) are curable if discovered early and treated by a doctor. However, venereal diseases can affect blood glucose control and lipids, among other things. Prevention is key. Anal and vaginal intercourse and oral sex should be avoided by anyone (heterosexuals or homosexuals) who is unsure of his or her sexual partners. Sexual partners who are intravenous drug users are especially high risk.

AIDS (acquired immune deficiency syndrome) is a sexually transmitted disease that is fatal. It's spread by the exchange of body fluids (semen, blood, menstrual blood, and vaginal secretions). Don't allow your partner's

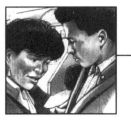

body fluids to enter your body. Body fluids can enter through the vagina, penis, anus, mouth, or any cut or open sore. AIDS is not a "gay" disease and it doesn't happen only to adults. Anyone can get it!

Herpes is a virus that can cause small blisters to appear on or around the mouth (Type I herpes) or the genitals (Type II herpes). It is transmitted by direct contact with the active virus. The first sign for the infected person is usually a tingling or itching sensation on the skin, followed by the appearance of blisters. The blisters eventually heal and disappear. Rarely is there active virus present without symptoms.

About 20 million people are infected with herpes. To avoid infection, don't touch the infected area as long as the virus is active. Always use condoms with spermicides to reduce risks.

Chlamydia infections are the most prevalent of all sexually transmitted infections. Chlamydia may be present without symptoms in either men or women and is often called silent for that reason. Because there are often no symptoms, sexual partners may be infected unwittingly. In men, symptoms include painful urination and watery discharge from the penis. In women, symptoms include itching and burning in the genitals, vaginal discharge, dull pelvic pain, and bleeding between menstrual periods. To prevent chlamydia, use condoms and diaphragms during intercourse.

Chlamydia is a serious bacterial infection that does not need to be reported to the health department. If you suspect problems, ask your doctor for a test. Chlamydia can be treated easily with antibiotics. Untreated chlamydia may lead to inflammation of the testicles in men and blockage and scarring of the fallopian tubes in women, all of which can cause sterility or infertility. Untreated chlamydia also poses a greater risk for spontaneous abortion and stillbirth and can be passed to babies during birth, putting them at risk for eye infections and pneumonia.

Gonorrhea ("clap") appears about two to six or more days after sexual relations with an infected person. If there are any noticeable symptoms, the first sign for both sexes is often a burning sensation when urinating. Pus may drip from the penis.

Syphilis appears from ten days to as long as three months after contact. The first sign is a single sore, usually around the genitals, followed by a rash on any part of the body. While these signs may disappear; they are soon replaced by fever, headache and sore throat.

Despite eventual disappearance of outward signs, untreated gonorrhea and syphilis infections remain active in the body and can cause sterility, blindness, insanity, and other crippling conditions. Syphilis can result in death.

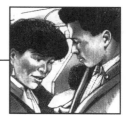

PREGNANCY

Having a baby as an adolescent is tough duty for the adolescent parents, yet probably even tougher on the baby. Trouble awaits if you haven't finished your own growth and if the pregnancy is not planned so that diabetes is under great control for three months before becoming pregnant and then during the pregnancy. Birth defects can happen. Diabetes complications may worsen during pregnancy. Will you have a long and healthy life in which to parent your child? These are risks you'll have to consider. The good news is that planned pregnancies with specialist medical care have become more and more successful. But it takes planning, effort, and money to pay the increased medical costs.

Symptoms of pregnancy include one or more missed periods in a row, tender breasts, morning nausea and vomiting, or unexplained insulin reactions in combination with any of the above.

If you're worried about pregnancy, or wonder if you're pregnant, see your doctor right away. You and your parents can discuss with the doctor all the options available regarding pregnancy and diabetes.

CONTRACEPTIVES (BIRTH CONTROL)

Talking about birth control with your parents may not be easy, but it is important. Most parents care deeply about the decisions their children make. Most teens want to be considered mature people. By bringing up the subject of contraception, you're taking responsibility for your feelings and actions. It can be the first step in building a more adult relationship with your parents and health care team.

It won't be easy and may not be successful. Your parents' first reaction may be a strong negative, which may be the only way they can react initially. They need time to think. On the other hand, they may not be surprised and may feel relieved. Be prepared for further talks, and don't push. Let your parents know you care about them and their opinions. Don't sound as if you're making an announcement—ask for their ideas.

If you can't talk to your parents, try another respected adult friend or relative, an older brother or sister, teachers, rabbi, or minister. You can visit a family planning clinic. If you are sexually active or plan to become sexually active, you need to talk about birth control options with your doctor.

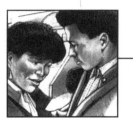

Major forms of birth control include the Pill; an intrauterine device (IUD); barrier methods such as a diaphragm, foam, sponges, and condoms; natural family planning; and other methods such as tubal ligation, rhythm, and so on.

Birth control pills are hormones that prevent ovulation and block implantation of fertilized eggs. They are 97 to 99% effective and require a pelvic examination and a doctor's prescription. They also tend to increase blood glucose levels and require more blood glucose monitoring. There may be more difficulties with yeast infections and mood changes, and there is a risk of vascular disease. Despite these complications, the Pill is the best choice for teenage girls.

Condoms with a lubricant containing spermicide Nonoxynal-9 protect both partners. Condoms (rubbers) should be held firmly in place when the penis is removed from the vagina. They are not reusable. See Chapter 26 for more information on pregnancy and birth control.

SEX FACTS TO REMEMBER

- Having sex makes babies unless you choose not to have a baby (by preventing the sperm from reaching the egg).
- Sperm can leave the penis before ejaculation (coming), so withdrawal is not a reliable form of birth control.
- Not having sex is the only way to prevent pregnancy 100% of the time. Many people don't have sex yet they fib about it.
- Douching, rhythm, suppositories, plastic wrap around the penis, and wishful thinking are not contraceptives. Repeating one hundred times "I can't get pregnant" is not a contraceptive. You can and you probably will.
- Not having sex protects us from sexually transmitted diseases and pregnancy. Not having sex also protects us emotionally.
- "I love you" is worth only as much as how it is expressed in day-to-day behavior.

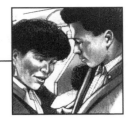

SEXUALITY ISSUES

Sex and sexuality are not the same thing. Sexuality is each person's unique maleness or femaleness. It's determined by many emotional and physical factors, such as:

- physical attractiveness
- personality
- perception of self
- life experiences
- values that are influenced by family, peers, culture, and religion
- expression of sexual feelings
- feelings for others
- ability to communicate
- ability to receive feelings

Sexuality doesn't just refer to sexual interaction with another person, it's an integrated part of yourself.

Diabetes can affect sexuality, both physically and emotionally, but people with diabetes still have healthy sexual lives. Diabetes does not affect sexual drive (*libido*), except secondarily to emotional factors. For example, diabetes may affect how people feel about themselves and how they interact with others, which will affect their sex lives. Several factors may affect sexual behavior in persons with diabetes and/or their partners. These include physical changes, potential complications (either from diabetes or from fear of pregnancy), self-esteem, fear of passing diabetes down to future generations, and the ability to give and take during a relationship.

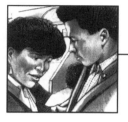

SUMMARY

Well, we covered a lot of ground with you. Most books about sex are written to please uptight parents, so few kids read them. Having read this far you've probably learned a lot more than you ever even thought you wanted to know about your body and sex. It's certainly a lot more than moonlight and roses and Prince Charming, isn't it? Yet relationships that grow in kindness, respect, and sharing and that appreciate the dignity of the people involved can result in mature committed relationships in which sexual intimacy is the salsa on the nachos. Think through how you want to handle sex in your life. Be proactive about decisions, whether they're about sex, your life's work, or your health.

This might be the longest letter you've ever received! We promise not to write another until you're 30. We wish you the best. You deserve it!

Love, *Marty and Broatch*

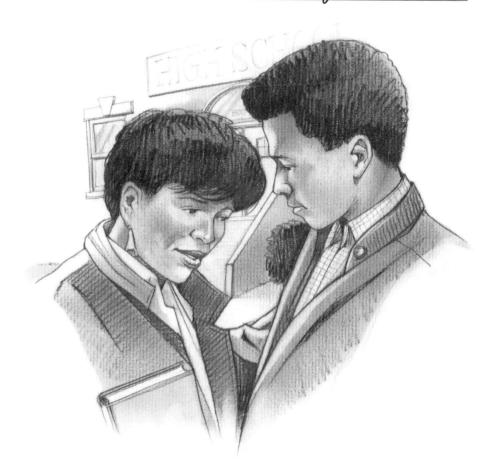

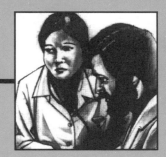

Finding The Light At The End Of The Tunnel

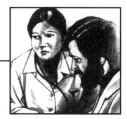

Research:
Can You Help?

For decades scientists and health care providers have been searching for a cure for diabetes and, until that's known, for better ways to manage diabetes. Their research has resulted in such innovations as insulin, self monitoring of blood glucose, laser therapy for retinopathy, glycohemoglobin testing, and other helpful treatment and management methods. However, none of these medical wonders would have been possible without the help of research study participants—people like you who have diabetes and were willing to help by testing the new treatments.

This chapter focuses on clinical trials, the phase of research studies that involves people. It provides guidelines to help you evaluate research studies and decide if you want to participate.

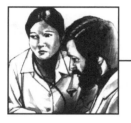

New treatments for diabetes aren't just created in test tubes. At first the ideas are examined through laboratory studies and tested on animals. If the results are encouraging, standards are set up for *clinical trials* with people.

Clinical trials are designed to answer certain questions about diabetes and come up with new and better ways to help those who have it. They study many different aspects of diabetes, including:

- diagnosis
- physical effects
- psychological effects
- treatment methods
- control methods
- prevention (of diabetes *and* its complications)

Clinical trials cannot be done without you, the person with diabetes. This is where your help is invaluable!

A PERSONAL DECISION

Whether or not to participate in research studies is an individual choice that should be made only after you understand both the possible risks and benefits. These vary from person to person and study to study. If you choose to participate, all research studies are required to inform you about these issues as part of a process called *informed consent*.

Informed consent means that everything involved in the clinical trial, including risks, benefits, and possible side effects, has to be explained to you by the health care providers conducting the trial. It's required for federally funded and regulated research. However, the final decision to participate is yours. Even after the consent form is signed, you still have the option to leave a study at any time.

SAFE AND SOUND

The need to regulate scientific research involving human subjects became evident after World War II. The Nuremberg Trials exposed many cases of suffering and death as a result of research conducted on Holocaust victims. As a result of the reports from these trials, the *Nuremberg Code* was adopted

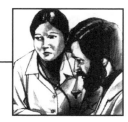

internationally to ensure that the rights of people participating in research would be protected. In brief, the Code's standards require that studies:

- obtain voluntary consent of the participant
- are meaningful and necessary and benefit society
- avoid unnecessary physical and mental suffering, injury, and risk of death
- never take a degree of risk that exceeds the humanitarian importance of the problem being studied
- are conducted by scientifically qualified persons in adequate facilities
- allow the subjects to quit if they can no longer continue

In the United States, the Department of Health and Human Services (HHS) has written standards and regulations for research based on the Nuremberg Code. It's absolutely essential that all research studies be carefully monitored for safety, ethics, and scientific standards.

THE CHOICE IS YOURS

The information below is a required part of written consent as designated by HHS. It's meant to help you decide if you wish to participate in a research study. Be sure these questions are answered for you before you decide to join a research study.

1. What's the purpose of the study?
2. What will be required of me if I join the study? What procedures will be done? How often and how much of my time will be required?
3. What discomforts, inconveniences, or risks might I expect? What are the side effects of the experimental method and how often do they occur?
4. What benefits will I receive?
5. What other treatments are available for my condition in addition to the experimental treatment? What are their potential benefits and risks?
6. Will there be costs to participate in the study? What direct (cash) or indirect (medical care, laboratory work, supplies, and so on) compensation will I receive?
7. Will the confidentiality of my medical records be preserved? Who besides the study team will review my medical records? How will the information gathered about me be handled?

463

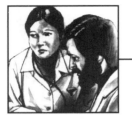

8. If the research results in injury to me, what can I expect in terms of treatment and who will pay for it?

9. If I choose to withdraw from the study early, or if I decline to participate, will my relationship with the research center be affected?

10. Whom may I contact if I have questions about the study once I've joined? Will I be given a plan, in writing, for reaching study staff 24 hours a day?

11. Whom may I contact (outside the research staff) if I have questions about my rights as a research participant?

In addition, these points can also help you make your decision.

- The research staff should be courteous, accessible, knowledgeable, and willing to answer your questions.

- You may want to speak with current study participants. Ask if it's possible.

- Find out how much experience the center has with the experimental treatment. In addition to the potential risks listed in the consent form, ask what the center's actual experience has been with the experimental method.

- Ask how much choice you have in selecting appointments. Think about how this will affect your personal schedule.

- Find out how you will be informed of test results done during the study and of the study's results.

- Ask how the study center will communicate with your doctor and how often.

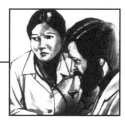

SUMMARY

Medical and scientific breakthroughs would not be possible without the research done in clinical trials. That's why you're so important. Research depends on human subjects, but participating in research is a highly personal decision. We hope that having the right information will make it an easier one for you.

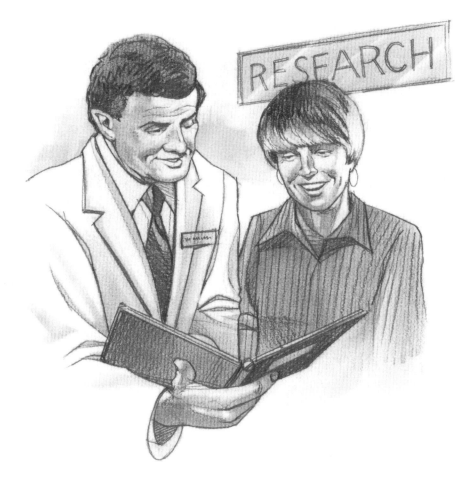

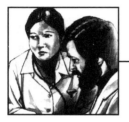

NOT SURE?
TAKE THIS TEST

People take part in research studies for various reasons. Answer these questions to discover what might motivate you to participate.

1. Would you like an opportunity to benefit from experimental treatment for a problem (such as neuropathic pain) for which you haven't found medical help?

2. Do you want to increase your knowledge of diabetes and help other people with diabetes, including members of your family who may have the potential to develop it?

3. Are you interested in receiving health care above and beyond what you normally receive for your diabetes?

4. Do you like to be an "explorer" or the first on the block with something new?

5. Do the financial benefits (free health care, supplies, cash) offered by studies appeal to you?

6. Would you like the chance to try a new health care team?

7. Do you like to share your opinions about diabetes care? This is especially important for studies that test devices such as syringes or meters, where consumer opinions can directly affect the design.

If you answered "yes" to any of these questions, you may wish to participate in diabetes research. It can be a win-win situation—you may benefit and so may other people with diabetes.

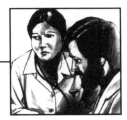

CHAPTER 35

Roger S. Mazze, PhD

Technology:
Its Role in Research and Diabetes Management

Several times each day people with diabetes use machines the size of pocket calculators (blood glucose meters) to test their blood glucose levels. The results are displayed on a small screen and then stored, along with date and time, in the machine's memory. This handy memory helps people more accurately record and track their blood glucose levels over time.

Technology like this has made it possible to achieve finer control of blood glucose levels and, ultimately, diabetes. Over the years, technology has changed the way diabetes is managed. Now that the importance of good blood glucose control has been established, technology is being developed, tested, and used that will help people gain the control they need to live *well* with diabetes. This chapter discusses how new technology, particularly computer technology, is being used and developed in diabetes research and management.

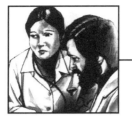

Diabetes management has come a long way since the discovery of insulin in the 1920s. Blood glucose meters have become common management tools, and more sophisticated tools are being developed and studied. With the help of computer technology, some people electronically send their blood glucose monitoring results to their doctors every few weeks. They connect their meters to phone modems to transfer the information to the doctor's office computer. The computer receives all the dates, times, and results, averages them, and prints them out to be studied later. The information is stored for later comparison. Such detailed records are helping people work with their health care teams to shape the best possible, individualized diabetes management plans.

Not everyone with diabetes, nor every health care professional, knows about these advances or values them. But computers are the wave of the future, and more and more people are choosing convenient, easy-to-use computer technology to help manage their diabetes and get the best possible results.

TECHNOLOGY WAVE

For more than a decade, researchers have been working on and trying out computer-based devices and programs for diabetes management. Equipment is now available that will help you gather, arrange, store, and report information about your diabetes. Putting this information together helps you understand your diabetes and decide how to better manage it. The focus is on things that affect management, such as blood glucose levels, insulin dose, food intake, activity level, psychological and social stress, and illness.

These efforts have contributed to a technological revolution in diabetes care and clinical research. For instance, *blood glucose meters* have changed the way people test and monitor blood glucose levels and make adjustments in daily care. The next wave of technology includes *patient management systems*, which involve all the areas of diabetes management mentioned above and the use of innovative *hand-held* computers. Hand-held computers help you record information about your diabetes. With computer hookups, you can transmit the information to your health care team. Then you and your health care team work together to program this information into a computer so it can be seen at the touch of a button. Together you use this information to make decisions about your diabetes management or changes in therapy.

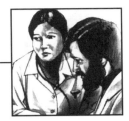

PROBLEMS WITH EARLY TECHNOLOGY

Development of blood glucose meters, using technology available ten years ago, was spurred by growing evidence that such information is important to diabetes management. As more advanced technology became available, the portable blood glucose meter underwent many changes and became smaller, more reliable, easier to use, and less costly.

Since early blood glucose meters could not record data, people had to record their test results and other information in logbooks. The first attempts at computerization included entering information from logbook records (such as insulin dose, blood glucose level, and caloric intake) into personal computers. The information was processed by computer programs specially designed to accept and analyze it. These programs also had the potential to integrate blood glucose levels, insulin dose used, food intake, and other data.

Initial research showed this method had two potentially serious flaws. First, there was the possibility for errors, intentional or unintentional, when people recorded their blood glucose values into a logbook. Second, there was a 10 to 20% chance that the person entering the information from patient logbooks onto the personal computer could make an error.

SOLVING THE PROBLEMS

To eliminate the first problem, a computer *microchip* was inserted into blood glucose meters to instantly record and store, or remember, all blood glucose values with corresponding time and date. This *memory* frees you from the task of recording the information and decreases the potential for a recording error to less than 1%.

To solve the second problem, a special computer cable was developed that can connect a blood glucose meter directly to a personal computer. Information from the meter's memory is transferred, or downloaded, to the computer and stored for later use. This *computer hookup* eliminates the possibility of a computer operator making an error while inputting the information.

Memory meters make it possible to collect accurate blood glucose data. At the press of a button, the meter can display the number of blood glucose tests done over a certain time, the range of the values, and the

469

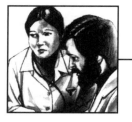

average. For instance, you might see that you tested 122 times this month, with results ranging from 60 mg/dl to 230 mg/dl and an average blood glucose value of 120 mg/dl.

Personal computer hookups help the health care team transmit information from meter to computer with no possibility for error. The information can then be summarized on a printout and arranged in various formats to provide a bird's-eye view of your blood glucose records—showing perhaps two months' worth of data in one graph or chart. The purpose is to show trends, averages, and timing problems with diabetes control and then work to help you improve.

For instance, you may know that your morning blood glucose levels are sometimes elevated, sometimes normal, and sometimes definitely low. By noticing this on the blood glucose printouts, your health care team can help you focus on the importance of consistency and timing of injections, food, and exercise to solve the problem. Or suppose you're having trouble with low or high blood glucose only on weekends. The health care team can quickly get a printout of the weekend records, try to pinpoint the problem, and come up with a potential solution.

In the past, such organized information on diabetes control was only possible through time-consuming and tedious hand calculations. The ease and efficiency offered by computer technology allow your health care team to spend less time with these calculations and more time with you.

THE WAVE OF THE FUTURE

While some researchers developed blood glucose meters with memory and computer hookups, others experimented with computers that would record data collected by people with diabetes and recommend changes in therapy. This involves the patient management systems mentioned earlier. These hand-held computers are small (about 8 inches long, 4 inches wide, 1 inch thick, and 14 ounces) and portable but have power and memory similar to some small, desktop personal computers.

Hand-held computers are programmed to take in information about insulin dose, glucose values, meal plan (calories, grams of carbohydrate), related illnesses, level of exercise, and level of stress. The computer program mathematically combines this information with standard information, such as the duration and action of insulin, the impact of high and/or low blood glucose values on the overall pattern, and individual

470

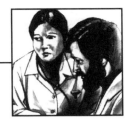

differences in response. In some systems, as more data is entered, the computer uses its artificial intelligence to "learn" from your experience.

Some hand-held computer systems are designed for health professional use, but eventually these may become commercially available for use by people with diabetes. Although the equipment (hardware) and programs that guide the equipment (software) are different, in principle they carry out the same functions. Most are designed for use by persons on multiple injections of mixed insulins or insulin pumps.

SUMMARY

It's hard to argue about the importance of using blood glucose monitoring information in diabetes management. Computer technology has made it faster and easier to evaluate large chunks of this information to help you. It can help you and your health care team determine whether complicated diabetes programs are for you. It can help you safely tighten your blood glucose control and independently evaluate your success. And it can help health care professionals develop new and better ways to manage diabetes. People who use hand-held computers with programs that recommend insulin adjustment can do better at collecting information on blood glucose control. As a result, better and more consistent diabetes control can be achieved.

As technology advances, the transfer of information will continue to improve. The next wave could see information being transferred back and forth between hand-held computers—from yours to your health care provider's and back. This would help the health care team evaluate whether the earlier recommendations programmed into your hand-held computer are working. Such a complete circle of information would truly benefit diabetes management for everyone.

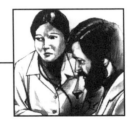

Research:
Providing Pieces
for the Diabetes Puzzle

More money is now being spent on diabetes research than ever before. Thousands of scientists, both in the United States and abroad, are devoting their careers and lives to diabetes. They are searching for ways to prevent, treat and, ultimately, cure diabetes. This chapter discusses some past research triumphs, as well as some of the research currently underway to accomplish these goals—research that provides hope for the future.

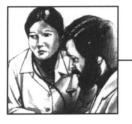

The improved outlook for persons with diabetes today is the result of endless hours spent by researchers. Researchers continue to identify persons at risk for developing diabetes in the hope that it can be prevented. They are continuously studying and evaluating better ways to treat diabetes and prevent its complications. And they are finding ways to provide better diabetes education so you can be actively involved in making decisions important to your health. The challenge to you is to *live well* while research continues to unravel the mysteries of diabetes.

PREVENTION

For years it has been known that diabetes can and does develop in members of the same family. However, the inheritance patterns were unclear and confusing. The realization that there is more than one type of diabetes cleared up some of this confusion. While the exact diabetes gene has not been detected, it is known that both Type I and Type II diabetes have genetic factors. Type II diabetes has the strongest genetic relationship, but Type I diabetes is also closely related to a trait found on one of the genes.

This gene, however, is not the only factor that determines who gets diabetes. It only places the person "at risk." Environment is also a factor. Environmental factors that may trigger the onset of diabetes include viral infections, chemicals, and/or stressful situations. An important research issue involves identifying persons who are genetically at risk for diabetes and then preventing environmental factors from triggering its onset. Although it is now possible to identify persons who are at risk for diabetes, prevention is still not possible.

When one or more environmental factors are present, the body's immune system makes proteins called *islet cell antibodies* to rid the body of the environmental intruder. A high level of islet cell antibodies is a sign that the body's immune system is gradually attacking the insulin-producing beta cells of the pancreas. Therefore, the presence of islet cell antibodies is the first indication that Type I diabetes may be developing. This is why Type I diabetes is believed to be an autoimmune disease (a process in which the body destroys its own tissue). In the past, it was thought that the onset of Type I diabetes was very rapid. We now know it may smolder for years before it suddenly erupts.

Studies are underway to see if certain immunosuppressive drugs may stop this process. (Immunosuppressives are drugs that prevent or diminish the immune response.) Although this therapy delays the onset of the

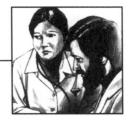

diabetes, these drugs have several undesirable side effects, some of which may damage the kidney or liver or may even increase the risk of certain cancers. As a result, these drugs are being used only at a few research centers.

Who develops Type II diabetes is even more closely related to genetic factors than Type I, although the genes related to Type II diabetes still have not been identified. Recently, researchers have become interested in an abnormal protein called amyloid (it's also called amylin) that is deposited in the pancreas of people with Type II diabetes. It's made and stored in the beta cells of the pancreas and is released into the bloodstream at the same time as insulin. People who have Type II diabetes have a higher amount of amylin than people who do not have diabetes. It is believed that amylin may affect both insulin secretion from the beta cell and the cell's use of insulin, which leads to insulin resistance. Since this is a major cause of Type II diabetes, a better understanding of what amyloid does and why it accumulates may help us understand the cause of Type II diabetes and, ultimately, its prevention.

TREATMENT ADVANCES

The discovery of insulin in 1921 by Banting and Best was followed by many improvements and purifications that enhanced the quality of insulin. However, in the late 1970s it appeared that the number of people needing insulin might exceed the amount projected to be available.

In response, Eli Lilly and a company called Genentech came up with an entirely new way to make insulin using *recombinant DNA technology (gene splicing)*. This technique allows genetic information (genes) to be transferred into bacteria, which gives it the information on how to make *human insulin*. The insulin made from this process is identical to the insulin made in the human pancreas.

Another company, Novo-Nordisk Pharmaceuticals, took a different approach. Using pork insulin and a naturally occurring enzyme, they converted the pork insulin into human insulin through a special chemical process. This human insulin is also structurally identical to the insulin produced by the pancreas. Because of the structure of the two human insulins, it seems reasonable to assume that using them might have some advantages. However, not enough time has passed to allow such a long-term evaluation.

The development of human insulin solved one of the problems of the future. Now that we have insulin identical to that manufactured by the

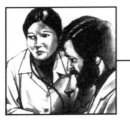

pancreas, the next logical step is to find a way to make it available to the entire body the same way the pancreas does.

Insulin Delivery

The current difficulty in blood glucose control lies in HOW insulin is delivered. Injecting insulin into the fat of the arms, legs, or trunk is very different from the way a pancreas carefully releases it directly into the bloodstream when it's needed. The *insulin pump* is one method that was developed to improve the delivery of insulin. The pump is a computerized device about the size of a deck of cards, with a reservoir for insulin connected to thin plastic tubing attached to a needle. The needle is placed under the skin, and insulin is delivered and carefully regulated according to a preprogrammed set of instructions. Pumps were popular for a few years, until it was shown that a program of three or four insulin injections a day by syringe could maintain blood glucose control just as well at a greatly reduced cost. Pumps also present some other problems. For instance, having one constantly attached to the body can be inconvenient when sleeping, showering, participating in athletic activities, and so on.

It is hoped that successful use of insulin pumps will lead to the development of an *artificial pancreas*. Such an instrument would consist of an insulin pump, a device that continually monitors blood glucose levels (a sensor), a small computer chip programmed to convert the amount of glucose in the blood to the amount of insulin required to keep it in a normal range, a storage space for insulin, and a power source capable of providing the necessary energy. Four of these components are currently developed and capable of performing the necessary tasks. Only the glucose sensor is missing, and many laboratories around the world are working on this problem. So it's possible that within the next few years, an artificial pancreas may become a reality.

Transplants

Newspapers constantly carry stories about kidney, liver, lung, and heart transplantation, so why not the pancreas? In 1967 Dr David L. Sutherland at the University of Minnesota performed the first modern pancreatic transplant. Of the first fourteen patients, only one did not need to inject insulin. Pancreas transplants have been done only in persons who need kidney transplants. More recently, such combined transplants have been quite successful. The transplanted pancreases have provided the necessary insulin, and a significant number of recipients have been able to stop injecting insulin. However, for this to be successful, some very powerful

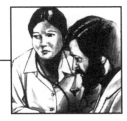

drugs must be taken daily. For persons who don't need a kidney transplant, the problem of associated kidney, liver, and possible cancer associated with these immunosuppressive drugs makes the risk of a pancreas transplant too great.

Since about one percent of the pancreas (the beta islet cells) is important to the release of insulin, some investigators have found ways to implant only the islet cells. However, once implanted they are susceptible to attack by the body's immune system, which destroys them. Instead of using immunosuppressive drugs to prevent this, researchers are studying development of a physical barrier, or a protective cover for the islet cells. It would have small holes, or pores, that would allow glucose to reach the islet cells, which in turn would secrete insulin that could flow out of the islet through the covering and into the blood stream. The substances that destroy the beta islet cells are very large, so they would not be able to enter the small holes in the covering and destroy the cell. The next few years will tell if this effort is successful.

Additional methods of insulin delivery currently being studied include taking it by mouth, spraying it into the nose, or stimulating its passage through the skin with the aid of an electric current. So far, the rate of absorption by these methods is too variable to be of use.

New Pills or Drugs

In Type II diabetes, oral agents or pills are often used to help keep blood glucose levels normal. New pills are constantly being developed and tested for this type of diabetes with increasing success.

Sometimes the damaged beta cells of the pancreas cannot respond immediately to the load of glucose absorbed after eating a meal. Some investigators are studying the effect of slowing down the passage of glucose through the intestine and into the bloodstream. Unfortunately, this approach often results in the production of large amounts of gas in the intestine, which may prove uncomfortable or embarrassing.

Another very active area of research involves finding drugs that could block the harmful effect of glucose on blood vessels. The major drugs being tested are called *aldose reductase inhibitors*. They work by blocking an enzyme called aldose reductase, which converts glucose into another sugar called sorbitol. Some studies have identified sorbitol as a substance that may be damaging blood vessels in the eyes, kidneys, and so on. If the drugs can inhibit or block this conversion, then damage may be prevented or minimized.

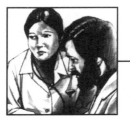

SUMMARY

The area of diabetes research is exciting right now. What is needed to solve many of the problems is time, money, and dedicated researchers. We have the dedicated researchers. We also have dedicated people who help raise money to support research. That leaves time. We must wait patiently for the research to answer and solve the problems related to the puzzle of diabetes.

There is a light at the end of the tunnel! But until we reach that light, you must continue learning to *live well* with your diabetes.

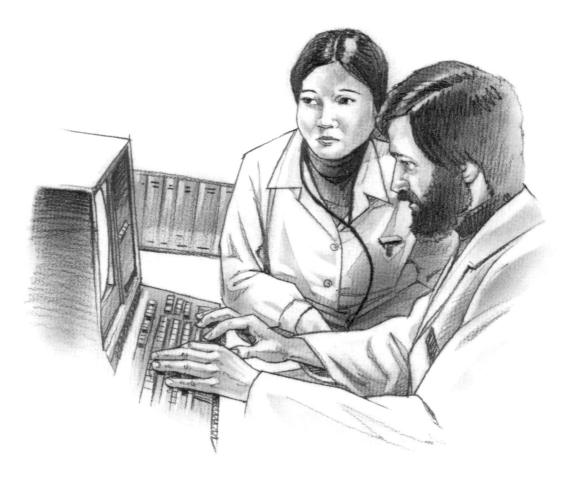

Appendix

Exchange Lists for Meal Planning

Each item in this list contains approximately 15 grams of carbohydrate, 3 grams of protein, a trace of fat, and 80 calories. Whole grain products average about 2 grams of fiber per serving. Some foods are higher in fiber. Those that contain 3 or more grams of fiber per serving are identified with the fiber symbol (*).

You can choose your starch exchanges from any of the items on this list. If you want to eat a starch food that is not on this list, the general rule is that:

- 1/2 cup of cereal, grain, or pasta is one serving
- 1 ounce of a bread product is one serving

Your dietitian can help you be more exact.

LIST 1. STARCH/BREAD EXCHANGES

Cereals/Grains/Pasta

Bran cereals, concentrated* (such as Bran Buds®, All Bran®)	1/3 cup
Bran cereals, flaked*	1/2 cup
Bulgur (cooked)	1/2 cup
Cooked cereals	1/2 cup
Cornmeal (dry)	2 1/2 Tbsp
Grapenuts®	3 Tbsp
Grits (cooked)	1/2 cup
Other ready-to-eat unsweetened cereals	3/4 cup
Pasta (cooked)	1/2 cup
Puffed cereal	1 1/2 cup
Rice, white or brown (cooked)	1/3 cup
Shredded wheat	1/2 cup
Wheat germ*	3 Tbsp

Dried Beans/Peas/Lentils

Beans and peas (cooked)* (such as kidney, white, split, blackeye)	1/3 cup
Lentils (cooked)*	1/3 cup
Baked beans	1/4 cup

Starchy Vegetables

Corn*	1/2 cup
Corn on cob (6 in. long)*	1
Lima beans*	1/2 cup
Peas, green (canned or frozen)*	1/2 cup

481

LIST 1. STARCH/BREAD EXCHANGES (CONTINUED)

Plantain*	1/2 cup
Potato, baked	1 small (3 oz)
Potato, mashed	1/2 cup
Squash, winter (acorn, butternut)*	1 cup
Yam, sweet potato (plain)	1/3 cup

Bread

Bagel	1/2 (1 oz)
Bread sticks, crisp (4 in. long x 1/2 in.)	2 (2/3 oz)
Croutons, low-fat	1 cup
English muffin	1/2
Frankfurter or hamburger bun	1/2 (1 oz)
Pita (6 in. across)	1/2
Plain roll, small	1 (1 oz)
Raisin, unfrosted	1 slice (1 oz)
Rye, pumpernickel	1 slice (1 oz)
Tortilla (6 in. across)	1
White (including French, Italian)	1 slice (1 oz)
Whole wheat	1 slice (1 oz)

Crackers/Snacks

Animal crackers	8
Graham crackers (2 1/2 in. square)	3
Matzoh	3/4 oz
Melba toast	5 slices
Oyster crackers	24
Popcorn (popped, no fat added)	3 cups
Pretzels	3/4 oz
Rye crisp* (2 in. x 3 1/2 in.)	4
Saltine-type crackers	6
Whole wheat crackers, no fat added* (crisp breads such as Finn®, Kavli®, Wasa®)	2–4 slices (3/4 oz)

Starch Foods Prepared with Fat
(Count as 1 starch/bread serving, plus 1 fat serving.)

Biscuit (2 1/2 in. across)	1
Chow mein noodles	1/2 cup
Corn bread (2-in. cube)	1 (2 oz)
Cracker, round butter type	6
French fried potatoes (2 in. to 3 1/2 in. long)	10 (1 1/2 oz)
Muffin (plain, small)	1
Pancake (4 in. across)	2
Stuffing, bread (prepared)	1/4 cup
Taco shell (6 in. across)	2
Waffle (4 1/2 in. square)	1
Whole wheat crackers, fat added* (such as Triscuits®)	4–6 (1 oz)

*3 grams or more of fiber per serving

Each serving of meat and substitutes on this list contains about 7 grams of protein. The amount of fat and number of calories vary, depending on what kind of meat or substitute you choose. The list is divided into three parts based on the amount of fat and calories: lean meat, medium-fat meat, and high-fat meat. One ounce (one meat exchange) of each of these includes:

	Carbohydrate (grams)	Protein (grams)	Fat (grams)	Calories
Lean	0	7	3	55
Medium-Fat	0	7	5	75
High-Fat	0	7	8	100

Try to use more lean and medium-fat meat, poultry, and fish in your meal plan. This will help decrease your fat intake, which may help decrease your risk for heart disease. The items from the high-fat group are high in saturated fat, cholestrol, and calories. Limit your choices from the high-fat group to three (3) times per week. Meat and substitutes do not contribute any fiber to your meal plan.

#400 mg or more of sodium if two or more exchanges are eaten
**400 mg or more of sodium per exchange

Tips

1. Bake, roast, broil, grill, or boil these foods rather than frying them with added fat.

2. Use a nonstick pan spray or a nonstick pan to brown or fry these foods.

3. Trim off visible fat before and after cooking.

4. Do not add flour, bread crumbs, coating mixes, or fat to these foods when preparing them.

5. Weigh meat after removing bones and fat and after cooking. Three ounces of cooked meat is about equal to 4 ounces of raw meat. Some examples of meat portions are:

- 2 ounces meat (2 meat exchanges) = 1 small chicken leg or thigh
  1/2 cup cottage cheese or tuna
- 3 ounces meat (3 meat exchanges) = 1 medium pork chop
  1 small hamburger
  1/2 of a whole chicken breast
  1 unbreaded fish fillet
  cooked meat, about the size of a deck of cards

6. Restaurants usually serve prime cuts of meat, which are high in fat and calories.

LIST 2.
MEAT EXCHANGES
(CONTINUED)

Lean Meat and Substitutes
(One exchange is equal to any one of the following items.)

Beef:	USDA Good or Choice grades of lean beef, such as round, sirloin, and flank steak; tenderloin; and chipped beef**	1 oz
Pork:	Lean pork, such as fresh ham; canned, cured or boiled ham**, Canadian bacon**, tenderloin	1 oz
Veal:	All cuts are lean except for veal cutlets (ground or cubed). Examples of lean veal are chops and roasts.	1 oz
Poultry:	Chicken, turkey, Cornish hen (without skin)	1 oz
Fish:	All fresh and frozen fish	1 oz
	Crab, lobster, scallops, shrimp, clams (fresh or canned in water)	2 oz
	Oysters	6 medium
	Tuna (canned in water)	1/4 cup
	Herring** (uncreamed or smoked)	1 oz
	Sardines (canned)	2 medium
Wild Game:	Venison, rabbit, squirrel	1 oz
	Pheasant, duck, goose (without skin)	1 oz
Cheese:	Any cottage cheese#	1/4 cup
	Grated parmesan	2 Tbsp
	Diet cheeses** (with less than 55 calories per ounce)	1 oz
Other:	95% fat-free luncheon meat**	1 oz
	Egg whites	3 whites
	Egg substitutes with less than 55 calories per 1/4 cup	1/4 cup

Medium-Fat Meat and Substitutes
(One exchange is equal to any one of the following items.)

Beef:	Most beef products fall into this category. Examples are: all ground beef, roast (rib, chick, rump), steak (cubed, Porterhouse, T-bone), and meatloaf	1 oz
Pork:	Most pork products fall into this category. Examples are: chops, loin roast, Boston butt, cutlets.	1 oz
Lamb:	Most lamb products fall into this category. Examples are: chops, leg, and roast.	1 oz

| Veal: | Cutlet (ground or cubed, unbreaded) | 1 oz |

Poultry:	Chicken (with skin), domestic duck or goose (well-drained of fat), ground turkey	1 oz
Fish:	Tuna# (canned in oil and drained)	1/4 cup
	Salmon# (canned)	1/4 cup
Cheese:	Skim- or part-skim-milk cheeses, such as:	
	Ricotta	1/4 cup
	Mozzarella	1 oz
	Diet cheeses ** (with 56–80 calories per ounce)	1 oz
Other:	86% fat-free luncheon meat#	1 oz
	Egg (high in cholesterol, limit to 3 per week)	1
	Egg substitutes with 56–80 calories per 1/4 cup	1/4 cup
	Tofu (2 1/2 in. x 2 3/4 in. x 1 in.)	4 oz
	Liver, heart, kidney, sweetbreads (high in cholesterol)	1 oz

High-Fat Meat and Substitutes

Remember, these items are high in saturated fat, cholesterol, and calories and should be used only three (3) times per week. (One exchange is equal to any one of the following items.)

Beef:	Most USDA Prime cuts of beef, such as ribs, corned beef#	1 oz
Pork:	Spareribs, ground pork, pork sausage** (patty or link)	1 oz
Lamb:	Patties (ground lamb)	1 oz
Fish:	Any fried fish product	1 oz
Cheese:	All regular cheeses, such as American,** Blue Cheddar,# Monterey Jack,# Swiss	1 oz
Other:	Luncheon meat,** such as bologna, salami, pimento loaf	1 oz
	Sausage,** such as Polish, Italian, smoked	1 oz
	Knockwurst**	1 oz
	Bratwurst#	1 oz
	Frankfurter** (turkey or chicken)	1 frank (10/lb)
	Peanut butter (contains unsaturated fat)	1 Tbsp

Count as one high-fat meat plus one fat exchange:

| | Frankfurter**(beef, pork, or combination) | 1 frank (10/lb) |

#400 mg or more of sodium if two or more exchanges are eaten
**400 mg or more of sodium per exchange

LIST 3. VEGETABLE EXCHANGES

Each vegetable serving on this list contains about 5 grams of carbohydrate, 2 grams of protein, and 25 calories. Vegetables contain 2 to 3 grams of dietary fiber. Vegetables that contain 400 mg of sodium per serving are identified with a ** symbol.

Vegetables are a good source of vitamins and minerals. Fresh and frozen vegetables have more vitamins and less added salt. Rinsing canned vegetables will remove much of the salt.

Unless otherwise noted, the serving size for vegetables (one vegetable exchange) is:

- 1/2 cup of cooked vegetables or vegetable juice
- 1 cup of raw vegetables

Artichoke (1/2 medium)
Asparagus
Beans (green, wax, Italian)
Bean sprouts
Beets
Broccoli
Brussels sprouts
Cabbage, cooked
Carrots
Cauliflower
Eggplant
Greens (collard, mustard, turnip)
Kohlrabi
Leeks
Mushrooms, cooked
Okra
Onions
Pea pods
Peppers (green)
Rutabaga
Sauerkraut**
Spinach, cooked
Summer squash (crookneck)
Tomato (one large)
Tomato/vegetable juice**
Turnips
Water chestnuts
Zucchini, cooked

Starchy vegetables such as corn, peas, and potatoes are found on the *Starch/Bread List*. For free vegetables, see *Free Food List*.

**400 mg or more of sodium per serving*

Each item on this list contains about 15 grams of carbohydrate and 60 calories. Fresh, frozen, and dried fruits have about 2 grams of fiber per serving. Fruits that have 3 or more grams of fiber per serving have a * symbol. Fruit juices contain very little dietary fiber.

Carbohydrate and calorie content for a fruit serving is based on the usual serving of the most commonly eaten fruits. Use fresh fruits or fruits frozen or canned without sugar added. Whole fruit is more filling than fruit juice and may be a better choice for those who are trying to lose weight. Unless otherwise noted, the serving size for one fruit serving is:

- 1/2 cup of fresh fruit or fruit juice
- 1/4 cup of dried fruit

Fresh, Frozen, and Unsweetened Canned Fruit

Apple (raw, 2 in. across)	1 apple
Applesauce (unsweetened)	1/2 cup
Apricots (medium, raw)	4 apricots
Apricots (canned)	1/2 cup, or 4 halves
Banana (9 in. long)	1/2 banana
Blackberries (raw)*	3/4 cup
Blueberries (raw)*	3/4 cup
Cantaloupe (5 in. across)	1/3 melon
(cubes)	1 cup
Cherries (large, raw)	12 cherries
Cherries (canned)	1/2 cup
Figs (raw, 2 in. across)	2 figs
Fruit cocktail (canned)	1/2 cup
Grapefruit (medium)	1/2 grapefruit
Grapefruit (segments)	3/4 cup
Grapes (small)	15 grapes
Honeydew melon (medium)	1/8 melon
(cubes)	1 cup
Kiwi (large)	1 Kiwi
Mandarin oranges	3/4 cup
Mango (small)	1/2 mango
Nectarine* (1 1/2 in. across)	1 nectarine
Orange (2 1/2 in. across)	1 orange
Papaya	1 cup
Peach (2 3/4 in. across)	1 peach or 3/4 cup
Peaches (canned)	1/2 cup, or 2 halves
Pear	1/2 large, or 1 small
Pears (canned)	1/2 cup or 2 halves
Persimmon (medium, native)	2 persimmons
Pineapple (raw)	3/4 cup
Pineapple (canned)	1/3 cup

LIST 4.
FRUIT EXCHANGES

LIST 4.
FRUIT EXCHANGES (CONTINUED)

Plum (raw, 2 in. across)	2 plums
Pomegranate*	1/2 pomegranate
Raspberries* (raw)	1 cup
Strawberries* (raw, whole)	1 1/4 cup
Tangerine* (2 1/2 in. across)	2 tangerines
Watermelon (cubes)	1 1/4 cup

Dried Fruit

Apples*	4 rings
Apricots*	7 halves
Dates	2 1/2 medium
Figs*	1 1/2
Prunes*	3 medium
Raisins	2 Tbsp

Fruit Juice

Apple juice/cider	1/2 cup
Cranberry juice cocktail	1/3 cup
Grapefruit juice	1/2 cup
Grape juice	1/3 cup
Orange juice	1/2 cup
Pineapple juice	1/2 cup
Prune juice	1/3 cup

3 grams or more of fiber per serving

LIST 5.
MILK EXCHANGES

Each serving of milk or milk products on this list contains about 12 grams of carbohydrate and 8 grams of protein. The amount of fat in milk is measured in percent (%) of butterfat. The calories vary, depending on what kind of milk you choose. The list is divided into three parts based on the amount of fat and calories: skim/very lowfat milk, lowfat milk, and whole milk. One serving (one milk exchange) of each of these includes:

	Carbohydrate (grams)	Protein (grams)	Fat (grams)	Calories
Skim/Very Lowfat	12	8	trace	90
Lowfat	12	8	5	12
Whole	12	8	8	150

Milk is the body's main source of calcium, the mineral needed for growth and repair of bones. Yogurt is also a good source of calcium. Yogurt and many dry or powdered milk products have different amounts of fat. If you have questions about a particular item, read the label to find out the fat and calorie content.

Milk is good to drink, but it can also be added to cereal and other foods. Many tasty dishes, such as sugar-free pudding, are made with milk (see the Combination Foods List). Add life to plain yogurt by adding one of your fruit servings to it.

Skim and Very Lowfat Milk

Skim milk	1 cup
1/2% milk	1 cup
1% milk	1 cup
Lowfat buttermilk	1 cup
Evaporated skim milk	1/2 cup
Dry nonfat milk	1/3 cup
Plain nonfat yogurt	8 oz

Lowfat Milk

2% milk	1 cup fluid
Plain lowfat yogurt (with added nonfat milk solids)	8 oz

Whole Milk

The whole milk group has much more fat per serving than the skim and lowfat groups. Whole milk has more than 3 1/4% butterfat. Try to limit your choices from the whole milk group as much as possible.

Whole milk	1 cup
Evaporated whole milk	1/2 cup
Whole plain yogurt	8 oz

Each serving on the fat list contains about 5 grams of fat and 45 calories.

These foods contain mostly fat, although some items may also contain a small amount of protein. All fats are high in calories and should be carefully measured. Everyone should modify fat intake by eating unsaturated fats instead of saturated fats. The sodium content of these foods varies widely. Check the label for sodium information.

Unsaturated Fats

Avocado	1/8 medium
Margarine	1 tsp
Margarine, diet#	1 Tbsp
Mayonnaise	1 tsp
Mayonnaise, reduced-calorie#	1 Tbsp

Nuts and Seeds:

Almonds, dry roasted	6 whole
Cashews, dry roasted	1 Tbsp

LIST 6.
FAT EXCHANGES
(CONTINUED)

Pecans	2 whole
Peanuts	20 small or 10 large
Walnuts	2 whole
Other nuts	1 Tbsp
Seeds, pine nuts, sunflower (without shells)	1 Tbsp
Pumpkin seeds	2 tsp
Oil (corn, cottonseed, safflower, soybean, sunflower, olive, canola, peanut)	1 tsp
Olives**	10 small or 5 large
Salad dressing, mayonnaise-type	2 tsp
Salad dressing, mayonnaise-type, reduced-calorie	1 Tbsp
Salad dressing (all varieties)#	1 Tbsp
Salad dressing, reduced-calorie**	2 Tbsp

(Two tablespoons of low-calorie salad dressing can be considered a free food)

Saturated Fats

Butter	1 tsp
Bacon#	1 slice
Chitterlings	1/2 ounce
Coconut, shredded	2 Tbsp
Coffee whitener, liquid	2 Tbsp
Coffee whitener, powder	4 tsp
Cream (light, coffee, table)	2 Tbsp
Cream, sour	2 Tbsp
Cream (heavy, whipping)	1 Tbsp
Cream cheese	1 Tbsp
Salt pork**	1/4 ounce

**400 mg or more of sodium per serving
#If more than one or two servings are eaten, these foods have 400 mg or more of sodium

A free food is any food or drink that contains less than 20 calories per serving. You can eat as much as you want of those items that have no serving size specified. You may eat two or three servings per day of those items that have a specific serving size. Be sure to spread them out through the day.

FREE FOODS

Miscellaneous:
Nonstick pan spray

Drinks:
Bouillon** or broth without fat
Bouillon, low-sodium
Carbonated drinks, sugar-free
Carbonated water
Club soda
Cocoa powder, unsweetened
  (1 Tbsp)
Coffee/Tea
Drink mixes, sugar-free
Tonic water, sugar-free

Fruit:
Cranberries, unsweetened
  (1/2 cup)
Rhubarb, unsweetened (1/2 cup)

Vegetables:
(raw, 1 cup)
Cabbage
Celery
Chinese cabbage*
Cucumber
Green onion
Hot peppers
Mushrooms
Radishes
Zucchini*

Salad greens:
Endive
Escarole
Lettuce
Romaine
Spinach

Sweet Substitutes:
Candy, hard, sugar-free
Gelatin, sugar-free
Gum, sugar-free
Jam/Jelly, sugar-free
  (less than 20 calories/2 tsp)
Pancake syrup, sugar-free
  (1 to 2 Tbsp)
Sugar substitutes
  (saccharin, aspartame)
Whipped topping (2 Tbsp)

Condiments:
Catsup (1 Tbsp)
Horseradish
Mustard
Pickles,** dill, unsweetened
Salad dressing, low-calorie
  (2 Tbsp)
Taco sauce (3 Tbsp)
Vinegar

FREE FOODS (CONTINUED)

Seasonings:

Seasonings can be very helpful in making food taste better. Be careful of how much sodium you use. Read the label and choose those seasonings that do not contain sodium or salt.

Basil (fresh)
Celery seeds
Cinnamon
Chili powder
Chives
Curry
Dill
Flavoring extracts
  (vanilla, almond, walnut,
  peppermint, butter, lemon, etc.)
Garlic

Garlic powder
Herbs
Hot pepper sauce
Lemon
Lemon juice
Lemon pepper
Lime
Lime juice
Mint
Onion powder
Oregano
Paprika
Pepper
Pimento
Spices
Soy sauce**
Soy sauce, low sodium ("lite")**
Winte, used in cooking (1/4 cup)
Worcestershire sauce

*3 grams or more of fiber per serving
**400 mg or more of sodium per serving

Much of the food we eat is mixed together in various combinations. These combination foods do not fit into only one exchange list. It can be quite hard to tell what's in a certain casserole dish or baked food item. This list of average values for some typical combination foods will help you fit these foods into your meal plan. Ask your dietitian for information about any other foods you'd like to eat. The *American Diabetes Association/American Dietetic Association Family Cookbooks* and the *American Diabetes Association Holiday Cookbook* have many recipes and further information about many foods, including combination foods. Check your library or local bookstore.

COMBINATION FOODS

Food	Amount	Exchanges
Casseroles, homemade	1 cup (8 oz)	2 starch, 2 medium-fat meat, 1 fat
Cheese pizza,** thin crust	1/4 of 15 oz or 1/4 of 10 in.	2 starch, 1 medium-fat meat, 1 fat
Chili with beans,** * (commercial)	1 cup (8 oz)	2 starch, 2 medium-fat meat, 2 fat
Chow mein** (without noodles or rice)	2 cups (16 oz)	1 starch, 2 vegetable, 2 lean meat
Macaroni and cheese**	1 cup (8 oz)	2 starch, 1 medium-fat meat, 2 fat
Soup:		
Bean** *	1 cup (8 oz)	1 starch, 1 vegetable, 1 lean meat
Chunky, all varieties**	1-10 3/4 oz can	1 starch, 1 vegetable, 1 medium-fat meat
Cream** (made with water)	1 cup (8 oz)	1 starch, 1 fat
Vegetable** or broth-type**	1 cup (8 oz)	1 starch
Spaghetti and meatballs** (canned)	1 cup (8 oz)	2 starch, 1 medium-fat meat, 1 fat
Sugar-free pudding (made with skim milk)	1/2 cup	1 starch
If beans are used as a meat substitute: Dried beans,* peas,* lentils*	1 cup (cooked)	2 starch, 1 lean meat

*3 grams or more of fiber per serving
**400 mg or more of sodium per serving

FOODS FOR OCCASIONAL USE

Moderate amounts of some foods can be used in your meal plan despite their sugar or fat content, as long as you can maintain blood glucose control. The following list includes average exchange values for some of these foods. Because they are concentrated sources of carbohydrate, you'll notice that portion sizes are very small. Check with your dietitian for advice on how often and when you can eat them.

Food	Amount	Exchanges
Angel food cake	1/12 cake	2 starch
Cake, no icing	1/l2 cake, or a 3 in. square	2 starch, 2 fat
Cookies	2 small (3/4 in.)	1 starch, 1 fat
Frozen yogurt	1/3 cup	1 starch
Gingersnaps	3	1 starch
Granola	1/4 cup	1 starch, 1 fat
Granola bars	1 small	1 starch, 1 fat
Ice cream, any flavor	1/2 cup	1 starch, 2 fat
Ice milk, any flavor	1/2 cup	1 starch, 1 fat
Sherbet, any flavor	1/4 cup	1 starch
Snack chips, all varieties#	1 oz	1 starch, 2 fat
Vanilla wafers	6 small	1 starch, 1 fat

#If more than one serving is eaten, these foods have 400 mg or more of sodium

The exchange lists are the basis of a meal planning system designed by a committee of the American Diabetes Association and the American Dietetic Association. While designed primarily for people with diabetes and others who must follow special diets, the exchange lists are based on principles of good nutrition that apply to everyone.

© 1986, American Diabetes Association, American Dietetic Association.

For details about exchange lists and for additional information on how to use the exchange system, read the IDC book *Exchanges for All Occasions* (see resource list at the back of the manual for more information).

Blood Glucose Monitoring Equipment Guide

METERS AND STRIPS

Company, Toll-free Number	Meter	Test Strip
Boehringer Mannheim Corporation 1-800-858-8072	Accu-Chek III	Chemstrip bG 50* for Accu-Chek III
	Accu-Chek Easy	Easy Test strips*
	Accu-Chek II Freedom (for the visually impaired)	Chemstrip bG 50 for Accu-Chek II
	Tracer II	Tracer bG*
Elco 1-800-3-DIRECT	Direct 30/30	No strips (sensor cartridge)
Home Diagnostics 1-800-DIASCAN	Diascan S	Diascan strips*
	Diascan SVM Audio Meter (for the visually impaired)	Diascan strips
LifeScan, Inc. 1-800-227-8862	Glucoscan 3000	Glucoscan strips
	One Touch	One Touch strips
	One Touch II	One Touch strips
MediSense, Inc. 1-800-527-3339	ExacTech	ExacTech glucose test strips
	Companion	
	Pen 2	Pen 2 Companion 2 Sensor Electrode
	Companion 2	Pen 2 Companion 2 Sensor Electrode

METERS AND STRIPS (CONTINUED)

Company, Toll-free Number	Meter	Test Strip
Miles, Inc. 1-800-348-8100	Glucometer II With Memory	Glucostix*
	Glucometer M	Glucostix*
	Glucometer 3	Glucofilm*
	Glucometer M+	Glucofilm*
Wampole Laboratories 1-800-525-6718	Answer	Answer strips

May also be read visually.

FINGER STICKING SUPPLIES

Company	Product
LifeScan, Inc.	Penlet II
Miles, Inc.	Glucolet
	Lancets: Dextro System Lancet
Palco	Auto-Lancet
Ulster Scientific, Inc.	Autolet Lite
	Lancets: Unilet Lite General Purpose Lancets
MediSense, Inc.	Lancets: Ultra TLC

URINE TESTING (FOR KETONES) SUPPLIES

Company	Product
Miles, Inc.	Ketostix (foil wrapped)
Boehringer Mannheim Corporation	Chemstrip K

Exchange Lists for Infant Foods**

Strained Vegetables		
Beets	1/2 (4.5 oz) jar	**VEGETABLE EXCHANGES**
Carrots	1/2 (4.5 oz) jar	
Creamed Spinach	1/2 (4.5 oz) jar	
Garden Vegetables	1/2 (4.5 oz) jar	
Green Beans	1/2 (4.5 oz) jar	
Mixed Vegetables	1/2 (4.5 oz) jar	
Peas	1/2 (4.5 oz) jar	
Squash	1/2 (4.5 oz) jar	
Vegetables and Meat (Bacon, Beef, Chicken, Ham, Lamb, Liver, Turkey)	1/2 (4.5 oz) jar	
Junior Vegetables		
Carrots	1/2 (7.5 oz) jar	
Squash	1/2 (7.5 oz) jar	

Strained Fruit		
Apple Blueberry	1 (4.5 oz) jar	**FRUIT EXCHANGES**
Applesauce	1 (4.5 oz) jar	
Applesauce and Apricots	1 (4.5 oz) jar	
Apricots with Tapioca	1 (4.5 oz) jar	
Bananas with Tapioca	1/2 (4.5 oz) jar	
Bananas with Pineapple and Tapioca	1 (4.5 oz) jar	
Peaches	1 (4.5 oz) jar	
Pears	1 (4.5 oz) jar	
Pears and Pineapple	1 (4.5 oz) jar	
Plums with Tapioca	1/2 (4.5 oz) jar	
Prunes with Tapioca	1/2 (4.5 oz) jar	

Source: *Nutrient Values - Gerber Products*, October 1988, Gerber Products Company, 445 State Street, Freemont, Michigan 49412.

FRUIT EXCHANGES (CONTINUED)

Mixed Cereal with Applesauce and Bananas	1 (4.5 oz) jar
Oatmeal with Applesauce and Bananas	1 (4.5 oz) jar
Rice with Applesauce and Bananas	1 (4.5 oz) jar

Junior Fruits

Apple blueberry	1 (6.0 oz) jar
Applesauce1 (6.0 oz) jar	
Apricots with Tapioca	1/2 (6.0 oz) jar
Bananas with Tapioca	1/2 (6.0 oz) jar
Peaches	1 (6.0 oz) jar
Pears and Pineapple	1 (6.0 oz) jar
Plums with Tapioca	1/2 (6.0 oz) jar
Pears	1 (6.0 oz) jar

Strained Juices

Apple, Orange, Pear, Mixed Fruit, Cherry, etc.	1 (4.2 oz) container

STARCH/BREAD EXCHANGES

Barley	6 Tbsp
High Protein	8 Tbsp
High Protein Cereal with Apple and Orange	6 Tbsp
Mixed	6 Tbsp
Mixed Cereal with Banana	6 Tbsp
Oatmeal	6 Tbsp
Oatmeal with Banana	6 Tbsp
Rice	6 Tbsp
Rice Cereal with Banana	6 Tbsp
Arrowroot Cookies	4
Animal Shaped Cookies	3
Pretzels	3
Teething Biscuits	3
Zwieback Toast	2
Strained Peas	1 (4.5 oz) jar
Strained Creamed Corn	1 (4.5 oz) jar
Strained Sweet Potatoes	1 (4.5 oz) jar
Junior Creamed Green Beans	1 (6.0 oz) jar
Junior Mixed Vegetables	1 (6.0 oz) jar
Junior Sweet Potatoes	1/2 (6.0 oz) jar

Lean Meat

Strained Meats

Beef	1/2 (2.5 oz) jar
Ham	1/2 (2.5 oz) jar
Lamb	1/2 (2.5 oz) jar
Pork	1/2 (2.5 oz) jar
Meat (Beef, Chicken, Ham, Veal with ˙Vegetables—omit 1 vegetable exchange)	1 (6.0 oz) jar

Junior Meats

Beef	1/2 (2.5 oz) jar
Ham	1/2 (2.5 oz) jar
Lamb	1/2 (2.5 oz) jar
Turkey	1/2 (2.5 oz) jar
Veal	1/2 (2.5 oz) jar

Medium-Fat Meat

Strained Chicken	1/2 (2.5 oz) jar
Junior Chicken	1/2 (2.5 oz) jar
Strained Turkey with Vegetables (omit 1 vegetable exchange)	1 (4.5 oz) jar
Junior Chicken with Vegetables (omit 1 vegetable exchange)	1 (4.5 oz) jar
Junior Turkey with Vegetables (omit 1 vegetable exchange)	1 (4.5 oz) jar
Meat Sticks	1 (2.5 oz) jar
Toddler Meat Dinners (omit 1 starch/bread exchange)	1 (6.25 oz) jar
Junior Vegetables and Meat (Beef, Chicken, Ham, Lamb, Liver, Turkey) (omit 1 starch/bread exchange)	1 (7.5 oz) jar

High-Fat Meat

Egg Yolks	4 Tbsp

MEAT EXCHANGES

MILK/FORMULA EXCHANGES*

	CHO/gm	Protein/gm	Fat/gm
Whole milk	12.0	8.0	9.0
Similac	17.0	3.6	8.8
Enfamil	16.8	3.6	9.0
SMA	17.3	3.6	8.6
Prosobee	16.3	4.8	8.6
Isomil	16.3	4.3	8.8

*Skim milk is not recommended for infants. The Milk/Formula Exchange is based on whole milk.

Resource List for Additional Information

Adding Fiber to Your Diet
Marion J. Franz, MS, RD, CDE
Explains the importance of fiber in the diet, the different types of fiber, and how to add fiber to the diet. Includes sample menus and average dietary fiber content of food groups.
16 pages, $3

Convenience Food Facts
Arlene Monk, RD; Marion J. Franz, MS, RD, CDE
Includes more than 1,500 popular name-brand processed foods from seventy-five companies to help you plan nutritious and easy-to-prepare meals. Features information on calories, carbohydrate, protein, fat, and sodium content of each food product.
216 pages, $8.95

Diabetes, Actively Staying Healthy (DASH): Your Game Plan for Diabetes and Exercise
Marion Franz, MS, RD, CDE; Jane Norstrom, MA
Valuable suggestions and guidelines for both young and old to help ensure performance, safety, and better health through exercise.
230 pages, $9.95

Diabetes and Alcohol
Marion J. Franz, MS, RD, CDE
Discusses the effects of alcohol on diabetes and explains precautions that must be taken if it is used.
4 pages, $1

Diabetes and Brief Illness
Marion Franz, MS, RD, CDE; Judy Ostrom Joynes, MA, RN, CDE
Self-care instructions and food suggestions to prevent ketoacidosis from developing during brief illness that disrupts normal eating.
8 pages, $2

Diabetes and Exercise
Marion J. Franz, MS, RD, CDE
Explains the general and diabetes-related benefits of exercise. Includes precautions for people with insulin-dependent diabetes as well as precautions and weight loss tips for people with noninsulin-dependent diabetes.
20 pages, $2.50

Diabetes and Impotence
Priscilla Hollander, MD
Up-to-date, anatomically illustrated explanation of why impotence occurs and how it can be diagnosed and treated.
6 pages, $2

Diabetes Record Book
International Diabetes Center
Handy pocket-size booklet for recording six months of daily glucose tests, insulin injections, and other information.
68 pages, $2.25

Emotional Adjustment to Diabetes
Randi Birk, MA, LP
Explains how emotions affect diabetes and the process of adjusting to diabetes.
16 pages, $2

Exchanges for All Occasions: Meeting the Challenge of Diabetes
Marion J. Franz, MS, RD, CDE
One of the few books available with the latest exchanges for meal planning. Will help you effectively use the exchange system in almost any situation. Includes meal planning suggestions for traveling, entertaining, camping, eating ethnic foods, school lunches, exercising, following a vegetarian diet, parties, and much more.
249 pages, $8.95

Fast Food Facts: Nutrition and Exchange Values for Fast-Food Restaurants (3rd Edition)
Marion J. Franz, MS, RD, CDE
The definitive guide to survival in the fast-food jungle. Newly revised and updated edition has nutrition information on more than 1,000 menu offerings from the thirty-two largest fast-food chains.
Trade edition (104 pages), $6.95
Pocket edition (173 pages), $4.95

Gestational Diabetes: Guidelines for a Safe Pregnancy and a Healthy Baby
Marion J. Franz, MS, RD, CDE; Nancy Cooper, RD, CDE; Lucy Mullen, RN, BS, CDE; Randi S. Birk, MA, LP; Priscilla Hollander, MD
Explains why gestational diabetes develops, how it's related to other types of diabetes, and what must be done to ensure a safe pregnancy and healthy baby and to prevent the development of permanent diabetes.
34 pages, $3.50

Intensified Insulin Management for You: A Personal Program for Advanced Diabetes Self Care
Priscilla Hollander, MD; Gay Castle, RD, CDE; Judy Ostrom Joynes, MA, RN, CDE; Joe Nelson, MA, LP
A road map for helping you understand and use an intensified insulin program under the guidance of your health care team. Advanced program focuses on emotional and intellectual goals as well as diet and exercise.
85 pages, $12

The Joy of Snacks: Good Nutrition for People Who Like to Snack
Nancy Cooper, RD, CDE
Nutritional guide to healthy eating between meals, with more than 200 recipes in twelve categories, including hearty snacks, popcorn, appetizers, muffins/breads, and a special chapter on children's recipes. Includes nutritional information as well as exchange values per serving for each recipe and for commercial snacks.
269 pages, $12.95

Managing Type II Diabetes: Your Invitation to a Healthier Lifestyle
Arlene Monk, RD, CDE; Sue Adolphson, RN, CDE; Priscilla Hollander, MD; Richard M. Bergenstal, MD
Interactive workbook on Type II diabetes facilitates problem solving, individualized meal plans, exercise plans, foot care, goal setting, what to look for in a health care team, and more.
170 pages, $9.95

Pass the Pepper Please!: Healthy Meal Planning for People on Sodium Restricted Diets
Diane Reader, RD, CDE; Marion Franz, MS, RD, CDE
Imaginative yet clear suggestions for cutting back on salt and lowering your blood pressure. Sodium intake can be reduced by 50% or more by choosing low-sodium foods, using salt substitutes, cutting back on processed foods, and dozens of other ways.
66 pages, $3.95

Recognizing and Treating Insulin Reactions
Judy Ostrom Joynes, MA, RN, CDE; Lucy Mullen, RN, BS, CDE; Joy Sandell, RN, BSN; Ellie Strock, RN, C, CDE
A guide to preventing, recognizing, and treating insulin reactions. Includes food suggestions and instructions as well as general guidelines for using glucagon to treat severe reactions.
4 pages, $1

502

Simplified Learning Series
Allison Nemanic, BA, RN, CDE; Gretchen Kauth Morin, RD, CDE; Judy Ostrom Joynes, MA, RN, CDE
Sixteen booklets, each covering a specific topic, written and designed for adults or children with low reading skills (evaluated at a third grade reading level). Developed in consultation with a literacy specialist. Preview pack contains one each of all sixteen booklets. Booklets also available separately in packs of one dozen only.
Preview pack, $19.95

A Step in Time: Diabetes Foot Care Awareness Series
Janet Swenson Lima, RN, MPH; Ronald H. Melincoff, DPM; Ellie Strock, RN, C, CDE; Stephen Powless, DPM
Well-illustrated, easy-to-understand explanation of why people with diabetes must take especially good care of their feet. Includes guidelines for daily care, prevention, and detection of problems.
18 pages, $2.95

Whole Parent/Whole Child: A Parent's Guide to Raising a Child With a Chronic Illness
Patricia M. Moynihan, RN, PNP, MPH; Broatch Haig, RD, CDE
What kind of parent are you now? What kind of parent do you want to be? How can you help your child with a chronic health problem lead the fullest possible life? Answers to these and other questions as well as practical parenting suggestions that really work.
180 pages, $9.95

Resources For Health Professionals

Diabetes Youth Curriculum: A Toolbox for Educators
Patricia M. Moynihan, RN, PNP, MPH; Barbara Balik, RN, MS; Sandra Eliason, MA; Broatch Haig, RD, CDE
Two volumes, the *Curriculum* and the *Resource and Activities Guide*, together provide health care professionals with a coordinated and innovative curriculum specifically developed for use with school-age children 6 to 16 years old.
Curriculum: 136 pages, $95
Resource and Activities Guide: 260 pages, $55

Challenge of Choice
Marion J. Franz, MS, RD, CDE; Betsy Kerr Hedding, RD, MPH
Slide show covers nutritional recommendations; how to reduce fat, sugar, and salt in the diet; how to increase carboyhdrate intake and fiber; and fad diets, supplements, and caffeine.
Slides: $85; cassette: $10

Diabetes and Impotence: A Concern for Couples
Priscilla Hollander, MD
Slide show covers how diabetes may cause impotence. A sensitive approach to a difficult subject.
Slides: $74; cassette: $10

Diabetes In Your School or Child Care Center
Broatch, RD, CDE; Becky Clasen, RN, BA, CDE; Martha Spencer, MD
Video for school personnel shows how to provide a safe and positive learning environment for the child with diabetes—without disrupting normal class routine.
1/2 in. VHS video: $75

Diabetes: The Light Grows Brighter
Marion J. Franz, MS, RD, CDE; Judy Ostrom Joynes, MA, RN, CDE; Donnell D. Etzwiler, MD; Priscilla Hollander, MD
Slide show and video explains diabetes and how it can be controlled and includes basic information on insulin, blood glucose monitoring, nutrition, emotional adjustment, exercise, and complications.
Slides: $98; cassette:$10; 1/2 in. VHS video: $95

Meal Planning With Exchange Lists
Marion J. Franz, MS, RD, CDE
Slide show and video explain the exchange lists and their practical application to meal planning. Includes beautiful food photography by General Mills, Inc.
Slides: $98; cassette: $10; 1/2 in. VHS video: $95

Guidelines for Managing Diabetes During Brief Illness
Marion J. Franz, MS, RD, CDE; Judy Ostrom Joynes, MA, RN, CDE
Slide show offers guidelines and food suggestions to help prevent the development of ketoacidosis in persons with diabetes during common brief illnesses.
Slides: $80; cassette $10

A Practical Guide to Insulin Injections:
Step by Step Instructions
Ellie Strock, RN, C, CDE
Helps your patients learn correct technique by providing step by step instructions on how to draw up, measure, and inject insulin. It also reviews types of insulin and syringes, storage of insulin, and injection sites.
Slides: $80; cassette: $10; 1/2 in. VHS video: $95

Shop Smart for Good Nutrition
Nancy Cooper, RD, CDE
Slide show and video offer tips and suggestions for
purchasing foods that meet the recommendations to reduce
fat, sugar, and salt in the diet. Includes information on
using food labels.
Slides: $98; cassette: $10; 1/2 in. VHS video: $95

A Step in Time: Diabetes Foot Care Awareness Series
Janet Swenson Lima, RN, MPH; Ronald H. Melincoff, DPM;
Ellie Strock, RN, C, CDE; Stephen Powless, DPM
Presentation combines photography and anatomical
illustrations to explain the whys and hows of foot care to
people with diabetes. A booklet by the same title is
available to be used a patient take-home guide.
Slides: $90; cassette: $10; 1/2 in. VHS video: $95;
flip-chart: $50

IDC books are published by Diabetes Center, Inc., in
Minneapolis, MN. All books and materials are available
nationwide and in Canada through leading bookstores.
If you can't find our books at your favorite bookstore,
contact us directly for a free catalog.

DCI Publishing
A Division of ChroniMed Inc.
PO Box 47945
Minneapolis, MN 55447-9727

IDC slide shows and videos are available from the
International Diabetes Center.

International Diabetes Center
5000 West 39th Street
Minneapolis, MN 55416
(612) 927-3393

Index

A

Acceptance, 111-12
Adjustments, insulin
  anticipatory, 345-46
  compensatory, 344-45
  for athletes, 365
  for travel across time zones, 379
Adolescence, 422-24, 445-58
  eating problems, 442-43
  meal planning, 436
  sexuality, 424, 445-58
Aerobic exercise, 53, 58-60, 225, 228
Alcohol, 23, 39, 204, 243, 314-18, 336, 387, 451
  guidelines for use, 315-18
Aldose reductase inhibitors, 242, 265, 477
Algorithms, insulin, 343-46, 352
Alpha cells, 9-10, 181
American College of Sports Medicine
  perceived exertion scale, 56-57
American Diabetes Association, 27-28
American Dietetic Association, 28
Amino acids, 25-26, 84
Anaerobic activities, 53
Anger, 105
Angina, 251
Arthritis, 242
Aspartame, 308
Atherosclerosis, 251-55
Athletes with diabetes, 363-73

B

Banting, Frederick, 10
Behavior change techniques. 214-17, 431
Behavior modification, 431
Bell's palsy, 261
Best, Charles, 10
Berson, Saul, 10-11
Beta blockers for hypertension, 253
Beta cells, 9, 84, 474-75, 477
Birth control, 358-60, 455-56
Bladder infection, 289, 385
Blood glucose, 10-11, 32, 66-67, 84
  changing levels, symptoms of, 13-15
  control, 18, 79-80, 202, 432
  effect of alcohol, 314-16
  effect of exercise, 51-52, 148-55, 221-30
  effect of medications, 333-40
  in pregnancy, 350-52
  monitoring goals, 78-79, 126, 129-30, 163
  relation to long-term problems, 242, 265
  setting goals for, 343-44

Blood glucose meters, 69-70, 74-75, 468-70, 495-96
  equipment guide, 495-96
Blood glucose monitoring, 32, 66-81, 129-30, 139-40, 149-54, 161-75, 205, 343-46, 415, 417, 419, 468-71
  during pregnancy, 351-52
  equipment guide, 495-96
  for athletes, 364-65
  for children, 400-01
  in gestational diabetes, 361
  in insulin intensification program, 343-46
  on vacation, 377
Blood pressure, high (hypertension), 41, 44, 51, 206-07, 210, 242-43, 252-53, 255, 281, 289-90, 293, 335
Blood pressure, low, 263
Blood vessel disease, 16-19, 198, 241-42, 250-57, 260, 263, 268-69, 297, 356
Body weight
  desirable, 211
  loss of, 36, 51, 210-18, 224
Brain, 14, 178-82, 253, 260
Breast-feeding, 358, 433-34

C

Calories, 23, 27-28, 33-44, 211-12, 222-24, 311, 314, 317-18, 352-53, 372, 481, 483, 486-89
  adjusting levels for weight loss, 211-12
  adult needs, 33-36
  children's needs, 36-39
  using calories through exercise (chart), 223
Camp, diabetes, 448-49
Carbohydrate, 12-15, 18, 24-28, 144-45, 152-53, 180, 186-87, 225, 311-13, 317-18, 366-68, 372, 386, 481, 483, 486-88
Cardiomyopathy, 252
Cardiovascular disease. *See* Heart disease
Career decisions, 449-50
Cataracts, 279
Children
  caloric needs, 36-39
  chapter for, 393-411
  detection of diabetes in, 15-17, 124
  eating habits, 428-43
  growth and development of, 17-18, 36-38, 162, 413-24
  teenagers and sexuality, 424, 445-58
Cholesterol, 22-23, 25, 27, 41-44, 51, 131, 206, 210, 222, 243, 255
Circulation problems, 198, 206, 227, 241, 250, 253-54

Clinical trials, participation in, 462-64, 465
Complications of diabetes, 10, 16-19
  early detection of, 244, 246-48
  immediate, or short-term, 16-17, 177-88
  long-term, 239-302 (see also specific problem areas, eg., heart disease)
Computer-based technology for diabetes management, 468-71
Contraception, 358-60, 455-56
C-peptide, 84
Crapo, Phyllis, 24

D

Dawn phenomenon, 166-67
Dehydration, 61, 155, 183-84, 186, 224, 366-67
Denial, 103
Dental care, 384, 451
Depression, 107
Diabetes
  complications of, 8, 10, 17-19, 177-88, 239-302
    detection of, 16-18
    emotional adjustment to, 101-12
    future outlook, 461-78
    history of, 9-11
    National Commission on, 8
    search for cure, 461-64
    statistics on, 8, 198
    types of, 15-18 (including table)
      gestational, 16-18, 360-61
      insulin-dependent (Type I), 15-18, 123-94
        causes of, 17-18, 127-28
        complications of, 17-18, 177-88
        diagnosis of 17-18, 124
        exercise, 147-59
        meal plan and nutrition, 126, 137-45
        symptoms of, 17-18, 124
        treatment of, 17-18, 123-34
      noninsulin-dependent (Type II), 15, 18, 197-235
        "adult-onset," 15, 198-201
        causes of, 18, 200-01
        complications of, 18, 239-302
        diagnosis of, 18, 201-02
        exercise, 221-30
        meal plan and nutrition, 209-18
        treatment, 18, 202-06
Diabetes pills, 18, 33, 185, 203-04, 336-37, 477
  side effects, 204
Dialysis, 291
Diet. See Meal plan

Dietary Guidelines for Americans, 23
Dietetic products, 310-11, 433
Driving, tips for people with diabetes, 386
Drugs. See Medications
Drugs, street, 387-88

E

Early detection of complications, 244
Eating habits, 212-17, 428-43
Education, 132-33, 240-44, 432
Electromyelogram, 264
Emergency treatment measures for severe hypoglycemia, 180-82
Emotional adjustment, 101-12
Energy, 12-15, 24-26, 76, 84, 183, 225
Ethnic incidence of Type II diabetes, 201
Exchange lists, 28-31, 34-35, 306-07, 312-13, 481-94, 497-500
  for infant foods, 497-500
Exercise, 49-62, 126, 271, 293, 332
  concerns for adolescents, 448
  for persons with Type I diabetes, 147-59
  heart rate during, 54-56
  insulin adjustments, 156-58, 365
  routine, in Type II diabetes, 221-30
  special considerations for athletes with diabetes, 363-73
Eye problems, 8, 16-18, 52, 131, 158, 198, 207, 241, 252, 261, 277-85

F

Family planning, 358-60, 455-56
Fat, 12-13, 18, 22-23, 25-28, 30, 41-44, 51, 76, 84, 183, 210-12, 225, 243, 271, 311-13, 372, 481, 483, 486, 488-90
  cholesterol. See Cholesterol
  monounsaturated, 41
  Omega, 3, 42
  saturated, 41
  unsaturated, or polyunsaturated, 41
Fear, 104-05
Feelings about diabetes, 101-12, 409-10, 421-24, 452-53
Fiber, 24, 29, 39-40, 481, 486-87
Flexibility for meals, 306-07
Flu shots, 241
Fluid replacement, 366-67
Fluorescein angiogram, 281
Food labels, 310-13
Foot problems and foot care, 52, 61, 227, 241, 267-75, 380
"Free" foods, 30, 311, 491-92
Fruit, 30, 487-88, 497-98
Future outlook, 461-78

G

Gangrene, 269
Gastroparesis, 262
Genetic factors, 200-01, 243, 255, 474-75
Gestational diabetes, 16-18, 360-61
Glucagon, 10, 181, 415-16
Glucose. *See* Blood glucose
Glucose tolerance test, 18, 201, 361
Glycogen, 26, 84, 148, 152, 366
Glycosylated hemoglobin, 78, 130, 149, 205-06, 244
Goal setting, 125-26
Good behavior, rewards for, 431
Growth and development, 17-18, 162, 241, 413-24
Guilt, 106

H

Health care plan
  for insulin-dependent diabetes (Type I), 123-34
  for noninsulin-dependent diabetes (Type II), 197-207
Health care team
  communicating with, 388
  early detection of complications, 244, 246-48
  involvement in prevention of complications, 257, 266, 275, 285, 293, 302
  routine visits with, 130-33
Health care visits, routine, 130-131, 206-07, 240, 244, 265
  regular follow-up to minimize complications, 244, 246-48
Heart disease, 8, 17-18, 41, 51-52, 148, 158, 206, 210, 222, 241, 243, 250-57, 263
Heart rate (pulse rate), 54-56, 59, 225, 263
  target rate during exercise, 55, 59, 225
Height-weight charts, 38, 435
Hemoglobin AIC test. *See* Glycosylated hemoglobin
Heredity (genetics, inheritance), 200-01, 243, 474-75
Holidays
  considerations for children, 433
  meal scheduling, 143-44
Humulin, 85
Hyperglycemia (high blood glucose), 183-85
  drug-induced, 334-36
  effect of exercise, 151-52

in infants, 416
Hypertension. *See* Blood pressure, high
Hypoglycemia
  caused by alcohol use, 314, 316
  described for children, 405-06
  drug-induced, 336-37
  effect of exercise, 150-51, 369
  effect of pregnancy, 355
  in children, 415-17
  prevention while traveling, 377-78
  risk during exercise, 226
  severe, 180-82
  side effects of oral agents, 204
  symptoms and treatment, 178-80

I

Illness, brief
  effect on food needs, 185
  management guidelines, 185-88
  replacement foods (table), 187
  sample sick-day menu, 186
  while traveling, 380
Immunosuppressives, 474-75, 477
Impotence, 296-300
Infants with diabetes, 433-35
  exchange lists, infant foods, 497-500
Infection, 241, 269, 289, 293, 354, 385
  preventive measures, 385
Informed consent, 462-64
Injection technique, 89-96
Injury, prevention, 386
Insulin
  discovery of, 10, 475
  injected, 15, 22, 33, 84-87, 127-30
    action times, 85-86
    adjustments for exercise, 152-58, 365
    concentration, 86
    pattern control, 161-75
    purity, 86
    sites for injection, 93-94
    source, 84-85
    technique, 89-96
  intensive therapy, 128-29, 144-45, 341-47
  molecular structure of, 11, 475
  produced by the body, 84-87
  relation to blood glucose levels, 13-15, 27
  role in the body, 9, 11-13, 26, 200
Insulin-dependent (Type I) diabetes. *See* Diabetes or Type I diabetes
Insulin intensification program, 341-47
Insulin pump, 129, 346-47, 476
Insulin reaction. *See* Hypoglycemia
Insulin receptor sites, 13, 199-200, 210
Insulin resistance, 200-03, 210, 475

International Diabetes Center, x-xi
Interpreting monitoring results, 164-74
Islet cell antibodies, 474
Islets of Langerhans, 9-10, 84

K

Ketoacidosis, 13-14, 76-77, 124, 183-85, 354, 385, 416
Ketones, 13-14, 76-78, 124, 183-84, 385, 416
Kidneys, 12, 17-18, 66-67, 76, 158, 206, 241, 252, 281, 287-93

L

Langerhans, Paul, 9
Laser treatments, 281-82
Lipids. *See* Cholesterol; Fat
Lipoproteins, 42

M

Macular edema, 281-82
Meal planning, 22-23, 28-44, 126, 138-44, 222, 305-19, 427-43
    during pregnancy, 352-53
    exchange lists, 481-94
    for athletes, 371
    sample meal plans and menus, 34-35
Meat, 30, 43, 483-85, 499
Medications, 227, 243, 251-53, 262
    effect on diabetes, 333-40, 387
    for painful neuropathies, 264-65
Menu, sick-day, 186
Menus, sample, 34-35
Mering, Joseph von, 10
Metabolism rate, 224
Meters, blood glucose, 69-70, 468-70
    equipment guide, 495-96
Milk, 30, 43, 488-89, 500
Minkowski, Oscar, 10
Motivation, 125-26, 130-33
    to establish and follow health care plan, 125-26, 130-33
    to exercise, 229
    to learn about diabetes, 1-4

N

National Commission on Diabetes, 8
National Diabetes Advisory Board, 8
National Institutes of Health, 162, 282
Nephrosis, 289
Nerve problem (neuropathy), 17-18, 52, 158, 198, 227, 241-42, 259-66, 268, 297

Nobel prize for Medicine, 10-11
Noninsulin-dependent (Type II) diabetes. *See* Diabetes or Type II diabetes
Nonprescription drugs
    effect on diabetes, 334, 337-40, 387
Novolin, 85
Nuremberg Code, 462-63
Nutrients, 23-27, 372
Nutrition, 21-45, 137-45, 209-18, 428-43
    during pregnancy, 352-53
    eating habits and problems of children, 428-43
    meal planning for Type I diabetes, 137-45
    meal planning for Type II diabetes, 209-18
Nutritional information on food labels, 311-13
Nutritional recommendations, 28

O

Obesity, 44, 52, 200-01, 204-06, 209-12, 217-18, 243, 255
Oral hypoglycemic agents. *See* Diabetes pills

P

Pain with peripheral neuropathies, 264-65
Pancreas, 9-10, 66, 84-85, 127, 181, 200, 203, 205, 342, 474-75
Parents, information for, 104-07, 132-33
    about children's eating habits, 427-43
    about children's growth and development, 413-24
Pattern diabetes control, 79-80, 161-75
Perceived exertion, 56-57, 225
Peripheral polyneuropathy and mononeuropathy, 263
Peripheral vascular disease, 254
Personality type, 329
Pneumonia shot, or pneumovax, 241
Postural hypotension, 263
Pregnancy, 16-17, 18, 162, 241, 349-61, 455
Prescription drugs. *See* Medications
Preventing complications, 241, 254-55, 257, 271, 290, 451
Proinsulin, 11, 84
Protein, 11-12, 18, 25-28, 84, 290, 293, 311-13, 372, 481, 483, 486-88
Proteinuria, 288-90
Psychological factors, 101-12, 298-300, 324-32, 423-24
Puberty, 451-52

R

Rebounding (Somogyi phenomenon), 166-68, 182-83
Recombinant DNA, 85, 475
Relaxation, 331-32
Renal threshold, 201
Research, 7-11, 461-78
Resources, 501-04
Restaurant meals, 306-07
Retinopathy, 281-82, 354
Rewarding good behavior, 431
Risk factors for heart and circulatory problems, 249-57

S

Saccharin, 308
Salt (sodium), 29, 44, 210, 290, 293
Sanger, Frederick, 11
Scheduling changes, 140-44
School, 420-24
  concerns for adolescents, 446-48
  informing personnel, 420-21
  parties and special events, 421
  provisions for glucose testing and snacks, 421
Self-monitoring blood glucose. *See* Blood glucose monitoring
Sexual concerns, 296-302
  for adolescents, 424, 445-58
  for adult men and women, 296-302
Sexually transmitted diseases, 453-54
Skin problems at injection sites, 93
Smoking, 41, 243, 254, 271, 387, 451
Snacks, 139, 150, 353, 370-71, 430
Sorbitol accumulation, 242, 477
Sports and diabetes, 363-73
Sports drinks, 367-69
Starch, 24, 29, 481-82, 498
Steiner, Donald, 11
Street drugs, 387-88
Stress, 51, 129, 205, 321-32
Stress hormones, 178, 180, 182, 185, 314, 323
Stress management, 321-32
Stretching exercises, 50, 60-61
Stroke, 18, 198, 241, 252-53
Sugar, 24
  alternative sweeteners, 307-10
Supplies for blood glucose monitoring, 68-70, 495-96
Support systems, 110-11, 226, 370
Sweeteners, 307-10
Syringes for insulin injection, 87-88, 97

T

Technology, in diabetes research and management, 467-71
Teen sexuality, 424, 445-58
Transplantation, 291-92, 476-77
Travel, 375-80
Triglycerides, 22-23, 27, 42, 51, 131, 206, 222, 243, 255
Type I diabetes, 123-88
  exercise, 147-59
  health care plan, 123-34
  immediate complications, 177-88
  nutrition, 137-45
  pattern control of blood glucose, 161-75
  symptoms of, 124
Type II diabetes, 197-230
  exercise, 221-30
  health care plan, 197-207
  nutrition, 209-18

U

Uremia, 289-90
Urine glucose testing, 76, 201-02
Urine ketone testing, 76-78, 130, 184-85
  supplies, 496
US Department of Health and Human Services, 463-64

V

Vegetables, 30, 486, 497
Venereal diseases. *See* Sexually transmitted diseases
Vision, blurred, 279-81
Vitamin supplements, 371
Vitrectomy, 283

W

Water, 366-67
Weight reduction, 36, 210-18, 224
Weight reduction programs, evaluation of, 217-18

Y

Yalow, Rosalyn, 10-11